The New Living Heart Diet

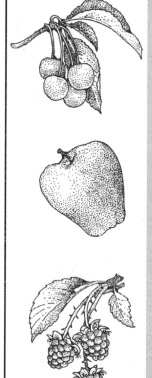

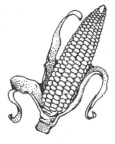

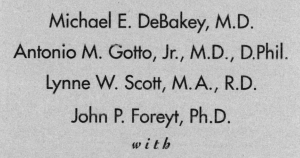

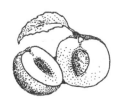

Michael E. DeBakey, M.D.

Antonio M. Gotto, Jr., M.D., D.Phil.

Lynne W. Scott, M.A., R.D.

John P. Foreyt, Ph.D.

with

Mary McMann, M.P.H., R.D.

Suzanne Jaax, M.S., R.D.

Suzanne Simpson, B.A.

Danièle Brauchi, R.D.

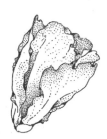

A FIRESIDE BOOK

PUBLISHED BY SIMON & SCHUSTER

New York London Toronto

Sydney Tokyo Singapore

F

FIRESIDE
Rockefeller Center
1230 Avenue of the Americas
New York, NY 10020

Neither this diet nor any other diet should be followed for medical
purposes without a physician's advice. Great care has been taken to
ensure the accuracy of all information presented in this volume. However, the authors cannot be held responsible for errors or for any consequences arising from the use of the information contained herein.

FIRESIDE and colophon are registered
trademarks of Simon & Schuster Inc.

DESIGNED BY BARBARA M. BACHMAN

Manufactured in the United States of America

10   9   8   7   6   5   4   3   2   1

Library of Congress Cataloging-in-Publication Data
The New living heart diet / Michael E. DeBakey . . . [et al.].
p.   cm.
"A Fireside book."
Includes index.
1. Heart—Diseases—Diet therapy.   I. DeBakey, Michael E.
(Michael Ellis), 1908–   .
RC684.D5L58   1996
641.5'631—dc20   95-40787
CIP

ISBN 0-684-81188-X

Contents

About the Authors

MICHAEL E. DEBAKEY, M.D., is an internationally acclaimed surgeon, medical educator, and medical statesman. As a medical student, he devised a pump that became an essential component of the heart–lung machine, which made open-heart surgery possible. He has devised numerous surgical instruments and diagnostic and therapeutic procedures for heart disease, including the first successful resection and graft replacement of an aneurysm of the thoracic aorta, first successful coronary artery bypass, first successful carotid endarterectomy, and first successful use of an artificial left ventricular assist device. He was also among the first to complete a successful heart transplant in the United States. In 1965 he was featured in the first telemedicine program, "Early Bird," which was beamed from Dr. DeBakey's operating room in Houston to an audience of surgeons and other physicians in Geneva. He is currently engaged in further development of this technology. For his contributions to medicine and humanity, Dr. DeBakey has been honored by heads of state throughout the world and has received more than forty honorary degrees. He is the recipient of the Lasker Award, the Presidential Medal of Freedom with distinction, and the Presidential Medal of Science. A prolific author and scholar, he has published more than 1,500 books, chapters, and articles. Formerly President and Chairman of the Department of Surgery at Baylor College of Medicine, he is currently its Chancellor and Distinguished Service Professor of Surgery, as well as Director of The DeBakey Heart Center and Senior Attending Surgeon at The Methodist Hospital.

ANTONIO M. GOTTO, JR., M.D., D.PHIL., is a blood lipid specialist and one of the world's leading researchers and educators in the prevention of coronary heart disease. He is a past president of the American Heart Association and is current President of the International Atherosclerosis Society as well as Scientific Director of The DeBakey Heart Center and Principal Investigator of the Baylor College of Medicine Specialized Center of Research in Atherosclerosis, a National Institutes of Health project. In addition, Dr. Gotto has served as a member of the National Heart, Lung, and Blood Advisory Council and on the National Diabetes Advisory Board. He is a member of the American Association of Rhodes Scholars and active in its selection process. Among his many awards and honors are the Gold Heart Award of the American Heart Association and the Order of the Lion of the Republic of Finland. Dr. Gotto is Distinguished Service Professor of Medicine and Chairman of the Department of Medicine at Baylor College of Medicine and Chief of the Internal Medicine Service at The Methodist Hospital, both of Houston, Texas.

LYNNE W. SCOTT, M.A., R.D., is Assistant Professor in the Department of Medicine and Director of the Diet Modification Clinic at Baylor College of Medicine and The Methodist Hospital. She serves as a member of the National Cholesterol Education Program Expert Panel on Blood Cholesterol Levels in Children and Adolescents. She is a registered dietitian and a clinical researcher investigating the effect of dietary components on blood cholesterol, and has published six books and forty-six articles in the area of nutrition. In addition, she serves on several national committees of the American Heart Association.

JOHN P. FOREYT, PH.D., a clinical psychologist, is Professor in the Department of Medicine at Baylor College of Medicine and Director of The DeBakey Heart Center's Nutrition Research Clinic. He has published thirteen books and more than 150 articles in the areas of behavior modification, cardiovascular risk reduction, obesity, and eating disorders.

MARY CAROLE MCMANN, M.P.H., R.D., is a registered dietitian in the Diet Modification Clinic at Baylor College of Medicine and The Methodist Hospital. She is a contributing author for four books in the Living Heart series and is Associate Editor of *Panic in the Pantry* (1992). She has written numerous magazine, newsletter, and newspaper articles on health-related subjects.

SUZANNE M. JAAX, M.S., R.D., is a registered dietitian in the Diet Modification Clinic at Baylor College of Medicine and The Methodist Hospital. She is involved in research on blood cholesterol, including the nutrition component of a study investigating regression of coronary atherosclerosis. She is also involved in a study investigating the effect of very low fat diets on skin cancer. She is a contributing author for four books in the Living Heart series.

SUZANNE SIMPSON, B.A., is Instructor in the Department of Medicine at Baylor College of Medicine. She edits books, chapters, and articles that present new information on blood lipids and coronary heart disease risk to physicians and patients. Her background in editing includes arts and letters as well as medicine.

DANIÈLE BRAUCHI, R.D., is a registered dietitian and a nutrition counselor at the Diet Modification Clinic at Baylor College of Medicine and The Methodist Hospital. She specializes in the dietary treatment of hyperlipidemia and is a contributing author for three books in the Living Heart series. She is a native of France and completed her degree and nutrition training in the United States.

Acknowledgments

It was a pleasure to work during the past year on *The New Living Heart Diet* with several of the same individuals who played key roles in preparing other books in the Living Heart series. We especially thank Myrthala Miranda-Guzman for her creativity in developing and testing recipes, and also for data entry for the Nutrient Content of Common Foods in the book's Appendix. Special thank-yous go to Laura Frey for typing the text and to Dorothy Hamilton and Angi Stewart for typing the recipes.

We also wish to express our gratitude to Jeremiah Stamler, M.D., Peter H. Jones, M.D., Joel Morrisett, Ph.D., Henry Pownall, Ph.D., Dale Spence, Ph.D., Doug House, M.Ed., J. Alan Herd, M.D., Stan Simpson, B.S., and Kay Dunn, Ph.D., for their technical and medical review of selected parts of the manuscript.

The authors are grateful to Dorothy Hamilton, Betty Smith, Sandi Smith, Shirley Canfield, and Shirley Mills for developing and testing recipes. We thank Rose Lee Westmoreland, Burniece Harding, Jenny Harding, Robert E. Sandfield, Dave Rex, R. D. Morton, L. T. Frazier, Jackie Hirschmann, and Jeffery Baker for contributing recipes for the book.

We are very grateful to Catherine Renteria for computer analysis of each recipe. We especially thank Mary Spitzer and Marieta Carlson, dietitians who are diabetes educators, for preparing exchanges for recipes in the book. The authors appreciate Kerrie Jara's invaluable editorial assistance, including her editing of the recipes, and Jesse Jou's editing of the index.

The authors express sincere appreciation to the readers of the original version of *The Living Heart Diet* for the valuable suggestions they made to us for this version.

Preface

Mortality from heart disease has continued to decrease in the United States since *The Living Heart Diet* was first published in 1984. Some of this improvement can be traced to advances in emergency treatment of heart attack victims. But also during this time, many Americans opted to make a number of lifestyle changes, including changes in diet and exercise habits, that help prevent and treat heart disease. In spite of these factors, cardiovascular diseases (diseases of the heart and arteries, such as coronary heart disease, stroke, and peripheral vascular disease) still cause almost half the deaths in the United States. It is estimated that 50 million Americans have high blood pressure, more than 11 million have coronary heart disease, and more than 3 million have had a stroke. One in every six men and one in every eight women age 45 and older have had either a heart attack or a stroke.

Although many Americans have changed the way they eat and how much exercise they get, many more have not. The public is often confused by the mixed messages about nutrition and health that appear in the media. Nutrition information that is widely accepted one day may not be accepted later. We revised *The Living Heart Diet* not only to provide up-to-date information for people already interested in improving their health but also to give people who have not yet made changes a simple way to begin. In addition to providing complete and accurate information about the relation between diet and heart disease, this book clarifies the link between following a healthier lifestyle, including diet and exercise, and the prevention or treatment of other common conditions or diseases, such as obesity, high blood pressure, and diabetes.

The New Living Heart Diet is intended to be both informative and practical. The book includes more than 300 heart-healthy recipes, as well as 24 menus each for breakfast, lunch, and dinner, which can be combined into several thousand daily menus. The extensive food table in the Appendix makes *The New Living Heart Diet* an unparalleled reference for health-conscious people.

Historically, the Living Heart series of books has grown in response to public interest and need. The series began in 1977, when *The Living Heart* first explored the nature of heart disease. It was followed seven years later by *The Living Heart Diet,* which became a *New York Times* best-seller; more than 1 million copies are in print. In 1992, the authors introduced *The Living Heart Brand Name Shopper's Guide,* which contained nutrient information on more than 5,000 supermarket foods and offered information on heart health; more than 441,000 copies of this book were printed. A second edition of *The Living Heart Brand Name Shopper's Guide* was published in 1993, and a third edition in 1995. *The Living Heart Guide to Eating Out,* which was published in 1993, listed values for calories, fat, saturated fat, and cholesterol for more than 1,600 foods from American, ethnic, and fast-food eating establishments; it also provided 160 tips for choosing restaurant foods lower in fat and sodium.

There are thousands of low-fat and fat-free foods available today that hadn't even been thought of when *The Living Heart Diet* was first published. Many restaurants now offer menu choices that are lower in fat and saturated fat. The requests and demands of informed consumers have made a profound difference in the foods that are available for anyone who wants to follow a lower-fat diet. But the fact remains that all the advances that have been made in the prevention of heart disease are useless until you take that first step, deciding to adopt a healthier lifestyle. There has never been a time when it was easier and simpler to follow a healthy diet than it is right now. Armed with the practical information in this book, you will be able to start your own journey toward better health.

Chapter 1

Risk Factors for
Coronary Heart Disease

In the United States cardiovascular disease kills close to 1 million people a year, or almost as many people as all other causes of death combined. Coronary heart disease (CHD) accounts for about one-half of the deaths due to cardiovascular disease and by itself kills nearly as many people as all cancers combined. Each year at least 250,000 Americans die of a heart attack before they are able to reach a hospital.

These statistics are frightening, but the good news is that much heart disease can be prevented. The keys are to improve eating patterns, control blood cholesterol levels, control blood pressure, not smoke, and stay physically active. CHD risk is lower for people who have better eating habits, better medical care, and more knowledge about health. Many studies have shown that the risk for death from heart attack is lower among the more educated than among the less educated. Education is vital in helping people understand how to take good care of themselves.

In this chapter Dr. Antonio M. Gotto, Jr., answers questions people frequently ask about what causes CHD and about what can be done to prevent or control this disease. If you do not have heart disease, this information can help you reduce your risk of its ever developing; if you do have heart disease, these answers can help you avoid further problems. Dr. Gotto is one of the world's leading researchers into the causes of CHD and a tireless educator about heart health. He is past national president of the American Heart Association.

What Is Coronary Heart Disease?

Dr. Gotto, what is coronary heart disease?

Coronary heart disease, also called coronary artery disease, is the development of atherosclerosis in the coronary arteries, that is, the arteries that supply blood to the heart muscle itself. Atherosclerosis is a buildup of fatty substances and cholesterol (that is, lipids), calcium, and other materials in the inner lining of an artery. The word is derived from Greek roots: *athero* (gruel or porridge) and *sclerosis* (hardening). This buildup, often called plaque, can be compared to the gradual blockage of pipes in a house by rust and scale.

Atherosclerosis develops in other arteries as well, for example, the aorta, which is the large vessel that carries blood away from the heart, and the cerebral, carotid, renal, and femoral arteries—that is, the arteries of the brain, neck, kidneys, and thighs. There are certain arteries and certain parts of the arteries that are more prone to this disease. Atherosclerosis is likely to develop at branch points of vessels and where arteries curve. "Mapping" atherosclerosis, or trying to understand why atherosclerosis develops exactly where it does, is a fascinating area of current research. Also, the artery walls themselves can thicken and harden, as opposed to the obstruction of the passage, or lumen. The general term *arteriosclerosis* is used to describe this thickening and hardening. Some hardening of the arteries normally occurs as we grow older.

Many people do not realize that the coronary arteries are fairly small. I think people often picture them as about the size of the aorta, which is about 1 inch wide as it descends from the heart. The major coronary arteries in adults are on average about $\frac{2}{16}$ to $\frac{3}{16}$ of an inch in diameter, measured on the inside of the vessel. They run along your heart, which is about the same size as your fist.

What causes atherosclerosis to develop?

Many people in the modern world live in a way that leads to atherosclerotic disease: they consume a diet high in saturated fat and get little or no exercise, for example, or they smoke. In many nonindustrialized countries people are more likely to die of infections than atherosclerotic disease. Atherosclerosis is a "modern" disease only insofar as rates of atherosclerosis are so high in modern, industrialized societies because of lifestyle. Evidence of atherosclerosis has been found in Egyptian mummies from the third millennium B.C. and in Peruvian remains from the first millennium B.C. There is preliminary evidence that arteriosclerosis affected the ancient man whose frozen body was recently found—some 5,300 years after his death—in the Alps.

The leading hypothesis about the exact mechanism of atherosclerosis is that the disease begins as a "response to injury." According to this hypothesis, damage to the endothelium, which is the layer of cells that lines the cavity of the blood vessel, allows cholesterol, platelets, fibrin, cellular debris, and calcium to be deposited in the artery wall. Three contributing causes of the injury to the vessel wall are

- Elevated levels of lipids in the blood

- High blood pressure

- Cigarette smoke

As local cells and platelets accumulate, they may produce growth factors that stimulate the abnormal proliferation of smooth muscle cells, a major component of atherosclerotic plaque. Oxidation may play a major role in the deposition of lipids in the artery wall.

No doubt genetic makeup, or heredity, plays a role in whether atherosclerotic plaque develops. Thus, there are both external risk factors, such as smoking and a diet high in saturated fat and cholesterol, and internal risk factors, such as genetic makeup, for atherosclerosis. We do not have to know the exact mechanism of a disease to be able to prevent it. For example, in the eighteenth century the British physician Edward Jenner was able to prevent smallpox by vaccination, long before anything was known about the role of infectious agents in general and viruses in particular in the development of disease; another eighteenth-century British physician, James Lind, was able to prevent and cure scurvy with citrus fruit long before there was any knowledge about vitamins and their role in disease prevention and cure.

How does atherosclerosis lead to a heart attack?

When a coronary artery becomes completely blocked, the blood it is supplying to the heart is cut off and part of the heart muscle may die. Physicians call this damage to heart muscle a myocardial infarction; it is commonly known as a heart attack. Currently, about 1½ million Americans a year have a heart attack, and about one-third of them die of the heart attack. Similarly, when an artery supplying blood to brain tissue is blocked by a clot, a stroke may occur, or when a vessel supplying blood to an arm or leg is blocked, the arm or leg may be damaged. Complete blockage of a blood vessel may occur when a blood clot forms at the atherosclerotic lesion's surface or when there is bleeding into the lesion. Clots rarely form in healthy arteries. Also, a spasm of a coronary artery, which momentarily narrows the vessel, can intensify the damage done by a blood clot. Rarely, spasm by itself leads to a heart attack.

Recent research has pointed to the composition of a lesion as a crucial factor in whether it ruptures. There is significant variability both between lesions and within individual lesions in composition. A major component of atherosclerosis is cholesterol, which is a lipid. The soft, lipid-rich component of plaque appears to be prone to rupturing. Also, atherosclerotic lesions are typically covered by a fibrous cap. These caps vary in thickness and strength, and lesions that have thin, weak caps appear more likely to rupture and to lead to a heart attack. However, we cannot yet predict with certainty which lesions will rupture and which won't, even when we know they are present.

Risk Factors

What is a "risk factor"?

A risk factor for a disease is defined as any habit or trait that can be used to predict an individual's probability of developing that disease. The concept of risk factors is a way to try to answer the question "Why do certain diseases develop in some people but not in others?"

We define risk factors by rigorous application of scientific and statistical methods. Habits and traits are examined in large and in varied populations against rates of disease. In addition to the statistical association, there must be a plausible way in which the risk factor could contribute to the development of the disease.

Many disease associations have been described by the ongoing Framingham Heart Study, begun in 1948 in Framingham, Massachusetts. In this study thousands of men and women were interviewed about their lifestyle habits and examined medically, then over the years the Framingham researchers followed up these individuals to see what health problems developed. The Framingham researchers match health characteristics with people's medical fates. It wasn't until fairly late in this century that it became clear to scientists, through work such as that in Framingham, that smoking was leading to cancers and to heart disease. Now everyone thinks it's obvious.

The concept of risk factors is particularly important when we do not know the exact mechanism of a disease. Even though we have not pinpointed how cancer develops, we know that a large proportion of lung cancer could be eliminated if people stopped smoking. Much skin cancer could be eliminated through decreased exposure to sunlight. And a great deal of heart disease could be eliminated if everyone improved his or her eating pattern (including following a diet low in saturated fat and cholesterol), kept blood pressure under control, and didn't smoke. For example, among the approximately 350,000 men who were screened as possible participants in the Multiple Risk Factor Intervention Trial (MRFIT), 3% were considered to be at low risk for CHD because of excellent blood cholesterol and blood pressure levels, no diabetes, no current smoking, and no personal history of heart attack. Sixteen years later these men had about one-tenth the CHD mortality rate of the rest of the men, and less than one-half the death rate from all causes.

What are the major risk factors for heart disease?

There are two groups of major risk factors for CHD: those that can be changed, and those that cannot be changed. The National Cholesterol Education Program, a program of the National Institutes of Health that issues guidelines for the assessment and treatment of elevated blood cholesterol, lists three major CHD risk factors that cannot be changed in an individual:

- Personal history of CHD or other atherosclerotic disease

- Age (45 years or older for men, 55 years or older for women, or in premature menopause without estrogen-replacement therapy)

- Family history of early CHD (heart attack or sudden coronary death before age 55 in father, brother, or son, or before age 65 in mother, sister, or daughter)

The National Cholesterol Education Program targets for intervention these factors that can be changed:

- Elevated blood level of low-density lipoprotein cholesterol (LDL-cholesterol, known as the "bad" cholesterol)

- High blood pressure

- Current cigarette smoking

- Diabetes mellitus

- Low blood level of high-density lipoprotein cholesterol (HDL-cholesterol, known as the "good" cholesterol)

- Obesity

- Physical inactivity

Each of these factors helps set the stage for a heart attack. You cannot change your personal or family history of cardiovascular disease—for example, whether you have had a heart attack or stroke, or whether your father had a heart attack. You cannot change your age. But LDL-cholesterol can be lowered and HDL-cholesterol can be raised, and high blood pressure and diabetes mellitus can be controlled. *You can change your eating pattern, control your weight, begin to exercise, and stop smoking—and if you smoke, stop today! You can help control your medical destiny.*

The list of CHD risk factors that can be changed is one of the most important lists you can have for taking care of your own and your family's health. People need to be just as serious about risk factors *before* they have a heart attack as after. The present book provides detailed information on lifestyle choices that will help you control your LDL-cholesterol, triglyceride, and HDL-cholesterol levels (Chapter 2), your weight (Chapter 3), and your blood pressure (Chapter 4). It also discusses exercise (Chapter 3) and managing diabetes (Chapter 5).

Just a few good lifestyle habits can contribute to good health in so many ways. For example, reduced fat intake, which includes a lower intake of saturated fat, can improve your blood lipid profile and can help you control your weight and thus your blood pressure, and all these factors can lower the likelihood that heart disease will develop. Also, excess weight creates extra work for your heart. A diet high in fat may contribute to the development of certain cancers, such as breast, prostate, and colon cancers. For reduced cancer risk, the American Cancer Society recommends that you not only reduce fat intake but also maintain a desirable weight, eat a varied diet (including a variety of fruits and vegetables and high-fiber foods), limit consumption of alcohol, and limit consumption of salt-cured, smoked, and nitrite-cured foods. So you can see that the "heart-healthy" diet described in this book fits well with dietary guidelines to help prevent cancer.

It seems that every day I see another risk factor for heart disease described in the newspaper or on television—for example, stress, drinking coffee, or not eating enough garlic. Why doesn't the National Cholesterol Education Program list these factors?

The National Cholesterol Education Program includes only factors that have been linked to CHD risk by extensive, strong data that have been rigorously analyzed. Many statistical and scientific criteria must be met before a factor is considered by experts to be a definite, independent risk factor for a disease. For some of the factors not listed, the findings from studies are inconsistent: some studies show increased risk, and others do not. In some cases, few data are available—perhaps findings from only small, preliminary studies or from studies that are poorly designed. Other risk factors will no doubt be accepted in the future, but not until strong data are available.

How much is my risk for heart disease increased if I have more than one risk factor?

This is a very important point. Two or more risk factors for CHD tend to multiply rather than simply add to risk. The MRFIT data showed that, on average, a male smoker with high total blood cholesterol (240 mg/dL or higher) and elevated diastolic blood pressure (90 mm Hg or higher) is 14 times as likely as a male nonsmoker with cholesterol and diastolic blood pressure below these limits to die of CHD during a six-year period. Similarly, reducing multiple risk factors should help dramatically lower risk for CHD.

When your physician estimates your individual risk for CHD, he or she will take many factors into account. Physicians look at you as a whole person, and your overall risk for CHD is what counts in risk estimation.

BLOOD LIPIDS

How do you know that elevated blood cholesterol is a risk factor for heart disease?

The recognition of elevated blood cholesterol as a major risk factor for CHD has a fascinating history. Here are some highlights:

- The Russian physician Nikolai Nikolaevich Anichkov before 1915 showed that cholesterol feeding would lead to the development of atherosclerosis in rabbits.

- The Seven Countries Study, begun in the 1950s by Ancel Keys, was a breakthrough study illuminating human risk. The study asked why the rates of CHD events such as heart attack were much lower in some countries, such as Italy, Greece, and Japan, than in others, such as Finland and the United States. Dr. Keys and his researchers looked at many factors, and the differences in saturated fat consumption and blood cholesterol levels emerged as crucial.

- The Ni-Hon-San Study and like studies showed that differences among countries in heart disease rates weren't simply genetic. The Ni-Hon-San researchers looked at the lifestyles and disease rates of Japanese men living in Japan (Nippon), Honolulu, and San Francisco. As the lifestyles became more "American" and the dietary fat and blood cholesterol levels rose, the rates of CHD events climbed, until longtime Japanese-Americans had the same CHD rates as any other men with a typical American lifestyle.

- The Framingham Heart Study and other observational population studies provided powerful data about how elevated cholesterol levels eventually contribute to higher rates of CHD.

- Many large clinical trials showed that lowering blood cholesterol would lower heart attack rates. These studies demonstrated that, in general, each 1% decrease in total blood cholesterol leads to about a 2% to 3% decrease in risk for CHD events such as heart attack.

Rare genetic diseases also shed some light on the role of blood cholesterol in risk for CHD. For example, in homozygous familial hypercholesterolemia, which occurs in only about 1 in 1 million people, cholesterol levels are extremely elevated—usually between 700 and 1,200 mg/dL—and angina pectoris (chest pain) and heart attacks may occur when patients are in their twenties or even earlier. People with this disease have no functional liver receptors for removing LDL particles from their bloodstream, and they have severe, widespread atherosclerosis when they are very young.

What are the different kinds of blood cholesterol and how do they influence risk for heart disease?

There is really only one cholesterol: it is a soft, fatlike substance found in all the cells of the body. It is a necessary component of cell membranes, some hormones, and other body components. Many people don't realize that usually the body can manufacture all the cholesterol it needs; it is not necessary to get cholesterol from the diet. Most of the body's own cholesterol is manufactured in the liver. Dietary cholesterol comes exclusively from animal products—egg yolk and organ meats are particularly rich in cholesterol. All types of meat, poultry, fish, and dairy products provide cholesterol; plant foods do not contain cholesterol. In a healthy individual who is eating some cholesterol, the body will manufacture less cholesterol.

The different "kinds" of blood cholesterol refer to how cholesterol is "packaged" for transport through the blood. Remember that the cholesterol manufactured in the liver or consumed in foods needs to reach the cells throughout the body that require it. Oil and water don't mix, so blood lipids (fat and fatlike substances) such as cholesterol and triglyceride are packaged by the body into special particles called lipoproteins. A lipoprotein is basically an oily droplet (the cholesterol and triglyceride) surrounded by a layer of proteins and other components:

$$\text{Lipid} + \text{protein} = \text{lipoprotein}$$

This packaging allows delivery of the lipids through the blood, which is water based.

Lipid deliveries are constantly being made through these different lipoproteins, or packages, in the bloodstream. These lipoproteins vary in size and density. Examples are

- Low-density lipoprotein (LDL, a fairly large particle)

- Very low density lipoprotein (VLDL, an even larger particle)

- High-density lipoprotein (HDL, a small particle)

Each lipoprotein has a specific job to do. The lipoprotein that delivers most of the cholesterol to cells is LDL; about 60% to 80% of cholesterol in the bloodstream is carried by LDL particles. The lipoprotein that is believed to carry excess cholesterol away from cells is HDL. Excess cholesterol is delivered to the liver for reuse or excretion from the body. When too much cholesterol remains circulating in the bloodstream, cholesterol may be deposited in the artery walls, leading to atherosclerosis. A high level of LDL particles in the blood is strongly associated with increased risk for CHD, as is a high level of total cholesterol.

The total cholesterol measurement your physician may order from the lab reveals the amount of cholesterol carried in all the various lipoproteins in the blood sample. An HDL-cholesterol value describes the cholesterol packaged in HDL particles. LDL-cholesterol is the cholesterol in the LDL particles. LDL-cholesterol is referred to as the "bad" cholesterol because an elevated level is strongly associated with the development of atherosclerosis. In contrast, high levels of HDL-cholesterol, the "good" cholesterol, are strongly associated with decreased risk for atherosclerosis. In most cases elevated total cholesterol reflects elevated LDL-cholesterol, but in some instances a high level of HDL-cholesterol leads to moderately elevated total cholesterol.

This metabolic description is extremely simplified but may help you understand the origins of some of the terms you will encounter when your blood lipids are assessed.

Can blood cholesterol be lowered too much?

Some recent reports have stated that very low blood cholesterol levels are associated with increased rates of certain diseases and outcomes, such as specific cancers and suicide. These results have largely been derived from analyses known as meta-analyses, in which many different studies, across different methodologies and populations, are analyzed as one study. Many researchers consider that some of these reports are flawed because of their method of combining results from heterogeneous studies and because of the studies selected. One "poorly done" large study that reaches an erroneous conclusion can negate a dozen well-done smaller studies. The National Cholesterol Education Program concluded that there is no convincing evidence that the proven benefits of cholesterol lowering are outweighed by any potential negative consequences. One missing link in establishing low blood cholesterol as a risk factor for disease is a plausible mechanism to account for adverse outcomes.

The low blood cholesterol levels that have been associated with increased rates of noncoronary diseases (total cholesterol levels well below 160 mg/dL) are not the levels achieved with cholesterol-lowering therapy in clinical trials (levels averaging around 230 mg/dL). In addition, some diseases themselves lead to low cholesterol levels. Very low cholesterol develops in some cancer patients in late-stage disease, and alcoholics sometimes have low cholesterol because of liver damage.

A key charge to the physician, however, is to "do no harm." Therefore, I hope this important issue will be investigated further. At present, however, there do not appear to be any convincing data that low cholesterol or cholesterol lowering is harmful.

What are triglycerides?

Triglycerides are another kind of lipid. Whereas cholesterol is used as a building block, triglycerides contain fatty acids that are used by the body for energy. They are delivered through the bloodstream so that their fatty acids can be used for muscle work or stored in fat (for future energy); in a lactating woman, triglycerides are also used in milk to provide energy to the infant. Lipoproteins that chiefly deliver triglycerides are the large chylomicron, manufactured in the intestinal wall using fats and cholesterol from food, and the VLDL, manufactured in the liver.

Most of the triglyceride measured in a fasting blood sample is carried in VLDL particles. Total cholesterol and HDL-cholesterol do not vary much on a daily basis, and their measurement does not require that you fast. The triglyceride level, however, fluctuates fairly widely depending on whether you have eaten recently. LDL-cholesterol is usually calculated rather than directly measured; calculating LDL-cholesterol requires values for total cholesterol, HDL-cholesterol, and triglyceride, so a fasting blood sample is required for accurate measurement of the triglyceride. (How to calculate LDL-cholesterol is shown on page 32.)

What is the relation of blood triglyceride level to the development of heart disease?

Whereas LDL-cholesterol and HDL-cholesterol levels are clearly related to CHD risk, the role of blood triglyceride levels in the development of CHD hasn't been definitely established. In many studies triglyceride elevation is associated with CHD. However, when other risk variables are taken into account—particularly HDL-cholesterol—the association sometimes becomes less clear. The close metabolic relation between the triglyceride-rich lipoproteins and HDL particles may make the statistical analyses misleading. Triglyceride levels and HDL-cholesterol levels typically stand in inverse relation: when triglyceride is elevated, HDL-cholesterol is low, in a seesaw effect.

Nevertheless, triglyceride-rich lipoproteins may, like LDL, cause lipid deposits to form in the artery wall. In addition, the combination of elevated LDL-cholesterol, low HDL-cholesterol, and elevated triglyceride has been associated with high CHD risk in some studies. The Framingham Heart Study has described high CHD risk in people with elevated triglyceride and low HDL-cholesterol. Very high triglyceride levels (greater than 1,000 mg/dL) are dangerous because they are associated with the development of pancreatitis, an inflammation of the pancreas that can be life-threatening.

What causes elevated LDL-cholesterol, low HDL-cholesterol, and elevated triglyceride?
In each instance, both genetic and environmental or lifestyle factors are usually at work.

- LDL-cholesterol elevation in our society is most often the result of excessive intake of dietary fats, particularly saturated fat, and cholesterol. Some diseases lead to elevated LDL-cholesterol, for example, a low level of thyroid hormone or chronic liver disease.

- Low HDL-cholesterol is often the result of physical inactivity, obesity, or smoking; it can result as well from diabetes mellitus.

- Triglyceride elevation can arise from a diet high in saturated fat and/or simple carbohydrate, obesity, excessive use of alcohol, use of estrogens, diabetes mellitus, or pregnancy, as well as other causes.

If you have elevated LDL-cholesterol, low HDL-cholesterol, or elevated triglyceride, or any combination of these, your physician will need to assess what may be causing the problem. A lipid problem arising strictly from a genetic problem is uncommon. Most people can control their blood lipid problems through diet, exercise, and weight control. Remember that a blood lipid problem can develop in anyone, regardless of age, gender, race, or ethnic background.

OTHER MAJOR RISK FACTORS
What lifestyle changes can help me avoid or control high blood pressure?
Key lifestyle changes to lower your blood pressure are

- Maintain a healthy weight.

- Reduce your salt and sodium intake.

- Avoid excess alcohol consumption.

- Become physically active based on your physician's advice.

Although some people have an inherited, or genetic, tendency toward high blood pressure, overweight and a sedentary lifestyle may convert borderline high blood pressure into overt high blood pressure. Preventing and treating high blood pressure is discussed in more detail later in this book (Chapter 4).

What is the best way for me to assess my family history of atherosclerotic disease?
A medical family tree will be very helpful to your physician. First, list everyone in your family, including parents, grandparents, sisters, brothers, aunts, uncles, cousins, and your children. Include people in earlier generations if you have any medical information about them. List only blood relatives. First-degree relatives are very important because they are the people with whom you share the most genes. First-degree relatives are:

- Parents

- Sisters

- Brothers

- Children

Next, for each relative list major illnesses and age at onset of these illnesses. For people who have died, list the cause of death if known and the age at death. Older relatives may be able to provide information, or you may be able to obtain medical records. A cause of death may be available from a death certificate. Just as in any family history, details are important. Were there unusual occupational exposures, or did the individuals smoke? Was high blood pressure or high blood cholesterol recorded? These details will be of interest to your physician. A brief, clear written report is most useful, and you can share it with other members of your family.

If you find out that you are at increased risk for heart disease because of your family history, you should consider appropriate lifestyle changes to reduce your overall risk. You can also help your children or other members of your family make changes to reduce their risk.

You emphasized the need to stop smoking, but I have found it hard to quit. Do you have any advice?

If you can make only one change in your life to improve your health, stop smoking. If you don't smoke, don't start. For young people we need to create an environment in which smoking is not encouraged by example or by philosophy.

I think most people are familiar with the health hazards of smoking, but the dangers bear repeating. Smoking is the single most important preventable cause of death in the United States. All told, it cuts about seven years off an individual's life.

- Smokers are at least twice as likely as nonsmokers to have a heart attack, and sudden cardiac death is two to four times more common among smokers. Smoking is estimated to be directly responsible for about 20% of all deaths from heart disease. Smoking is also a major risk factor for peripheral vascular disease, in which blood vessels that carry blood to the arms or legs are narrowed. Peripheral vascular disease can result in damage to or even loss of an arm or a leg.

- Even light smokers are at increased risk for CHD, stroke, lung cancer and certain other cancers, and many other diseases such as emphysema and chronic bronchitis. Cigarette smoking is responsible for about 90% of lung cancer cases and for about 30% of all cancer deaths.

- Secondhand smoke can harm family members, co-workers, and others who breathe the cigarette smoker's smoke. Teenagers whose parents smoke are more likely to start smoking. Pregnant women who smoke are more likely to miscarry and also more likely to deliver babies low in birth weight.

A more complete list of the health hazards would take pages. The good news is that your body starts to repair itself almost immediately when you quit smoking, unless irreversible damage has been done. The benefits of quitting apply to both men and women of all ages. Within two to three years of quitting smoking, ex-smokers have about the same level of risk for heart attack as people who have never smoked. This decline in risk has been seen regardless of the number of cigarettes that were smoked in the past or the duration of the habit. Quitting also decreases risk for lung cancer (and the other cancers associated with smoking), stroke, peripheral vascular disease, chronic lung diseases, and respiratory diseases. Lung function increases up to 30%, circulation improves, the senses of smell and taste are enhanced, and the body's overall energy increases. These points provide excellent incentives for quitting.

Nevertheless, quitting smoking can be very difficult. Smokers must overcome both physiological and psychological withdrawal. Probably the key to quitting is making up your mind to do it. Ask yourself these questions: How much do I smoke? Why do I smoke? What are my chief obstacles to quitting? Set a firm quit date, and choose a method of quitting. Many people who successfully quit smoking stopped "cold turkey," but a gradual approach is fine as well. Some people have had success with individual or group counseling programs, and nicotine chewing gum or nicotine patches have been helpful for some. There is no one right way to stop smoking. Here are some tips from the American Cancer Society:

- Change your smoking routines—for example, switch to tea, juice, or sparkling water if you usually smoke when you drink a cup of coffee, or avoid alcohol if you smoke when you have an alcoholic drink. Spend time in places where smoking is prohibited.

- If you are not stopping cold turkey, switch to a brand of cigarettes you don't like.

- Keep busy. Exercise will help you relax.

- If you miss having something in your mouth, try carrot sticks, gum, or a toothpick. If you miss having something in your hand, hold a pencil or a marble.

- Ask a friend or family member to support you psychologically in your efforts to quit. Think positive thoughts.

- If you do lapse and smoke a cigarette, don't give up. Just start again.

- Reward yourself for not smoking—for example, purchase a new pair of walking shoes with the money you save by not buying cigarettes, or treat yourself to a movie.

Many people worry about the possibility of weight gain with smoking cessation. Studies have shown that about one-third of people gain weight when they quit smoking, in part because their senses of taste and smell improve and they are able to enjoy food more. Appetite usually improves as health improves. Also, quitting smokers may use food as a reward, and they may crave having something in their mouth. However, the average weight gain after quitting smoking is only 5 pounds, and the benefits of smoking cessation far exceed any risk from a small weight gain.

The Living Heart Diet can be an important part of stopping smoking because it can help you avoid weight gain and replace unhealthy habits with healthy habits. To help avoid weight gain, eat a well-balanced diet that is low in fat. Have low-fat snacks such as carrot sticks, raisins, apples, and celery available for oral substitutes, and avoid spicy or sugary foods that may make you crave a cigarette. Drink plenty of water (six to eight glasses per day). Regular physical activity, which is emphasized by the Living Heart Diet, is another important aspect of improving your health; in addition to other health benefits, exercise helps you stay busy and relax. Incorporate exercise in your life after talking to your physician about what level of exercise is right for you.

Many excellent free publications are available to help people quit smoking. To obtain them, you can call

- The American Cancer Society at 800-227-2345
- The Cancer Information Service of the National Cancer Institute at 800-4-CANCER (800-422-6237)

Also, you may check your telephone directory to get in touch with a local chapter of the American Cancer Society, American Heart Association, or American Lung Association, or your local or state health department.

To what extent does diabetes mellitus increase risk for heart disease?
Atherosclerotic disease is the cause of death in 75% to 80% of adults with diabetes. Risk for CHD is doubled in diabetic men and quadrupled in diabetic women compared with their nondiabetic counterparts.

Diabetics tend to have multiple risk factors for atherosclerotic disease, such as high blood pressure, low HDL-cholesterol, and overweight. These risk factors, however, do not account for all the increased risk for CHD in diabetics; we do not know why diabetes itself further increases the risk, but the question is under investigation. It is particularly important that individuals with diabetes adhere to all the recommendations for reducing risk for CHD. Additional research on atherosclerotic risk in people with diabetes should be a priority. Diabetes is discussed in more detail later in the book (Chapter 5).

If You Already Have Coronary Heart Disease

How will I know if I have coronary atherosclerosis? What is the first symptom?
Unfortunately, you probably won't know you have atherosclerosis in your coronary arteries until you have chest pain or a heart attack. Atherosclerosis is a silent disease for many years. It generally begins in childhood, and there is a long phase during which there are no symptoms and the plaques

are generated. The earliest lesions are yellowish "fatty streaks," which are found in children. By young adulthood some of these have evolved into fibrous plaques. As time passes, many of the fibrous plaques become ulcerated or calcified.

Atherosclerotic disease is very common in our society because of our lifestyle, and physicians generally consider middle-aged American adults who do not have atherosclerosis to be the exception rather than the rule.

Can't a physician tell if I have coronary atherosclerosis by making an angiogram?

Yes, atherosclerosis can be visualized by angiography, a procedure in which a dye is injected into the bloodstream and a radiograph, or x-ray image, is made. But angiography cannot be used as a screening tool, that is, to look for atherosclerosis in people without symptoms, because it is expensive and carries certain risks for the patient.

Perhaps someday we shall be able to visualize atherosclerosis routinely by using a noninvasive imaging technique such as ultrasound. The use of ultrasound to look for atherosclerosis in the carotid (neck) arteries may prove to be helpful in detecting early coronary atherosclerosis. Some researchers are using methods to detect calcium buildup in blood vessels—for example, by fast computed tomography, or CT scanning—as a way of diagnosing CHD when symptoms are not present. Also, positron-emission tomography, or PET scanning, can be used to determine whether the heart tissue is well supplied with blood. Poor blood supply may indicate the presence of narrowed vessels. This approach is a noninvasive one but is currently considered experimental.

Is it true that if I have already had a diagnosis of coronary atherosclerosis or atherosclerotic disease, there's not much I can do about risk factors to avoid a heart attack?

Not at all! Clinical studies of lowering blood cholesterol, for example, have shown excellent results for lowering rates of CHD events in people who have already had atherosclerotic disease. In fact, success in reducing heart attack rates has been roughly comparable between cholesterol-lowering trials in people who have had CHD and people who have not had CHD. Data from at least two large studies with long-term follow-up—MRFIT and the Coronary Drug Project—demonstrate unequivocally that blood cholesterol, blood pressure, the presence of diabetes, and cigarette smoking still relate to CHD risk for people recovered from an acute heart attack. *Risk-reduction strategies are particularly important in people known to be at high risk because they have atherosclerotic disease.* In a recently reported large study in men and women with a history of heart attack or angina, patients who lowered their cholesterol with diet and a drug called a statin (see Chapter 2, page 64) not only had 42% fewer fatal heart attacks but also had a 30% lower overall death rate after five years compared with patients who received a placebo. These findings have been confirmed by the combined results of four smaller studies using another statin. In these studies, patients who were treated with diet and the statin had 62% fewer heart attacks and 46% fewer deaths after an average of two years compared with patients treated with diet plus placebo. Benefit was seen in both men and women, patients above and below 65 years of age, and patients without a history of high blood pressure or heart attack.

Of course, some people will need intervention such as coronary artery bypass surgery or angioplasty to restore circulation or blood supply to the heart. Your physician may want you to take aspirin or a beta-blocker drug to reduce risk for a heart attack. You will need to discuss these options with your physician.

Is atherosclerosis reversible? Once I have a certain amount of blockage in my arteries, will I have that amount of blockage—or more—for the rest of my life?
Until quite recently, atherosclerosis was viewed as an irreversible process. But now studies in both animals and humans have shown that the process can be slowed, stopped, or even reversed. A number of clinical trials in which LDL-cholesterol was aggressively lowered by using dietary intervention and/or lipid-lowering drugs have shown a decrease of plaque in a small percentage of patients. In many more patients plaque was stabilized or its progression was slowed. As I mentioned before, the lipid-rich part of an atherosclerotic lesion, because it is soft and unstable, is more likely to rupture. New research suggests that cholesterol-lowering therapy can cause these soft, lipid-rich areas of the plaque to shrink.

Equally exciting is the finding that these results seem to translate into greater-than-expected reductions in clinical CHD events such as heart attacks. Because of such findings, the National Cholesterol Education Program has set a lower LDL-cholesterol goal for people known to have atherosclerotic disease than for people without atherosclerotic disease. (The categories for desirable, borderline-high, and high LDL-cholesterol are shown on page 33.)

Special Groups

Are women at risk for heart disease?
Many people do not realize that CHD is the leading cause of death among women in the United States, as well as in many other industrialized nations. The development of symptomatic CHD is somewhat delayed in women: about 6 to 10 years later than the development of CHD in men, on average. So the difference between men and women in heart disease risk is really a question of *when* women are likely to get heart disease, as opposed to *whether* they are likely to have it. Before menopause, women who are not diabetic have a relative protection from CHD. Postmenopausal estrogen-replacement therapy appears to reduce risk for CHD.

Much research into heart disease has been conducted exclusively or predominantly in men, in part because CHD occurs at a relatively young age in men—that is, there is a high rate of disease in a fairly healthy age group, making the research somewhat easier and less expensive. Additional research into heart disease in women is greatly needed, and many large research programs are now beginning, including the Women's Health Initiative of the National Institutes of Health.

Women appear to have all the same risk factors for CHD as men, although it is possible that some factors, such as diabetes and blood HDL-cholesterol and triglyceride levels, play a more important role in women. Vigilant management of CHD risk in women is imperative. Some studies have shown that women fare less well than men after a heart attack: that women are more likely to die because of the heart attack and more likely to have another heart attack. It is important to know that oral contraceptive use can greatly increase risk for CHD among women who smoke. (Estrogen-replacement therapy and the blood lipid changes that occur with menopause are discussed on pages 65–66.)

Are risk factors important for older people?

Four of five people in the United States who die of a heart attack are 65 years of age or older. Heart disease or stroke affects about one in six American men and one in seven American women aged 45 to 64, and that ratio for each sex soars to one in three after age 64.

The major risk factors for CHD continue to operate beyond age 60 and even beyond age 70 in both sexes, although the risk relation may cease to apply in the very old. In the Kaiser Permanente Coronary Heart Disease in the Elderly Study, risk for CHD death attributable to elevated blood cholesterol increased fivefold between the ages of 60 and 79 in men. Some elderly people have mildly to moderately elevated blood cholesterol because their HDL-cholesterol (the "good" cholesterol) is increased, in which case no cholesterol-lowering therapy is needed. In other elderly people a blood lipid problem develops because their thyroid gland is no longer very active; the physician can test for this problem by measuring thyroid-stimulating hormone.

Should the elderly be treated for high blood cholesterol?

The elderly should not be excluded from cholesterol-lowering therapy simply because of their age. High-risk but otherwise healthy older people are candidates for lipid-lowering therapy.

Dietary intervention should be carefully individualized to accommodate established food preferences. Malnutrition should be watched for because many elderly people are isolated or have limited incomes or coexisting illnesses. The elderly should undertake regular physical activity if possible, but there is no evidence that slight overweight needs to be corrected in this age group. Lipid-lowering drugs are appropriate in many elderly patients at high risk for CHD because of high cholesterol.

Should I have my children's blood cholesterol measured? At what age should management of risk factors begin?

Children and adolescents with elevated blood cholesterol levels are more likely than their peers in the general population to have high blood cholesterol as adults. Remember that it is known that atherosclerosis begins in childhood. It is recommended that all healthy Americans 2 years of age and older follow a heart-healthy diet that is low in fat, saturated fat, and cholesterol. (See pages 35–37.) Before age 2, however, more calories as fat are needed for growth and development.

The National Cholesterol Education Program recommends that a blood test for cholesterol be performed only in children who are at high risk—for example, who have a parent with high cholesterol or a family history of early cardiovascular disease. A physician may also wish to order a test for cholesterol in a child or adolescent for whom the family history is unobtainable or other risk is present—for example, smoking, overweight, diabetes, high blood pressure, or excess fat consumption. Such lipid screening in children is usually performed after age 2 years. (See page 34 for classifications of cholesterol levels in children and adolescents.)

Eating a diet low in fat, saturated fat, and cholesterol—with adequate calories for growth and development—and participating in physical activity are emphasized for children and adolescents in the age group of 2 to 19 years. Parents play a very important role in influencing heart-healthy behavior from an early age. The best way for children to learn good eating and physical-activity habits is to see their parents following these good habits. Also, parents should be active in making sure their children's schools support heart-healthy eating patterns, especially in school breakfast and lunch programs. Parents can influence advertisers and food manufacturers not only through their purchasing power but also through writing letters to the advertisers and manufacturers.

A recent scientific report underscores why it is important to manage risk factors as early as possible. For the report researchers tracked until 1991 the health of men who were members of the 1949 to 1964 graduating classes of Johns Hopkins Medical School. The mean age of the physicians at the time of the report was 60 years. It turned out that the men's blood cholesterol levels when they were in medical school correlated not only with how many of the men later were stricken by cardiovascular disease but also with how many died. Risk for heart attack was five times higher for the 25% of the men who had the highest cholesterol levels compared with the 25% who had the lowest cholesterol. A difference of 36 mg/dL in initial cholesterol level was significantly associated with risk for death *before age 50*. Blood cholesterol above optimal is indeed a particularly serious risk factor when present in young adulthood or earlier.

For all the risk factors for heart disease, you want to break the chain of causation as early as possible. *The key to prevention is starting early.*

Additional Questions

Will my genes protect me? My grandfather ate bacon and eggs every day of his life and lived to be 85 years old!

It seems everyone has a story like this; there is always an exception to the rule. The *New England Journal of Medicine* published the documented case of an 88-year-old man who was in good health and had normal blood cholesterol levels despite eating 25 eggs every day for 15 years. The man ate the eggs because he had a compulsive disorder. That's an enormous amount of dietary cholesterol, but the man was resistant to the cholesterol. I was asked by the journal to write an editorial to accompany the report, to elaborate on what might have been happening metabolically in such an unusual case. And that's the point: the case is unusual.

Statistics show that nearly all heavy smokers will have a serious consequence of smoking: cancer, CHD, aneurysm, emphysema, or one of many other serious disorders. Yet there is, say, the one person in ten whose health is little affected or not affected by smoking. Why take a chance with your most valuable asset—your health?

Perhaps someday we shall have genetic "magic bullets" that will allow us to eat whatever we like and not gain weight or have CHD. But I believe such therapy is years away, if it is ever developed.

Could I worry less about my diet if I took an aspirin every day or a vitamin E supplement?
Absolutely not. Taking aspirin or vitamin E cannot substitute for following a low-fat, low-cholesterol diet or quitting smoking in reducing CHD risk. The lifestyle interventions we recommend are therapies against established major risk factors for CHD. Eating a heart-healthy diet, exercising, and not smoking are fundamental to good health.

It appears from current evidence, which is still fairly preliminary, that taking one 325-milligram aspirin tablet every day or on alternate days can reduce the rate of heart attacks in some groups of people. But you should not take aspirin in this way without discussing it with your physician. Aspirin is a drug and, like any drug, has side effects in some people. There is not enough evidence to support the routine recommendation of antioxidants such as vitamin E for the prevention of CHD. (Vitamin E and other antioxidants are discussed on pages 171–77.)

Dr. Gotto, do you believe progress is being made in moving toward a heart-healthy diet and lower rates of heart disease in this country?
It's not a matter of belief but a matter of fact. In 1993 the Centers for Disease Control and Prevention (the CDC) released its findings from the first phase of the National Health and Nutrition Examination Surveys (NHANES) for 1988 to 1991. This large survey of Americans was first conducted in 1960 to 1962 and followed up in 1971 to 1974, 1976 to 1980, and 1988 to 1991.

Between 1960 and 1991 the average blood cholesterol decreased from 220 to 205 mg/dL in people aged 20 to 74 years. That means we are nearing the "Healthy People 2000" goal of 200 mg/dL. The decline was seen across all total cholesterol levels and all age–sex groups, and more than one-half of the change was seen in 1976 to 1991. The 1980s were a period of extensive nutrition education, health-promotion activities, decreased consumption of certain high-fat foods, increased use of lipid-lowering diet and drugs, and intensive efforts by the National Cholesterol Education Program. Public concern about heart-healthy eating has grown stronger each year. The changes in total cholesterol levels correspond with decreased CHD death rates: 54% between 1963 and 1990, accounting for 49% of the decline in overall death rate in this country. The CHD death rate dropped 31% from 1984 to 1992.

Still, there is much more to be done. The NHANES data show that 27% of women and 32% of men in the United States require dietary intervention because of their blood cholesterol levels. As many as 12.7 million American adults might require lipid-lowering drugs by current national cholesterol guidelines. Forty percent of adults require fasting lipid analysis (determination of total cholesterol, HDL-cholesterol, triglyceride, and LDL-cholesterol) by current guidelines. CHD, despite our gains against it, remains overwhelmingly the leading single cause of death in the United States; it is a formidable adversary.

Chapter 2

The Living Heart Diet in Preventing and Treating High Cholesterol and Triglyceride Levels

It is estimated that one of every three American adults needs to make dietary changes to lower blood cholesterol. The focus of this chapter is on diet—the Living Heart Diet—to lower cholesterol and triglyceride levels. First, however, you are given the opportunity to become familiar with the measurement of blood cholesterol and triglyceride and with the levels that are considered desirable or elevated. More information on how total cholesterol, low-density lipoprotein cholesterol (LDL-cholesterol), high-density lipoprotein cholesterol (HDL-cholesterol), and triglyceride levels affect coronary heart disease (CHD) risk is provided in Chapter 1. The dietary methods for lowering cholesterol and triglyceride levels are on pages 35–50. Since many people have questions about the medications used for lowering cholesterol and triglyceride, a section on this topic is included, beginning on page 62.

Detection and Evaluation

All adults (20 years of age and older) should have their total cholesterol measured at least every five years. In addition, the blood test should include HDL-cholesterol. Both measurements are ideally made at the time of a visit to a physician. Total cholesterol and HDL-cholesterol may be measured in a nonfasting blood sample. For many people, however, such as those at increased risk for heart disease or who already have heart disease, a fasting blood sample must be taken so that triglyceride can be measured and LDL-cholesterol calculated (see below). Also, your physician may prefer to have all the information from this "full lipid profile" even if you are not at increased risk for heart disease. He or she will advise you if you need a full lipid profile more often than every 5 years.

There are several things you can do before your nonfasting or fasting blood test to help assure its accuracy:

- Do not change what you usually eat. Changes in what you eat and drink can make the test results different from what your lipid levels typically are and give your physician inaccurate information on which to base his or her recommendations. For example, if you follow a very low fat diet for several weeks before the test, your blood cholesterol reading may be "falsely low," and your physician will not be basing his or her recommendations on what your cholesterol levels are the rest of the time. If you have had extensive dental work and have not been able to eat typically, or if you have been on vacation and consumed more food and alcohol than usual, ask your physician if you can wait a couple of weeks before having the test done.

- If a fasting blood sample is needed, fast for 12 hours before the test—this means nothing to eat or drink except plain water. The total cholesterol and HDL-cholesterol readings from the test will be accurate if you have eaten, but the triglyceride reading will not be accurate. If you have had anything to eat during the 12 hours preceding a test for triglyceride, request that the test be rescheduled. Most people find it easiest to have a blood test in the morning, after fasting overnight. You can usually wait to take most medications until after the test; to be sure, check with your physician.

- You should be sitting for at least 5 minutes before your blood is drawn, and the tourniquet should be on your arm for as brief a period as possible.

Usually, laboratories do not measure LDL-cholesterol directly; the value for LDL-cholesterol is calculated by using the values for total cholesterol, HDL-cholesterol, and triglyceride. The following formula works if the triglyceride level is below 400 milligrams per deciliter (mg/dL); if it is higher, your physician will need to order a special blood test to determine your LDL-cholesterol.

Formula for Calculating LDL-Cholesterol*

LDL-cholesterol = total cholesterol − HDL-cholesterol − (triglyceride ÷ 5)

All measurements are in mg/dL.

CLASSIFICATION OF CHOLESTEROL AND TRIGLYCERIDE LEVELS

If an individual is known to have CHD or other atherosclerotic disease (for example, if he or she has had a heart attack, stroke, angioplasty, or coronary artery bypass surgery), LDL-cholesterol is always determined. The LDL-cholesterol level gives a better estimate of CHD risk than total cholesterol. The goal for LDL-cholesterol is lower in patients with atherosclerotic disease than in patients who are not known to have atherosclerotic disease. Patients with atherosclerotic disease are at high risk for a CHD event, such as a heart attack, and clinical studies have shown that aggressively lowering LDL-cholesterol can slow, halt, or sometimes even reverse the progression of atherosclerotic disease (plaque) in the arteries.

The following tables show classifications of total cholesterol, LDL-cholesterol, HDL-cholesterol, and triglyceride levels for adults, children, and adolescents.

CLASSIFICATION OF LDL-CHOLESTEROL LEVELS IN ADULTS KNOWN TO HAVE ATHEROSCLEROTIC DISEASE

Acceptable LDL-cholesterol	100 mg/dL or less
Higher-than-acceptable LDL-cholesterol	More than 100 mg/dL

For individuals who do *not* have evidence of atherosclerotic disease, total cholesterol along with HDL-cholesterol may be used as a first estimate of risk. As noted above, LDL-cholesterol classifications are different according to whether an individual is known to have atherosclerotic disease.

CLASSIFICATION OF TOTAL CHOLESTEROL AND LDL-CHOLESTEROL LEVELS IN ADULTS WITHOUT EVIDENCE OF ATHEROSCLEROTIC DISEASE

Total cholesterol	
Desirable	Less than 200 mg/dL
Borderline-high	200–239 mg/dL
High	240 mg/dL or greater
LDL-cholesterol	
Desirable	Less than 130 mg/dL
Borderline-high	130–159 mg/dL
High	160 mg/dL or greater

Classifications of HDL-cholesterol and triglyceride in all adults are as follows:

CLASSIFICATION OF HDL-CHOLESTEROL LEVELS FOR ALL ADULTS

HDL-cholesterol	
Low (increased CHD risk)	Below 35 mg/dL
Acceptable	35 mg/dL or greater
High (protective level of HDL)	60 mg/dL or greater

CLASSIFICATION OF TRIGLYCERIDE LEVELS FOR ALL ADULTS

Triglyceride	
Normal	Less than 200 mg/dL
Borderline-high	200–400 mg/dL
High	400–1,000 mg/dL
Very high	1,000 mg/dL or greater

Total cholesterol and LDL-cholesterol classifications for children and adolescents are lower than for adults:

CLASSIFICATION OF TOTAL CHOLESTEROL AND LDL-CHOLESTEROL LEVELS IN CHILDREN AND ADOLESCENTS (2–19 YEARS)

Total cholesterol	
Acceptable	Less than 170 mg/dL
Borderline	170–199 mg/dL
High	200 mg/dL or greater
LDL-cholesterol	
Acceptable	Less than 110 mg/dL
Borderline	110–129 mg/dL
High	130 mg/dL or greater

In children and adolescents, a triglyceride level of more than 150 mg/dL is considered quite elevated. The approximate level for moderately elevated triglyceride is 120 mg/dL in boys and 130 mg/dL in girls. Low HDL-cholesterol in children and adolescents is the same as in adults: less than 35 mg/dL.

It is important to bear in mind that the classifications shown in the tables above for adults, children, and adolescents are general guidelines, not magic levels above or below which CHD risk suddenly increases or decreases. Risk exists across a range of values, without exact points at which risk either is or is not present. For example, an HDL-cholesterol level of 38 mg/dL is relatively low (particularly for a woman, since women tend to have higher HDL-cholesterol values than men on average), and an HDL-cholesterol level of 55 mg/dL is relatively high (particularly for a man). Your physician will look at your entire lipid profile in assessing your individual CHD risk.

For people of all ages and for both sexes, risk for CHD increases as the values for total cholesterol and LDL-cholesterol increase—the higher the cholesterol, the higher the risk for heart disease. For example, an adult with a total blood cholesterol level of 240 mg/dL has about twice the risk for

CHD of someone with a blood cholesterol level of 200 mg/dL. Data collected on 361,662 men in the Multiple Risk Factors Intervention Trial (MRFIT) showed that the group of men with a total blood cholesterol of about 300 mg/dL had more than five times more deaths from heart disease than the men with a total cholesterol of about 150 mg/dL.

Goals to Remember

The "H" in HDL-cholesterol means you want your level to be *High*.

The "L" in LDL-cholesterol means you want your level to be *Low*.

Individuals who have a cholesterol level in the "desirable" range still need to follow the guidelines of the Living Heart Diet and to reduce any other risk factors for CHD (see list on pages 16 and 17). Even if a person's total cholesterol is low (less than 160 mg/dL), he or she should still follow recommendations for the general public for prevention of heart disease, such as selecting foods low in fat, saturated fat, and cholesterol.

UNITS OF MEASURE FOR BLOOD CHOLESTEROL AND TRIGLYCERIDE

In some scientific and laboratory reports, blood cholesterol and triglyceride values are given in millimoles per liter (mmol/L), which is international terminology. For information on converting mmol/L to mg/dL, see pages 366–67 in the Appendix.

Controlling Cholesterol and Triglyceride Levels Through Diet

Dietary modification, weight control, and increased physical activity are lifestyle changes recommended for

- Prevention: to maintain desirable levels of blood cholesterol and triglyceride and help reduce risk for heart disease

- Treatment: to lower elevated levels of total cholesterol, LDL-cholesterol, and triglyceride, and to raise the level of HDL-cholesterol

The same type of eating pattern (diet) is recommended for both prevention and treatment of high blood cholesterol and triglyceride levels; this basic eating pattern is called the Step I Diet.

STEP I DIET

The Step I Diet is recommended both for the general population (age 2 years and older) and for individuals with elevated blood levels of cholesterol. This cholesterol-lowering diet is not necessarily a weight loss diet; that is, it is not "dieting" in the popular sense and includes all calorie levels. However, the Step I Diet does emphasize achieving and maintaining a desirable body weight (see pages 358–59). Nondietary recommendations for lifestyle changes to reduce risk for CHD also include regular physical activity (see pages 78–87) and stopping smoking (see pages 23–25). Patients with known CHD or other atherosclerotic disease always begin with the Step II Diet (see below).

The primary goal of the Step I Diet is to reduce risk for CHD by lowering levels of total cholesterol and LDL-cholesterol in the blood. This is accomplished by a well-balanced, nutritious diet that

- Decreases saturated fat intake

- Decreases dietary cholesterol intake

- Controls body weight (including initiating weight loss in overweight individuals and maintaining a desirable weight)

STEP I DIET

Calories	A level to achieve and maintain desirable weight
Total fat	30% or less of calories
Saturated fat	8–10% of calories
Polyunsaturated fat	Up to 10% of calories
Monounsaturated fat	Up to 15% of calories
Carbohydrate	55% or more of calories
Protein	Approximately 15% of calories
Cholesterol	Less than 300 mg per day

For people who drink alcoholic beverages, the recommendation is for a maximum of two drinks per day (see page 60 for the definition of one drink). Women should not drink alcoholic beverages during pregnancy because of the increased risk for birth defects.

Emphasis in the Step I Diet is on selecting foods that are low in fat as a means of reducing saturated fat intake and controlling calories. The Step I Diet is well balanced, includes a wide variety of foods that are low in fat and saturated fat, and provides adequate amounts of vitamins and minerals. Methods for implementing the Step I Diet start on page 41. The table on page 43 shows the number of grams of fat equal to 30% of calories and the number of grams of saturated fat equal to 10% of calories at several calorie levels. The Living Heart Diet food lists and suggested serving sizes, which can be used with the Step I Diet, appear in the Appendix, starting on page 345. These food lists are consistent with the Food Pyramid even though the foods are divided into slightly different groupings. For example, the Food Pyramid combines fats and sugars in one group, and the food lists have one group for fats and oils and another for sweets and alcohol. A discussion of the dietary components (such as calories, fat, and sodium) is on pages 50–62. The Step I Diet can be implemented in a stepwise fashion. A detailed discussion of how to go about lowering cholesterol and triglyceride levels by diet appears on pages 41–50.

FOODS TO CHOOSE FOR THE STEP I AND STEP II DIETS*

Food Group	Servings
Meat, poultry, fish (lean)	5 to 6 oz (cooked) per day
Eggs	No more than 4 yolks per week on Step I No more than 2 yolks per week on Step II
Dairy Products (fat-free or low-fat)	2 to 3 servings per day
Fats & oils	No more than 6 to 8 teaspoons per day
Bread, cereal, pasta, & starchy vegetables	6 or more servings per day
Vegetables	3 to 5 servings per day
Fruits	2 to 4 servings per day
Sweets & alcohol	No more than 2 alcoholic drinks per day (see page 60); sweets allowed in moderation (according to calorie level)

*Lists of specific foods and serving sizes are in the Appendix, on pages 345 to 355.

The Step I Diet combined with increased physical activity can result in other beneficial effects besides reduced risk of CHD through lower LDL-cholesterol:

- Lower levels of triglyceride

- Higher levels of HDL-cholesterol

- Lower blood pressure as the result of weight reduction and decreased salt/sodium and alcohol intake

- Improved glucose tolerance as the result of weight reduction

In addition, a low intake of saturated fat has been shown to reduce risk for the sudden formation of a blood clot that can clog an artery. Laboratory and population data indicate that the fruits, vegetables, grain products, and fish that are an important part of a diet low in saturated fat may also confer health benefits unrelated to cholesterol lowering. Among the food components suggested to have such benefit are antioxidants, fiber, and phytochemicals. There are increasing data indicating that regular and sustained moderate physical activity provides protection against CHD death.

ADDITIONAL CHANGES TO RAISE HDL-CHOLESTEROL LEVELS

There is no specific dietary treatment to increase HDL-cholesterol; however, the Step I Diet is usually recommended. In addition to the Step I Diet, the following lifestyle changes should receive special emphasis:

- Weight loss, if overweight

- Regular moderate exercise

- Smoking cessation

Low levels of HDL-cholesterol are often associated with high triglyceride levels; therefore, the changes recommended to increase HDL-cholesterol are similar to the recommendations for decreasing triglyceride levels listed in the following section. To increase HDL-cholesterol, you should follow a diet low in fat and saturated fat, achieve a desirable body weight, engage in regular moderate exercise, and stop smoking.

ADDITIONAL CHANGES TO LOWER TRIGLYCERIDE LEVELS

The lifestyle modifications that are the primary treatment for an elevated triglyceride level are consistent with the Step I Diet and other changes recommended to lower total cholesterol and LDL-cholesterol and increase HDL-cholesterol. For triglyceride lowering, special emphasis is placed on the following lifestyle components:

- Controlling body weight

- Restricting alcohol use

- Eating a diet low in saturated fat and cholesterol

- Exercising regularly

- Decreasing intake of simple carbohydrate (if intake is very high)

- Stopping smoking

For overweight individuals who have an elevated triglyceride level, weight control is the most important part of the treatment program (see pages 67–88). As weight is lost, the triglyceride level usually goes down. The weight-loss program should include selection of foods low in total fat, saturated fat, and cholesterol and should be combined with regular physical activity (see pages 78–87). For triglyceride lowering, alcohol intake should be limited to no more than two drinks per day. (The amount of alcohol considered as one drink is shown on page 60.) Some people are very sensitive to alcohol, and any amount increases the triglyceride level; these people need to avoid all alcoholic beverages. This particularly applies to individuals with triglyceride higher than 500 mg/dL.

For some people a high intake of carbohydrate, particularly the "refined" carbohydrate found in sweetened foods, causes an elevation of triglyceride level. Refined carbohydrate is found in foods with a high content of sugar, syrup, or high-fructose sweeteners, used in foods such as soft drinks, desserts, and candy.

Individuals with very high triglyceride levels are at risk for developing acute pancreatitis, an inflammation of the pancreas that can be life-threatening. Development of pancreatitis is more likely at triglyceride levels above 1,000 mg/dL. Very high levels of triglyceride usually occur when an individual has inherited a tendency to have high triglyceride, has diabetes mellitus, is obese, uses alcohol to excess, or takes certain prescription medications. Individuals with a very high triglyceride level should follow a diet with only 10% to 20% of calories from fat. Information on very low fat diets is on page 40.

STEP II DIET

If following the Step I Diet does not reduce blood cholesterol to the goal level, the patient should progress to the Step II Diet. Also, as noted above, all patients with a history of heart attack or other atherosclerotic disease begin therapy with the Step II Diet. *The Step II Diet is the same as the Step I Diet with two exceptions: (1) saturated fat intake is reduced to less than 7% of calories, and (2) dietary cholesterol is reduced to less than 200 mg per day.* The changes necessary to reduce saturated fat intake from 8% to 10% of calories (Step I Diet) to less than 7% of calories include selecting leaner meats, eating less meat, poultry, and fish, and substituting fat-free dairy products for low-fat dairy products. In the Step II Diet, dietary cholesterol is reduced by limiting the consumption of egg yolks to no more than one per week and decreasing the amount of meat eaten. The table on page 43 shows the number of grams of saturated fat equal to 7% of calories at several calorie levels.

If good adherence to the Step II Diet does not lower LDL-cholesterol to the goal level (see page 33), the patient may need to progress to a diet with no more than 20% of calories from total fat (discussed on page 40), or cholesterol-lowering drugs may be considered (see page 62).

EXPECTATIONS WITH THE STEP I AND STEP II DIETS

The levels to which the Step I and Step II Diets can lower total cholesterol and LDL-cholesterol vary according to several factors: (1) composition of the individual's "typical" diet before starting the Step I or Step II Diet, (2) adherence to the diet, (3) individual biologic responsiveness to dietary changes, and (4) amount of weight loss, if overweight. The Step I Diet usually lowers total cholesterol 3% to 14%, although some people lower their cholesterol level up to 25%. The Step II Diet should lower total cholesterol an additional 3% to 7%, depending on the extent to which saturated fat and dietary cholesterol are restricted.

The typical American diet provides 13% to 14% of calories from saturated fat, compared with 8% to 10% of calories from saturated fat in the Step I Diet. Generally, people who have a high intake of saturated fat when they start the diet will have a greater lowering of LDL-cholesterol than those who already have an intake with 8% to 10% of calories from saturated fat.

Adherence to the diet is an important factor in determining response. People who follow the guidelines of the diet only part of the time will not lower their LDL-cholesterol as much as those who follow it consistently. For example, someone who follows the diet when eating at home but does not follow it when eating out cannot expect as much cholesterol lowering as if he or she followed it all the time.

Biologic responsiveness to dietary changes varies from person to person. But even those people who have an inherited tendency toward high blood cholesterol can achieve some cholesterol lowering by diet, although usually not down to their goal level. In this situation it may be necessary to take a medication (see pages 62–66) in addition to following the diet and making other lifestyle changes. There is no way to predict your individual responsiveness to diet without actually following the diet.

Weight reduction improves LDL-cholesterol response to a low-fat, low-cholesterol diet. For example, obese people who have a very high intake of saturated fat can often lower their total cholesterol by 25% with diet and weight reduction. This degree of cholesterol lowering is as great as can be expected from some cholesterol-lowering medications. Normalization of weight in obese people can often in itself reduce triglyceride to normal levels; in addition, weight loss in overweight individuals increases HDL-cholesterol.

It has been proposed by some researchers that changes in cholesterol and triglyceride levels have a greater beneficial effect on heart disease if produced by diet rather than by drugs; however, this hypothesis has not been tested in a controlled clinical trial. If all Americans lowered their cholesterol levels by 5% to 7% with diet alone, the result could be a 10% to 15% reduction in CHD in this country. That would mean 100,000 to 150,000 fewer new cases of CHD each year as a result of diet—a safe, inexpensive, natural approach.

VERY LOW FAT DIET

For some people, it may be necessary to reduce further the percentage of calories from total fat from about 30% to 20% to achieve the desired level of LDL-cholesterol. Some health authorities prefer a diet providing no more than 20% of calories from fat to maximize the reductions in saturated fat and calories. The reduction in saturated fat should help lower LDL-cholesterol, and consuming fewer calories should help facilitate weight loss. The benefit of restricting fat intake to this level has been shown in several clinical studies. Information on implementing a diet with no more than 20% of calories from fat begins on page 44.

Implementing a Diet to Lower Cholesterol and Triglyceride Levels

Changing your eating habits to lower cholesterol and/or triglyceride levels is not a simple process. One way to help ensure success is to go through the same steps that registered dietitians use with their patients to help them make lifestyle changes: assessment, goal setting, method selection, and follow-up and maintenance. Each of these steps is described here as well as on pages 69–78 of Chapter 3; however, the steps can be helpful whether or not you need to lose weight. The information on the steps listed below is specifically designed to help you lower cholesterol and triglyceride levels.

ASSESSMENT

It is important to assess your present eating habits before starting to make changes. Start by answering the following questions about your food intake (if you need to lose weight, answer the additional questions on page 69).

1. How often do you eat foods high in fat? (These foods are often also high in saturated fat.)

2. What low-fat foods do you enjoy eating at home and away from home?

3. How often do you eat food cooked away from home (fast food, restaurant, deli, carry-out, etc.)?

4. How much alcohol do you drink?

The best way to assess what you are eating is to keep a food diary and record everything you eat and drink for several days (see pages 47–48). Then add up the calories, grams of fat, and grams of saturated fat provided by these foods. For a more accurate assessment, ask a registered dietitian to do a computerized nutrient analysis to determine your exact intake of calories, fat, saturated fat, and cholesterol (including the percentages of calories from fat and saturated fat), as well as vitamins and minerals. To be useful, the food diary must be a detailed and accurate record of every item you eat or drink and the amount consumed.

GOALS

Based on your assessment of your current eating habits, you can set realistic, short-term goals for changing both the type and amount of food you eat. It is better first to set goals based on changing *types* of foods and later to work on the amounts. The emphasis is on selecting lower-fat foods; both saturated fat and calories are decreased when you substitute lower-fat for higher-fat foods. Selecting leaner meats and selecting lower-fat dairy products are usually the most effective dietary changes for lowering blood cholesterol. The goals for lowering fat intake are on page 43.

You also need to set goals for physical activity. For both diet and physical activity, set goals for yourself that can be implemented gradually. *You do not have to change everything at once to start receiving benefits from changes you make.*

METHODS

Three methods are helpful for lowering blood cholesterol and triglyceride levels.

1. Counting grams of fat and saturated fat

2. Selecting low-fat foods

3. Counting servings of food from each food group

Each method is effective—there is not a "best" that applies to everyone. Your choice will depend largely on which method appeals to you and the amount of structure you prefer. The first method is described in detail here. The second and third methods, which are as effective for reducing weight as for lowering blood levels of cholesterol and triglyceride, are described in detail in Chapter 3, "The Living Heart Diet in Weight Control."

Selecting low-fat foods is the least structured of the three methods. It consists of identifying high-fat foods that you typically eat and substituting lower-fat foods for them (see pages 72–73). Counting servings of food from each food group is a more structured approach. For this method, the table on page 74 provides the number of servings from each of nine food groups allowed at several calorie levels; detailed descriptions of each food group begin on page 345 in the Appendix. With this method you consume approximately the same number of calories and amounts of fat, carbohydrate, and protein each day.

The Living Heart Diet recipes (which begin on page 207) are moderately low in calories, fat, saturated fat, and cholesterol; this nutrient information, plus amounts of carbohydrate, sodium, and fiber, is provided for each recipe. The menus in this book can be used with the methods for implementing a diet low in fat, saturated fat, and cholesterol.

COUNTING GRAMS OF FAT AND SATURATED FAT IN THE STEP I OR STEP II DIET – Counting grams of fat and saturated fat allows you to monitor the grams of fat and saturated fat in the foods you eat. This method is excellent for lowering blood cholesterol and triglyceride levels. Whether you lose weight while using this method will depend on how many fat-free and low-fat foods you eat that are high in calories; for example, the calories in fat-free desserts add up quickly. If low-fat and fat-free foods are eaten in excess, they can cause weight gain.

To use the "counting grams of fat and saturated fat" method, you will first need to estimate the calories you require each day (see pages 356–59). Once you have estimated your calorie needs, use the table below to find the number of grams of fat equal to 30% of calories; your goal is to consume that amount of fat *or less*. If you are on the Step I Diet, use the column showing grams of saturated fat equal to 10% of calories and consume *no more than* the grams that are listed. If you are on the

Step II Diet, use the column showing grams of saturated fat equal to 7% of calories and consume *fewer* grams than are listed.

MAXIMUM GRAMS OF FAT AND SATURATED FAT AT SELECTED CALORIE LEVELS

Calorie Level	Grams of Fat Equal to 30% of Calories	Grams of Saturated Fat Equal to 10% of Calories	Grams of Saturated Fat Equal to 7% of Calories
1,200	40	13	9
1,300	43	14	10
1,400	47	16	11
1,500	50	17	12
1,600	53	18	12
1,700	57	19	13
1,800	60	20	14
1,900	63	21	15
2,000	67	22	16
2,100	70	23	16
2,200	73	24	17
2,300	77	26	18
2,400	80	27	19
2,500	83	28	19
2,600	87	29	20
2,700	90	30	21
2,800	93	31	22
2,900	97	32	23
3,000	100	33	23

The "counting grams of fat and saturated fat" method consists of your listing all the foods in the amounts eaten each day with the grams of fat and saturated fat they contain. You may wish to make copies of the food diary form on page 47 to use for recording your food intake. The total grams of fat and saturated fat should not go over the maximum number of grams shown in the table above.

Be sure to list all the foods and beverages consumed each day, along with any fat used in cooking, such as margarine used to season vegetables and oil used to cook meat. You can find the fat and saturated fat content of many common foods in the following places:

- General foods: Nutrient Content of Common Foods, beginning on page 372 in the Appendix

- Commercial foods: Nutrition Facts portion of food labels

- Alcoholic beverages: page 371 in the Appendix

- Ethnic and American restaurant foods and fast foods: the Appendix, beginning on page 369 in the Appendix; about 1,600 others are listed in *The Living Heart Guide to Eating Out,* another book in our series (see order form on the last page of this book)

The Living Heart Diet menus, which begin on page 186, provide the calories, fat, saturated fat, and cholesterol for 24 breakfasts, 24 lunches, and 24 dinners.

The "counting grams of fat and saturated fat" method allows you to use a technique called *compensating.* This technique gives you the flexibility to eat many of your favorite foods even if they are high in fat and saturated fat. The technique works because you "compensate" for the high-fat foods you eat by selecting other foods that are very low in fat. By keeping a written record of the grams of fat and saturated fat in foods you eat, you can stay under your recommended maximum intakes for the day.

COUNTING GRAMS OF FAT IN A VERY LOW FAT DIET – You will need to do some careful planning if your physician has recommended a very low fat diet with either 20% or 10% of calories from fat. The method for following a very low fat diet is the same as that described above for the Step I and Step II Diets but with the following exceptions:

- The maximum grams of fat consumed are lower (see the table below).

- It is *not* necessary to count grams of saturated fat; when the total fat is very low, the saturated fat is automatically low.

GRAMS OF FAT EQUAL TO 20% AND 10% OF CALORIES

Calorie Level	Grams of Fat Equal to 20% of Calories	Grams of Fat Equal to 10% of Calories
1,200	27	13
1,300	29	14
1,400	31	16
1,500	33	17

(continued)

Calorie Level	Grams of Fat Equal to 20% of Calories	Grams of Fat Equal to 10% of Calories
1,600	36	18
1,700	38	19
1,800	40	20
1,900	42	21
2,000	44	22
2,100	47	23
2,200	49	24
2,300	51	26
2,400	53	27
2,500	56	28
2,600	58	29
2,700	60	30
2,800	62	31
2,900	64	32
3,000	67	33

Special attention should be given to each of the food groups to decrease total fat to 20% or 10% of calories:

Meat, poultry, and fish: Choose only the leanest cuts of meat, poultry without skin, and fish (see pages 345–46 in the Appendix). These meats are often labeled "extra lean" (5 grams of fat per 3.5 ounces, or 100 grams, of cooked meat) in supermarkets. A diet providing 20% of calories from fat can include 5 ounces of cooked meat per day as long as it is extra lean, with emphasis on the lowest-fat fish and on the white meat of chicken and turkey. If meat containing more fat is eaten, the amount will need to be reduced. If you decrease your level of fat to 10% of calories, meat must be limited to no more than 3 ounces cooked each day. It is usually helpful to combine smaller amounts of meat with other foods, such as pasta, rice, or vegetables. Dried beans and peas can be substituted for meat as a source of protein. Some people following a diet that is very low in fat find it easier to select a vegetarian style of eating (see Chapter 6 on vegetarian diet).

Eggs: Limit egg yolks to one per week; egg whites are not limited.

Dairy products: Adults need to consume two to four servings per day of fat-free (skim) dairy products, which are a major source of calcium. The amounts of dairy products considered a serving are on page 348 of the Appendix.

Fats and oils: Small amounts of unsaturated oil (see pages 348–49 of the Appendix) may be included. If a spread is used, it should be a fat-free, diet, or reduced-fat type. Salad dressings and sandwich spreads should be fat free.

Bread, cereal, pasta, and starchy vegetables: Include six or more servings daily (see pages 349–51 of the Appendix).

Vegetables: Select three or more servings of vegetables each day (see pages 351–52 of the Appendix).

Fruits: Select two or more servings of fruit each day (see pages 352–53 of the Appendix).

Sweets and alcohol: Choose only those sweets that contain very little or no fat. If you drink alcoholic beverages, the number should be limited to no more than two drinks per day. (The amount considered as one drink is on page 60, and tables showing the calories and fat in alcoholic drinks are on pages 370–71 in the Appendix.)

Free foods: See pages 354–55 in the Appendix.

Food Diary

Name_____

Day_____ Date_____

Exercise_____

GOALS: _____ grams fat

_____ grams sat. fat

Write ONE food item on each line.

Time & Place	Amount	Food—How Prepared	Fat g	Sat. Fat g
		Totals for day		

Sample Food Diary

Food Diary

Name Pat Doe   GOALS: 53   grams fat

Day Wednesday   Date 9/7   18   grams sat. fat

Exercise walked 2 miles in 35 minutes

Write ONE food item on each line.

Time & Place	Amount	Food—How Prepared	Fat g	Sat. Fat g
7 am	¾ cup	orange juice	0	0
home	1 cup	cornflakes	0	0
	1 cup	1% low-fat milk (½ cup on cereal)	3	2
	2 slices	toast, white	2	0
	1 tbsp	margarine, tub (reduced fat)	7	1
12 noon	2 slices	bread, whole-wheat	6	2
cafe	2 oz	roast beef, lean	5	2
	1 tbsp	mustard	0	0
	1 slice	American cheese	7	4
	2 cups	tossed salad	0	0
	2 tbsp	French dressing, low-calorie	2	0
	1 cup	frozen yogurt, low-fat	3	2
	1 glass	iced tea, plain	0	0
6 pm	4 oz	chicken breast, roasted w/o skin	4	1
home	1 cup	spaghetti w/tomato sauce	1	0
	1 cup	broccoli	0	0
	1	dinner roll	2	1
	1 tbsp	margarine (reduced fat)	7	1
	2	fig bar cookies	2	0
	1 glass	iced tea, plain	0	0
		Totals for day	51	16

Values rounded to nearest whole number.

FOLLOW-UP AND MAINTENANCE

Each person's blood lipid response to the Step I Diet should be determined at 4 to 6 weeks after starting the diet and again at 3 months. The table below can be used to determine if the LDL-cholesterol treatment goal has been achieved at follow-up. The goals take into account the presence of CHD or other atherosclerotic disease and the number of major risk factors present (listed on pages 16–17). The table includes values for both total cholesterol and LDL-cholesterol because your physician may order a test that measures only total cholesterol at some of your clinic visits.

GOALS FOR BLOOD CHOLESTEROL AT FOLLOW-UP*

Patient Category	Goal for LDL-Cholesterol	Goal for Total Cholesterol
Without CHD		
With fewer than 2 other risk factors	Less than 160 mg/dL	Less than 240 mg/dL
With 2 or more other risk factors	Less than 130 mg/dL	Less than 200 mg/dL
With CHD	100 mg/dL or less	

Goals apply whether the diet is Step I or Step II.

For a person who has CHD or other atherosclerotic disease, the goal for LDL-cholesterol is much lower (100 mg/dL or less) than for a person without heart disease. The goal is lower because the risk for having a CHD event, such as a heart attack, is greater for those who have atherosclerotic disease than for those who do not.

If your goal for lowering LDL-cholesterol *has been met* at 3 months, you should continue following the fat-modified diet and return regularly to your physician for long-term monitoring. Long-term monitoring consists of follow-up with the physician at least four times the first year and twice yearly for the following years.

If at 3 months your cholesterol *has not come down* enough to meet your goal level, ask your physician for the name of a registered dietitian who can help you with your diet. Your cholesterol should be rechecked at 4 to 6 weeks and again at 3 months.

One way you can evaluate your adherence to the Step I Diet or Step II Diet is to complete the MEDFICTS food assessment tool found on page 360 of the Appendix. Although MEDFICTS does not give you the exact calories you have eaten or the percent of calories from fat, it can help you evaluate how carefully you are following the Step I or Step II Diet. Directions for scoring appear on page 361.

If you have carefully followed the Step I Diet and your LDL-cholesterol has not decreased to your goal level, you should ask your physician to have a registered dietitian help you progress to the

Step II Diet. If following the Step II Diet still does not result in adequate cholesterol lowering, your physician may advise you to follow a very low fat diet providing no more than 20% of calories from fat (see page 40, as noted above).

Keeping detailed food records increases your awareness of the foods you eat and therefore can help you make better food choices. Food records are very useful to a registered dietitian who is trying to assess your adherence to the Step I or Step II Diet or to a very low fat diet. A dietitian can evaluate your food records through estimation, or he or she can obtain a more accurate picture of your eating habits through computer analysis of 3 to 4 days of food records.

Dietary Components

The information in this section about basic dietary components can be useful to you in planning a diet to lower blood cholesterol and triglyceride levels as well as body weight. The major dietary components considered here are calories, total fat, saturated fat, monounsaturated fat, polyunsaturated fat, cholesterol, carbohydrate, fiber, protein, alcohol, vitamins, minerals, sodium, and caffeine. Sugars are discussed in Chapter 5 on managing diabetes.

CALORIES

Obesity, which results from excessive calorie intake, can raise total cholesterol, LDL-cholesterol, triglyceride, blood pressure, and blood glucose levels and can lower HDL-cholesterol. Weight reduction is an important step in improving these conditions. Weight reduction is most successful when achieved by a combination of calorie restriction and regular physical activity (exercise). A discussion of what you should weigh and the number of calories you need daily starts on page 356. Information on weight control and physical activity is in Chapter 3.

Sources of calories in the diet are carbohydrate, protein, fat, and alcohol. Fat is the most concentrated source of calories, providing more than twice as many calories per gram as carbohydrate or protein. In practical terms, a teaspoon of oil (pure fat) has more than twice the calories of the same amount of sugar (pure carbohydrate).

SOURCES OF CALORIES

Fat	9 calories per gram
Carbohydrate	4 calories per gram
Protein	4 calories per gram
Alcohol	7 calories per gram

Decreasing your intake of fat is the most efficient way to lower calories. The table starting on page 372 of the Appendix shows the calorie content of many common foods.

TOTAL FAT

The Step I and Step II Diets limit fat intake to no more than 30% of calories. Two primary reasons for limiting fat in the diet are to decrease calories, thereby lowering body weight, and to decrease saturated fat in order to lower total cholesterol and LDL-cholesterol.

The guideline of limiting fat to no more than 30% of calories means accounting for all the fat being consumed. This includes fat that naturally occurs in food (meats and dairy products), fat used in food preparation (cakes, cookies, candies, sauces, and salad dressings), and fat added to food at the table (spread on bread). As discussed on pages 42–43, the maximum amount of fat recommended for you depends on your calorie intake. For example, at 1,500 calories per day you should have a maximum of 50 grams of fat, whereas at 2,000 calories you may have up to 67 grams of fat.

There are at least three ways to look at fat content of foods: (1) calories from fat, (2) percent of calories from fat, and (3) percent fat by weight.

- *Calories from fat* refers to the number of calories provided by fat in one serving of a food. The calories-from-fat value is calculated by multiplying the number of grams of fat in one serving by 9 (the calories in each gram of fat). For example, a 570-caloric slice of cheesecake that contains 40 grams of fat provides 360 calories from fat ($40 \times 9 = 360$). The Food and Drug Administration (FDA) requires manufacturers to print the calories from fat in the Nutrition Facts portion of food labels.

- *Percent of calories from fat* is calculated by dividing the calories from fat by the total calories in the food. For example, the slice of cheesecake described above provides 360 calories from fat and 570 total calories. Divide 360 by 570 (and multiply by 100 to get percent) to find the percent of calories from fat in the cheesecake, which is 63%. *It is important to note that percent of calories from fat should not be used to evaluate whether individual foods are appropriate in a cholesterol-lowering eating plan.* The guideline of 30% of calories from fat refers to all the food eaten in a day and not to individual foods or meals. Applying "30% of calories from fat" to single foods in an attempt to evaluate them will lead to the exclusion of many foods that are often included in limited amounts in a well-balanced cholesterol-lowering eating plan. Examples of these foods include oil and margarine (100% of calories from fat), eggs (64% of calories from fat), regular salad dressing (85% to 100% of calories from fat), dark chicken meat without the skin (43% of calories from fat), salmon (36% of calories from fat), and turkey ham (34% of calories from fat).

- *Percent fat by weight* is often confused with percent of calories from fat. Percent fat simply means the amount of fat by weight (in grams) in a specified amount (100 grams) of a food. Percent fat is used only to describe the amount of fat in a single food. For example, "2%-fat milk" means that 2% of the weight of the milk is fat; each 100 grams of milk (a little less than ½ cup) contains 2 grams of fat. Other examples of foods for which percent fat is often given are 10% fat ground meat and 4%-fat cottage cheese. Another way to state fat content by weight is by listing "percent fat free." When a label states that a product is 90% fat free, this is the same as saying that it is 10% fat by weight. Both ways of stating percent fat are accurate.

FATS AND OILS – Fat has a number of important functions in the body. It is the most concentrated source of calories, providing more than twice the calories of carbohydrate or protein. Fat spares protein so that protein can be used to build and repair tissue instead of being used for energy. It helps with the transportation and absorption of the fat-soluble vitamins (A, D, E, and K). Fat slows down the rate at which food leaves the stomach and produces a feeling of satiety (fullness) after a meal. Fat adds to the palatability of food.

Fats at room temperature range in consistency from liquid to solid. In dietetics fats that are solid are referred to as fats, and those that are liquid are referred to as oils. However, "fat" can be used to refer to both liquid and solid forms, and that is how it is used in this book.

Fats are divided into three types, based on their chemical structure, specifically, the number of double bonds they contain. Saturated fatty acids contain no double bonds. Monounsaturated fatty acids have one double bond in the fatty acid chain, and polyunsaturated fatty acids have two or more double bonds. Each fat naturally found in food is made up of a combination of these three types of fatty acids. For example, olive oil, which is often described as a monounsaturated fat, also contains both saturated and polyunsaturated fatty acids. The following table shows the specific fatty acids found in common food sources.

FATTY ACID CONTENT OF COMMON FATS

| Fat Source (100 g) | Saturated | | | | Monounsaturated | Polyunsaturated |
	Lauric g	Myristic g	Palmitic g	Stearic g	Oleic g	Linoleic g
Beef fat	0.9	3.7	24.9	18.9	36.0	3.1
Butter	2.3	8.2	21.3	9.8	20.4	1.8
Canola oil	—	—	3.1	1.2	29.2	17.5
Chicken fat	0.1	0.9	21.6	6.0	37.3	19.5
Cocoa butter	—	0.1	25.4	33.2	32.6	2.8
Coconut oil	44.6	16.8	8.2	2.8	5.8	1.8
Corn oil	0.0	0.0	10.9	1.8	24.2	58.0
Lard	0.2	1.3	23.8	13.5	41.2	10.2
Olive oil	—	0.0	11.0	2.2	72.5	7.9
Palm kernel oil	47.0	16.4	8.1	2.8	11.4	1.6
Palm oil	0.1	1.0	43.5	4.3	36.6	9.1
Peanut oil	—	0.1	9.4	2.2	44.8	32.0
Safflower oil	—	0.1	6.2	2.2	11.7	74.1

(continued)

Fat Source (100 g)	Saturated				Monounsaturated	Polyunsaturated
	Lauric g	Myristic g	Palmitic g	Stearic g	Oleic g	Linoleic g
Soybean oil (partially hydrogenated)	—	0.1	9.8	5.0	42.5	43.9
Sunflower oil	—	—	5.9	4.5	19.5	65.7

Adapted from USDA, Composition of Foods, *Agriculture Handbook series no. 8 (Washington, D.C.: USDA, 1976–1992).*
— = No data available.

SATURATED FAT

The primary dietary factor that raises total cholesterol and LDL-cholesterol is saturated fat, that is, saturated fatty acids. The specific saturated fatty acids that raise cholesterol are lauric (12 carbon atoms in the fatty acid chain), myristic (14-carbon chain), and palmitic (16-carbon chain). The table below includes common sources of fat, listed from lowest to highest in saturated fat.

COMPOSITION OF COMMON FATS

Fat Source (1 tablespoon)	Saturated Fat g	Monounsaturated Fat g	Polyunsaturated Fat g
Canola oil	0.8	8.4	4.2
Safflower oil (oleic acid over 70%)	0.8	10.2	1.9
Safflower oil	1.2	1.6	10.1
Walnut oil	1.2	3.1	8.6
Sunflower oil	1.4	2.7	8.9
Corn oil	1.7	3.3	8.0
Olive oil	1.8	9.9	1.1
Soybean oil	2.0	3.2	7.9
Margarine, corn oil (tub)	2.1	4.5	4.5
Peanut oil	2.3	6.2	4.3
Margarine, soybean oil (stick)	2.4	5.4	3.0
Chicken fat	3.8	5.7	2.7
Beef fat	6.4	5.3	0.5
Butter	7.2	3.3	0.4

Adapted from USDA, Composition of Foods, *Agriculture Handbook series no. 8 (Washington, D.C.: USDA, 1976–1992).*

The public is often confused by reports of research studies that deal with the effect of single fatty acids on LDL-cholesterol. For example, stearic acid (18-carbon chain) is a saturated fatty acid that does not raise or lower LDL-cholesterol. Although beef fat, lard, and cocoa butter (the fat in chocolate) are high in stearic acid, they also contain palmitic acid and other fatty acids that do raise LDL-cholesterol (see table on pages 52–53).

Saturated fats are found in all foods of animal origin and in certain plant oils. In the American diet about two-thirds of the saturated fat consumed comes from animal fats. The animal fats include butterfat (in butter, whole milk, cheese, cream, sour cream, and ice cream) and fat from meat (beef, pork, lamb, and poultry). The plant oils that are high in saturated fat are palm oil, coconut oil, and palm kernel oil (tropical oils). When food manufacturers decreased their use of tropical oils, they replaced most of them with hydrogenated fats.

HYDROGENATION AND *TRANS* FATTY ACIDS – Hydrogenation of polyunsaturated fats is a process by which double bonds in the fatty acid chains are replaced with single bonds. This process increases the melting points of oils and frequently converts them from a liquid to a solid state at room temperature. Hydrogenation increases the amount of saturated fat present; however, the most abundant saturated fatty acid usually formed by hydrogenation is stearic acid, which does not raise blood levels of LDL-cholesterol. Hydrogenation of polyunsaturated fatty acids often produces monounsaturated fatty acids; one of these is the naturally occurring oleic acid, which has *cis* geometry, and another is the unnatural elaidic acid, which has *trans* geometry. *Trans* fatty acids also occur naturally in the fat of beef and dairy products. Recent research indicates that *trans* fatty acids have almost the same cholesterol-raising effect as saturated fatty acids, and analyses of the diets of more than 85,000 nurses surveyed as part of the Nurses' Health Study indicate that hydrogenated vegetable oils may contribute to the occurrence of CHD.

It is estimated that *trans* fatty acids contribute 3% to 7% of the fat consumed in the American diet. Most of the tropical oils (palm, palm kernel, and coconut) used in processed foods have now been replaced by partially hydrogenated fats that contain *trans* fatty acids. Major food sources of *trans* fatty acids identified in the Nurses' Health Study included margarine, cookies, cake, and white bread. The best ways to decrease your intake of *trans* fatty acids are to decrease your total fat intake and to decrease your use of fats that are hydrogenated.

The more hydrogenated a fat is, the harder it becomes and the more *trans* fatty acids it contains. For example, shortening is higher in *trans* fatty acids than margarine, and stick margarine is higher than soft (tub and squeeze) margarine. Reduced-fat margarines are even lower in *trans* fatty acids than soft margarines because they contain less total fat; fat-free margarines contain no *trans* fatty acids. Margarine that is soft, reduced in fat, or fat free is a much better choice than butter. Oil is even lower in *trans* fatty acids than margarine, and unhydrogenated oils are extremely low in *trans* fatty acids.

Since the *trans* fatty acid content of food is not currently a required part of food labeling, there is no way to know the exact amount present in a food. If a food is labeled "low fat," it cannot have a significant *trans* fatty acid content because the total fat is low. The only Nutrient Content Claim that is part of food labeling and has *trans* as part of its definition is "saturated fat free" (page 134). For a food to be labeled saturated fat free, it must have less than 0.5 gram of *trans* fatty acids per serving. The best way to determine which foods contain *trans* fatty acids is to read the list of ingredients. If a food contains a hydrogenated or partially hydrogenated fat, it likely contains some *trans* fatty acids.

MONOUNSATURATED FAT

Foods high in monounsaturated fat help lower LDL-cholesterol when they are substituted for foods high in saturated fat in the diet. The most concentrated sources of monounsaturated fat are olive oil, canola oil, peanut oil, and the high-oleic form of safflower oil, as seen on page 53. Other sources of monounsaturated fat in the American diet are avocados, nuts (especially hazelnuts, pecans, and macadamia nuts), and the fat in beef and pork (which also contain saturated fat).

The current American diet derives 14% to 16% of its calories from monounsaturated fat, which is the same as the recommendation for both the Step I and Step II Diets. However, much of the monounsaturated fat in the American diet comes from animal foods, such as meat fat, and foods prepared with shortening and butter; all of these are also high in saturated fat. These foods need to be replaced in the diet with foods lower in saturated fat to lower LDL-cholesterol. Therefore, an oil, such as olive or canola, that is low in saturated fat and high in monounsaturated fat should be the fat used for food preparation. Of course, monounsaturated fats (like all fats) are a concentrated source of calories, and care must be taken not to increase calories above a person's needs.

THE MEDITERRANEAN DIET AND THE FRENCH PARADOX – The Mediterranean diet has traditionally been the best example of an eating pattern in which the main source of fat is high in monounsaturated fatty acids. Interest in the Mediterranean diet first began as the result of data collected in the 1950s and 1960s that showed a low rate of CHD in Crete (one of the Greek islands) at a time when the diet there contained 35% to 40% of calories from fat, a level comparable to the American diet. Data also showed that the CHD rate in southern Italy, where the fat intake was 25% to 27% of calories, was lower than in Japan, where on average 11% of calories were from fat. One common feature of the Cretan and Italian diets was their primary fat source: olive oil, rich in monounsaturated fatty acids.

Compared with the American diet, the traditional Mediterranean diet contained less butter, cream, whole milk, red meat, and eggs, and more cheese, seafood, fruit, vegetables, beans, whole grains, and olive oil. However, the eating pattern in some of these areas has changed over the last 30 years. There has been a trend toward a higher intake of fat and saturated fat, primarily through increased consumption of meat and dairy products. For example, between 1960 and 1991 in Crete the intake of monounsaturated fat decreased from 29% of calories to 23%, and saturated fat increased from 8% of calories to 10%. In Greece there was a 29% increase in the death rate from cardiovascular disease in the twenty years between the period 1960 to 1964 and the period 1980 to 1984. Data from 1989 indicate a death rate for men from cardiovascular disease in Greece of 432 per 100,000 population; this is only slightly lower than the rate of 456 per 100,000 in the United States.

Studies of CHD in various parts of the world have focused attention on CHD rates in southern Europe, which are much lower than in the United States, and especially in France, which has lower CHD rates than other Mediterranean countries such as Greece, Italy, and Spain. The low CHD rate in France has puzzled researchers because the French diet is similar to the U.S. diet in amounts of fat and saturated fat; in addition, the average blood cholesterol and blood pressure levels in France are higher than in the United States, the rate of obesity is comparable, and the rate of smoking is higher. A number of possible explanations have been offered for this "French paradox," but no answer has been found. One possible explanation of the French paradox is that the red wine drunk with meals may provide some type of protection against CHD (see page 60 for discussion of alcohol and heart disease). It is not clear whether the possible protection afforded by moderate alcohol intake is due to alcohol's ability to increase the HDL-cholesterol level; the antioxidant effect on LDL-cholesterol of substances such as phenols in red wine (see pages 171–77 for discussion of antioxidants); or the effect of alcohol on reducing the coagulation of platelets, a step that reduces the tendency to form blood clots. Some researchers have suggested that the French paradox does not really exist, and that heart disease rates are higher in northern France than in southern France, where the diet is Mediterranean.

CHD is a complex disease for which there are multiple risk factors; to date, the French paradox has provided more questions than answers. Some researchers believe that there is no French paradox and that changes in the French diet, such as increased fat intake (from 29% of calories in the early 1960s to 39% in the late 1980s) and decreased alcohol intake, are too recent to have had an effect on CHD rates. CHD takes many years to develop; perhaps the CHD rates have not had time to reflect the change in diet. The diet in the United States has been high in saturated fat since the 1950s. It is possible that in a few years the changing diet in France may increase CHD rates until they are similar to those in other countries with high intakes of fat and saturated fat.

POLYUNSATURATED FAT

Polyunsaturated fat helps lower LDL-cholesterol when it is substituted for saturated fat in the diet. There are two major types of polyunsaturated fatty acids: omega-6 fatty acids and omega-3 fatty acids. Omega-6 fatty acids are made up primarily of linoleic acid. Most vegetable oils, including corn, safflower, sunflower, and soybean, are high in linoleic acid (as shown in the table on pages 52–53).

Fish and fish oils are the major sources of omega-3 fatty acids, primarily as eicosapentaenoic acid and docosahexaenoic acid. High-fat varieties of finfish are better sources of omega-3 fatty acids than low-fat finfish and shellfish (see the following table). Fish that live in cold water (for example, mackerel and salmon) are higher in omega-3 fatty acids than those that live in warm water (for example, flounder and redfish). For the fish that live in frigid waters, omega-3 fatty acids act like antifreeze to keep their bodies pliable.

CONTENT OF TOTAL FAT, OMEGA-3 FATTY ACIDS, AND CHOLESTEROL OF SELECTED FISH

Fish (3 oz)	Total Fat g	Omega-3 Fatty Acids* g	Cholesterol mg
Finfish: cooked by dry heat			
Mackerel, Atlantic	15.1	1.0	64
Salmon, sockeye	9.3	1.0	74
Swordfish	4.4	0.7	43
Trout, rainbow	3.7	0.6	62
Halibut	2.5	0.4	35
Tuna, white (canned in water)	2.1	0.6	35
Redfish	1.8	0.3	46
Flounder	1.3	0.4	58
Haddock	0.8	0.2	63
Cod, Atlantic	0.7	0.1	47
Shellfish: cooked by moist heat			
Clam	1.7	0.2	57
Crab, blue	1.5	0.4	85
Crayfish	1.2	0.2	151
Shrimp	0.9	0.3	166
Lobster, northern	0.5	0.1	61

Adapted from USDA, Composition of Foods, *Agriculture Handbook series no. 8 (Washington, D.C.: USDA, 1976–1992).*
*Omega-3 fatty acids include eicosapentaenoic acid and docosahexaenoic acid.

Omega-3 fatty acids have only a minor effect in lowering LDL-cholesterol; however, they are much more effective in lowering triglyceride level. Some recent research suggests that consuming at least two portions of fatty fish per week reduces mortality in men who have had a heart attack. Taking a fish oil supplement is not recommended unless prescribed and monitored by a physician.

DIETARY CHOLESTEROL

Dietary cholesterol raises the level of cholesterol in the blood of many people. Individuals differ in the extent to which consuming cholesterol raises their blood cholesterol level. Dietary cholesterol may also contribute to the ability of saturated fat to increase blood levels of LDL-cholesterol. In the diet for the general population it is recommended that dietary cholesterol be limited to less than 300 mg per day—the level recommended in the Step I Diet. For those people who do not achieve sufficient blood cholesterol reduction at this level of cholesterol restriction, and for people with known atherosclerotic disease, the recommendation is limitation of dietary cholesterol to no more than 200 mg per day (Step II Diet).

Dietary cholesterol is found only in animal foods—egg yolk, meat, poultry, fish, and dairy products. Egg yolk is the most concentrated source of dietary cholesterol; an average egg yolk contains 213 mg. Cholesterol is found in both the lean and fat portions of all types of meat: beef, pork, veal, lamb, poultry, game, and fish. Some shellfish (primarily shrimp and crayfish) are higher in cholesterol than other meats; however, since they are low in fat, they can be included in an eating plan within the recommended cholesterol level. Organ meats, such as liver, brain, and sweetbread, are very high in cholesterol; if eaten at all, their use should be limited to a small serving occasionally.

Your eating pattern will average less than 300 mg of cholesterol per day when you limit (1) meat, poultry, and fish to no more than 6 ounces cooked per day, (2) egg yolks to three per week, and (3) dairy products to low-fat and fat-free varieties. The cholesterol content of common foods is listed in the Appendix, starting on page 372.

Many people trying to lower their blood cholesterol stop eating beef because of a mistaken idea that it is too high in dietary cholesterol. Recent research, however, has shown that an eating pattern low in fat, saturated fat, and cholesterol that contains lean beef is just as effective in lowering blood cholesterol as a similar eating pattern in which the only meat is chicken or a combination of fish and chicken.

CARBOHYDRATE

It is recommended on the Step I and Step II Diets that at least 55% of calories come from carbohydrate. Complex carbohydrate, such as that found in beans, bread, cereal, pasta, potatoes, rice, and vegetables, is preferred. Other naturally occurring carbohydrate is found in fruit and milk. All of these foods are good sources of vitamins and minerals; with the exception of milk, these foods also provide fiber. The term "refined" carbohydrate refers to the sugar, syrup, and high-fructose sweeteners found in many products, such as cakes, candies, pastries, and soft drinks.

It is recommended that when fat intake is reduced to 30% or less of calories to help lower blood cholesterol levels, the fat calories be replaced primarily by complex carbohydrate. Replacing saturated fat in the diet with carbohydrate, monounsaturated fat, or polyunsaturated fat results in about the same lowering of LDL-cholesterol. When fat is reduced to much below 30% of calories and replaced with carbohydrate, there is a tendency for the triglyceride level to rise and the HDL-cholesterol level to fall. Some experts believe that when HDL-cholesterol goes down as a result of such dietary changes, the reduction is harmless; however, more research is needed in this area. When fat reduction is undertaken primarily for weight loss, fat calories should not be replaced; the total calories consumed should be at a lower level.

FIBER

Fiber is a type of carbohydrate that the body cannot digest; it does not provide calories. Fiber is of two types—soluble and insoluble—which have different effects in the body. Consumption of soluble fiber is associated with some lowering of blood cholesterol. Good sources of soluble fiber include oat cereals, dried beans, legumes, guar gums, barley, pectins (from fruit), and psyllium. The addition of 2 ounces of an oat cereal (oatmeal or oat bran) daily to an eating pattern low in total fat and saturated fat lowers blood cholesterol by an additional 2% to 3%.

Insoluble fiber, such as that found in wheat bran, helps increase bulk in the stool and promotes regular bowel habits but does not help reduce cholesterol levels. Consuming large amounts of insoluble fiber can lead to bloating, flatulence, and increased bowel movements; it may also result in reduced intestinal absorption of calcium and other nutrients.

The recommended intake of fiber for adults is 20 to 30 grams per day; about one-fourth (5 to 7 grams) of the total fiber should be of the soluble type. Consumption of six or more servings of grain products and five or more servings of fruits and vegetables per day should provide adequate dietary fiber. The fiber in food is a combination of both soluble and insoluble fiber, as shown in the following table.

FIBER CONTENT OF SELECTED FOODS

Food	Total Fiber g	Soluble Fiber g	Insoluble Fiber g	Calories
100% wheat bran cereal (¾ cup)	14.0	1.2	12.8	106
Pinto beans, cooked (¾ cup)	9.0	2.8	6.2	177
Corn, cooked (¾ cup)	2.3	0.3	2.0	100
Oat bran muffin (1 medium)*	1.0	0.5	0.5	142
Apple with skin (1 medium)	2.8	1.0	1.8	81
Oat bran, cooked (¾ cup)	4.0	2.0	2.0	68
Oatmeal, cooked (¾ cup)	2.7	1.4	1.3	109

Adapted from Nutrition Data System, University of Minnesota, Minneapolis.
*Fat content is 6 g; other foods in table contain less than 2 g fat each.

PROTEIN

The recommended intake of protein in the Step I and Step II Diets is about 15% of calories. Both animal and vegetable sources of protein are appropriate in a healthy diet, as long as the foods are low in saturated fat. For more information on protein, see Chapter 6, on vegetarian diet, which starts on page 116.

Some experts believe that eating a very high protein diet for many years may not be healthy. When fat in the diet is decreased, the calories should not be replaced with high-protein foods; it is important to keep protein at approximately 15% of calories. If weight loss is not needed, calories from fat can be replaced with carbohydrate.

ALCOHOL

It has been noted in population studies that people with a moderate alcohol intake have lower rates of CHD than nondrinkers. These observations have led to numerous research studies designed to identify any effects of alcohol on risk factors for CHD. The results of these studies are not in general agreement. Some research supports the hypothesis that red wine is the only type of alcoholic drink that is protective (see the discussion of the French paradox on pages 55–56). Some researchers believe that a compound found in the skins of the grapes used to make red wine is responsible. More recently, several studies have shown that an alcohol intake (whether from wine, beer, or spirits) not exceeding two drinks per day (see below) increases HDL-cholesterol ("good" cholesterol) and may decrease a person's tendency to form blood clots that can block an artery narrowed by plaque in atherosclerosis.

However, consumption of alcohol for the purpose of reducing CHD risk is not recommended for several very good reasons. Although alcohol does not affect LDL-cholesterol levels in most people, it raises triglyceride levels in some. It is a source of calories and can contribute to weight gain. (Calorie content and alcohol content of alcoholic beverages are in the Appendix on pages 370–71.) Nondrinkers are not advised to begin using alcohol; it is difficult, if not impossible, to predict which beginning drinkers will graduate from moderate to heavy alcohol use, with all its harmful results. High alcohol intake can lead to a number of serious disorders, including cirrhosis and other liver damage, and has negative psychological and social consequences. Women should not drink alcoholic beverages during pregnancy because of the risk for birth defects. Alcohol use is associated with increased motor vehicle accidents. Anyone who does drink is advised to do so in moderation; moderate alcohol intake is defined as no more than two drinks per day. One drink is defined as:

- 12 fluid ounces of regular or light beer

- 5 fluid ounces of table wine

- 3 fluid ounces of fortified wine, such as sherry, port, marsala, or Madeira

- 1½ fluid ounces (a jigger) of 80-proof liquor or 1 fluid ounce of 100-proof liquor such as bourbon, rum, gin, vodka, or Scotch

VITAMINS

The Step I and Step II Diets can provide adequate amounts of all the vitamins needed for good health. Researchers are investigating whether additional amounts of antioxidants, such as vitamins C and E and beta-carotene (a precursor of vitamin A), have a protective effect against heart disease. There is not enough evidence at the time of printing this book to recommend taking supplements of antioxidants to protect against heart disease. However, the best food sources of vitamin C and beta-carotene are deep-yellow vegetables and fruits, especially citrus fruits, and dark-green vegetables (see pages 173–77 for lists of food sources of antioxidants and their values). It is recommended that five or more servings of fruits and vegetables be consumed each day. The best food sources of vitamin E are vegetable oils and margarines made from them; other sources include wheat germ, nuts, and green leafy vegetables. Additional information on antioxidants is on pages 171–72. Vitamins and minerals are the subject of Chapter 9.

MINERALS

As a rule, most people can get sufficient minerals by eating a balanced diet and do not need to take a mineral supplement. One exception may be calcium intake in women; a sufficient intake of calcium is important for a woman throughout her life to help avoid developing osteoporosis after menopause. Dairy products are the best source of calcium in the diet; fat-free or low-fat milk, yogurt, and cheese contain as much calcium as high-fat varieties. The calcium content of selected foods is shown on page 183.

Some research has suggested that high levels of iron stored in the body are linked to increased risk for heart disease; however, other research studies have failed to demonstrate this association. There is little chance of getting too much iron from food, but taking iron supplements can easily result in consumption of more than the recommended level (see page 178). For example, the Recommended Dietary Allowance (RDA) per day for iron is 10 mg for females ages 11 through 50 years, and 15 mg for males 19 years and older and for females 51 years and older. Most multiple vitamin and mineral supplements contain 18 mg of iron; typical single-nutrient iron supplements contain 30 to 65 mg.

SODIUM

One mineral that deserves special attention is sodium. Sodium intake is associated with blood pressure levels. Moderate salt restriction, which will usually lower blood pressure and thus reduce risk for heart disease (high blood pressure is a major risk factor for heart disease), is recommended for all healthy adults. The level of sodium recommended by the National High Blood Pressure Education Program is a maximum of 2,400 mg per day. The American Heart Association recommends a slightly higher level—no more than 3,000 mg per day. Additional information on sodium begins on page 93 in Chapter 4.

CAFFEINE

Caffeine is addictive and has recently been defined as a substance that can cause dependence. Caffeine is found in coffee, tea, many carbonated soft drinks (both regular and sugar free), chocolate, some pain medications, diet pills, and preparations to keep you awake. The median daily intake of caffeine is 357 mg. Caffeine is a stimulant. For some people it can cause an increase in appetite, particularly between meals; this increase in appetite can result in consumption of excess calories, which can lead to weight gain.

The effect of drinking coffee on blood cholesterol has been investigated. Although several studies suggest that drinking large amounts of coffee, especially boiled, unfiltered coffee, increases blood cholesterol, the findings are unclear. Cigarette smoking appears to be an aggravating factor. In other words, increases in blood cholesterol with heavy consumption of coffee appear to be more likely in smokers than nonsmokers.

COMMON FOOD SOURCES OF CAFFEINE

Source	Caffeine mg*
Coffee (6 fl oz)	
Brewed, drip	105
Instant	60
Tea (6 fl oz)	
Brewed	35
Instant	25
Cola (12 fl oz)	
Regular	35
Diet	50
Chocolate	
Semisweet (3 oz)	60
Milk chocolate candy (3 oz)	15

Adapted from Nutrition Data System, University of Minnesota, Minneapolis.
*Values rounded to the nearest 5 mg.

Drugs to Lower Cholesterol and Triglyceride Levels

When patients at high risk for CHD are unable to reach their goals for blood lipids with the lifestyle modifications of a low-fat eating pattern, exercise, and weight control, medications that improve lipid levels may be prescribed. These drugs are always given in addition to lifestyle modifications, never as a replacement for them. In other words, if your physician recommends that you begin lipid-lowering medication, you need to continue your lifestyle efforts with as much or even more vigor than before. Changes in lifestyle may enable you to take a lower dose of a drug, which reduces the risk for side effects from the drug. Bear in mind that the lifestyle modifications that improve your blood lipid levels also improve your health in many other ways.

In most cases in which lipid-lowering drugs are necessary, the drug therapy must be long-term or lifelong. Just as blood pressure medications can control but cannot cure high blood pressure, lipid-lowering medications can control but do not cure blood lipid elevations. Abnormal blood lipids or blood pressure should be controlled with diet and exercise when at all possible. If a drug is necessary in addition to diet and exercise, your physician will consider many factors to decide which drug or drugs are right for you—for example, your overall risk for CHD, your lipid goals, your age, and your medical history. A variety of safe and effective drugs for controlling blood lipid levels are available. The drugs differ in their effects on the major lipids, so your physician has a varied "arsenal" for different lipid targets.

The available lipid-lowering drugs fall into five classes: (1) nicotinic acid, (2) bile-acid resins, (3) HMG-CoA reductase inhibitors, (4) fibric-acid derivatives, and (5) probucol. The National Cholesterol Education Program notes that physicians may also consider using estrogen-replacement therapy to help control moderate LDL-cholesterol elevation in postmenopausal women. The major actions and side effects of the five classes of lipid-lowering drugs, as well as estrogen-replacement therapy (which is not classified by the FDA as a lipid-lowering drug), are described below. These drugs may be given as single agents or in drug combinations by your physician. Probucol, as noted below, is rarely used.

The drug names used below are all generic names; if you know only the trade name of the drug you are taking, check the drug packaging or ask your pharmacist or physician for the generic name.

NICOTINIC ACID

Nicotinic acid, or niacin, is a B vitamin that is very effective for lowering LDL-cholesterol ("bad" cholesterol), lowering triglyceride, and raising HDL-cholesterol ("good" cholesterol). Thus, it is useful in most lipid disorders, and it has the advantage of being a relatively inexpensive drug. Nicotinamide is sometimes called niacin but does not lower cholesterol; the two should not be confused.

Many patients experience uncomfortable side effects with the use of nicotinic acid, including tingling, warm feelings, headaches, nausea, gas, and heartburn. Nicotinic acid may also cause diarrhea, fatigue, itching, or a rash. Taking an aspirin (or, if necessary, ibuprofen instead of aspirin) 30 minutes before a dose of nicotinic acid or taking the drug while you have food in your stomach can lessen the side effects. Side effects are more likely to occur when you first begin taking nicotinic acid or when the dosage is increased. Your physician will probably begin nicotinic acid at a low dose and gradually increase it, so that your body can get used to the drug.

Nicotinic acid is prepared in both immediate-release and slow-release forms. However, the slow-release form may increase risk for liver toxicity and is not approved by the FDA for treatment of cholesterol disorders. Nicotinic acid is not used in patients with chronic liver disease, and it is usually not used in patients with diabetes mellitus because it can worsen glucose intolerance. While taking nicotinic acid, you will need routine blood tests to make sure that other side effects are not occurring; be sure to obtain these tests as scheduled by your physician.

BILE-ACID RESINS

Bile-acid resins are also called bile-acid sequestrants or simply resins. Those available in the United States are cholestyramine and colestipol. The resins are chiefly active in lowering LDL-cholesterol ("bad" cholesterol). They may slightly increase HDL-cholesterol ("good" cholesterol), but they can sometimes also increase triglyceride. More often they have no effect on blood triglyceride level.

The resins are particularly safe drugs because their direct actions occur only in the intestines; they do not enter the bloodstream. They bind bile acids in the intestines and are eliminated in the stool. Some symptoms associated with bile-acid resins are constipation, bloating, gas, and heartburn. Increasing consumption of fluids and fiber can help relieve constipation if it occurs, and trying to avoid swallowing air when taking the resin can help prevent gas. Also, mixing the scoops or packets of resin with noncarbonated rather than carbonated liquids helps prevent belching. Side effects usually lessen over time.

Resins can interfere with the absorption in the intestine of other medications. It is important that you check with your physician about when to take other medications if you are taking a resin. Patients with a history of severe constipation or a triglyceride level higher than 500 mg/dL should not take bile-acid resins.

HMG-CoA REDUCTASE INHIBITORS

HMG-CoA reductase inhibitors, or statins, are the newest class of approved lipid-lowering drugs. Approved agents in the United States are fluvastatin, lovastatin, pravastatin, and simvastatin; other statins are under development. All the statins work in a similar way, by interfering with a key step in the body's manufacturing of cholesterol. The HMG-CoA reductase inhibitors as a class achieve the greatest reductions in LDL-cholesterol. They have the added benefits of moderately lowering triglyceride and moderately increasing HDL-cholesterol. They are easy to take and have good safety histories.

Rare side effects have included inflammation of muscles, called myositis, so alert your physician if you experience any unexplained muscle weakness or pain while taking a statin.

HMG-CoA reductase inhibitors are not used in patients with liver disease or women who are pregnant, likely to become pregnant, or breast-feeding. As with any drug, your physician will consider other factors (such as other drugs you are taking) and potential side effects in deciding whether a statin is the best lipid-lowering drug for you. Your physician will need to take routine blood tests to monitor your liver enzymes before you begin taking a statin and periodically thereafter.

FIBRIC-ACID DERIVATIVES

Fibric-acid derivatives, or fibrates, are well-tolerated drugs that have major effects in lowering triglyceride and raising HDL-cholesterol ("good" cholesterol). Their effect on LDL-cholesterol ("bad" cholesterol) is variable; they can substantially lower LDL-cholesterol, but in some cases they may even raise LDL-cholesterol, depending on the triglyceride level. Fibrates available in the United States at the time of this printing are gemfibrozil and clofibrate, although clofibrate is rarely used in this country.

Fibrates are not used in patients with liver or severe kidney disease or in patients with gallbladder disease. Your physician will need to use routine blood tests to monitor your liver enzyme levels during therapy with a fibrate. Side effects such as nausea, diarrhea, or the development of gallstones are rare.

PROBUCOL

Probucol is rarely used, although it is somewhat more likely to be used in combination-drug therapy than as a single drug. It moderately lowers LDL-cholesterol but in addition substantially lowers HDL-cholesterol. It usually has no effect on triglyceride level. Side effects are uncommon and usually of short duration; they are chiefly gastrointestinal (for example, diarrhea, abdominal pain, gas, nausea, and vomiting). Patients who take probucol must be monitored by electrocardiograms (ECGs) because some reports of side effects involving the heart have been made. In addition, probucol (like vitamin C or E) has antioxidant properties (see pages 171–72).

ESTROGEN-REPLACEMENT THERAPY

Postmenopausal estrogen-replacement therapy is chiefly prescribed to reduce the symptoms of menopause (for example, "hot flashes") and to lessen risk for the development of osteoporosis. However, physicians may also choose to prescribe oral estrogen-replacement therapy to improve the blood lipid profile, since it moderately lowers LDL-cholesterol and moderately raises HDL-cholesterol.

Premenopausal women who are not diabetic are relatively protected from CHD compared with men in their age group. After menopause the rate of heart disease gradually rises in women until women and men have about the same rate of heart disease. Changes in lipid levels probably account at least in part for the increase in heart disease after menopause. At menopause, LDL-cholesterol levels rise sharply and may thereafter exceed levels in men. Also at menopause, HDL-cholesterol levels may decrease somewhat, but they generally remain higher in women throughout life. Triglyceride levels gradually rise in both males and females after puberty but at a slower rate in women; in middle age they may decrease in men yet continue to rise in women.

Many researchers believe that the apparent benefit of oral estrogen-replacement therapy on risk for CHD is related to the beneficial effects of the estrogen on the blood lipid profile. Evidence from many large population studies supports the concept that oral estrogen-replacement therapy given after menopause (whether the menopause is natural or surgical) reduces risk for CHD. In 10-year findings from the Nurses' Health Study, current estrogen use was associated with about a 50% decrease in risk for CHD as well as a 50% decrease in risk for death from any cardiovascular cause, such as stroke.

Such results, however, are considered preliminary because they need confirmation from randomized studies designed from the outset to examine this question. One such study, begun in 1995, is the Women's Health Initiative, which will include the largest clinical trial ever conducted in the United States. The Women's Health Initiative, which is a project of the National Institutes of Health, is focusing on CHD, breast and colorectal cancer, and osteoporosis and will assess the value of estrogen-replacement therapy, dietary patterns, and supplementation with calcium and vitamin D in preventing these conditions.

In addition to decreasing LDL-cholesterol and increasing HDL-cholesterol, oral estrogen may also increase triglyceride. The effect of increasing the triglyceride level is particularly likely in women who already have elevated triglyceride. A physician may choose not to prescribe oral estrogen in a woman with elevated triglyceride. When oral estrogen is given, the physician will monitor the triglyceride level. As with any drug, the physician must consider many pros and cons in deciding whether oral estrogen is the best choice for a particular patient. Estrogen-replacement therapy that is administered through routes other than the oral route (for example, as a skin patch or cream) does not appear to have the same beneficial effects on blood lipids or CHD risk. Also, nonoral estrogen would not be expected to increase the triglyceride level.

It is important to take estrogen only when it is really needed. Estrogen given alone increases risk for cancer of the uterus. Women who have not undergone hysterectomy (removal of the uterus) are given hormone-replacement therapy that includes not only estrogen but also progestin. This combination of hormones reduces or even eliminates the increased risk for uterine cancer from estrogen administration. Less consistent evidence implicates estrogen use in increased risk for breast cancer; adherence to standard recommendations for breast cancer screening is prudent. Estrogen also increases risk for the development of gallbladder disease needing surgery and can cause such problems as nausea and vomiting, breast tenderness or enlargement, and enlargement of benign tumors of the uterus. So even though estrogen has important uses, it has risks as well. You and your physician must carefully assess the ratio of risk to benefit to decide if estrogen use is the right choice for you.

Chapter 3

The Living Heart Diet in Weight Control

One-third of U.S. adults are obese, that is, 20% or more above their desirable weight. This figure does not include the many people who are overweight—who have 10 or 15 pounds that they cannot seem to lose but who are not heavy enough to be considered obese.

Nancy, age 35, is a typical example of someone who has had a constant struggle with "those stubborn 15 pounds." Nancy first began gaining weight while at college; she went from 127 pounds (slim for her height of 5 feet 6 inches) in high school to 135 pounds by college graduation. Nancy lost and regained 8 to 10 pounds several times before stabilizing at 145 pounds after her second pregnancy. The news that her older sister, who is 40 pounds over her desirable weight, had developed diabetes made Nancy decide to get serious about losing weight.

By working with a registered dietitian to plan a practical low-fat eating plan and adopting a moderate exercise program recommended by her physician, in three months Nancy succeeded in reducing her weight to 130 pounds.

She did not use a structured diet plan but primarily substituted foods lower in fat and calories for some of her favorite high-fat and high-calorie foods. First, Nancy talked to her husband and children and asked for their support in the changes she was going to make, some of which would affect the entire family. To make the transition easier for all of them, she made fairly small changes one at a time. For example, Nancy began by trading her usual breakfast of high-fat granola cereal with whole milk for raisin bran with ½% low-fat milk. Banning snack foods entirely didn't seem practical, so she gradually began to replace high-fat cookies, ice cream, and corn chips with graham crackers, low-fat frozen yogurt, and baked tortilla chips. The tuna salad she usually prepared for quick sandwich meals is now made with water-packed tuna and low-fat mayonnaise. Instead of serving a fried meat, such as fried chicken or chicken-fried steak, for dinner almost every night, Nancy prepares baked or grilled skinless chicken breasts, broiled fish, or lean roast or serves a meatless meal several nights a week with only an occasional lightly pan-fried meat. She now uses a low-fat or fat-free dressing on salads. In addition, Nancy began a daily walking program with a neighbor; after six weeks she added three sessions per week of doing sit-ups and working out with light hand weights.

Nancy's program is a long-term lifestyle change, not like the "quick-fix" approaches she had used in the past. Many of her previous methods had resulted in weight loss; however, as soon as she returned to her usual eating pattern, the weight was regained even more quickly than it had been lost.

Body Weight and Risk for Disease

Nancy is typical of millions of Americans who "halfway" diet much of the time. It is estimated that from 30 to 40 billion dollars are spent each year in the United States on weight-loss treatments. Obesity affects so many people and is a factor in the development of so many disorders that it has been called the number-one public health problem in the United States. Health problems associated with obesity include diabetes mellitus, high blood pressure, elevations of blood cholesterol and triglyceride, atherosclerosis, heart attack, stroke, sleep apnea (episodes of stopped breathing during sleep that last for several seconds), gallbladder disease, gout, and certain cancers. Weight loss in overweight people helps lower blood pressure and levels of cholesterol and triglyceride in the blood.

Obesity is a chronic disease that has many causes; it is more complicated than simply lacking self-control and eating too much. Because obesity has complex causes, there has been little long-term success in treating it. It is estimated that 95% of the people who lose weight gain it back within 3 to 5 years.

WAIST-TO-HIP RATIO

As far as risk for heart disease is concerned, where fat is located in the body may be as important as how much excess fat is present. Weight loss is very important for individuals who may not appear to be overweight according to height–weight tables but who carry excess fat within the abdomen (characterized by a potbelly or apple shape). These individuals are at special risk for developing cardiovascular disease and certain of its risk factors, such as elevated blood levels of cholesterol and triglyceride and high blood pressure. The degree of abdominal obesity is usually expressed as a waist-to-hip ratio, which is determined by dividing the size of the waist by the size of the hips. A desirable waist-to-hip ratio for men is less than 0.9; for women it is less than 0.8. For example, a woman who has a waist measurement of 26 inches and a hip measurement of 38 inches has a waist-to-hip ratio of 0.7 (26 ÷ 38 = 0.7); if her hips stayed the same size but her waist increased to 34 inches, her waist-to-hip ratio would become 0.9, reflecting an unhealthy level of fatness in the abdomen. Of course, people who are too large in both the waist and hips may have an acceptable waist-to-hip ratio but still be at increased risk for disease because of their degree of overweight.

How to Lose Weight

The Living Heart Diet is designed to help you lose weight and keep it off. It is compatible with lowering blood cholesterol, triglyceride, and blood pressure. It consists of permanent lifestyle changes that include both healthy, low-fat eating and increased physical activity—a "nondieting" approach. This approach to weight loss is not highly restrictive or regimented; however, it provides enough structure to help you make changes in your eating and exercise habits that will enable you to lose weight. The nondieting approach emphasizes identifying the habits you have that prevent you from losing weight and working to change them. This section of the chapter discusses changes in what you eat.

Changing habits is not a simple process. One way to help ensure success is to follow the same process that registered dietitians use with patients to help them make dietary changes. These steps are:

- Assessment
- Goal setting
- Selection of methods
- Follow-up and maintenance

ASSESSMENT

The first step in making dietary changes is to assess honestly what you are presently eating and how much physical activity you do on a regular basis. Begin by answering the following questions:

1. What high-calorie foods do you eat?
2. What low-calorie foods do you like?
3. How many meals and snacks do you typically eat each day?
4. How many meals are eaten away from home?
5. What types of restaurants do you choose when eating out?
6. How much alcohol do you drink?
7. Do you binge on food? How often? When?
8. Do you exercise? If so, what kind of exercise do you do?
9. If you exercise, how long are your exercise sessions? How often do you exercise?

It is also important to think about your past "successes" and "failures" in weight loss. For example, in the past which techniques helped you lose weight and maintain that weight loss? How much support do you have at home and away from home? What do you expect to be the most difficult part of making dietary changes? What is motivating you to make changes in your diet and physical activity now?

Another way to assess what you are eating is to keep a diary in which you record everything you eat and drink for several days. You can then use the information starting on page 372 of the Appendix to add up your calories.

GOALS

It is important to set realistic, short-term goals based on your assessment of your current eating habits. The assessment helps you see what changes you need to make and helps you identify which ones you are willing to work on.

People who are overweight often set unrealistic goals that are difficult to achieve and almost impossible to maintain. For example, choosing a severe calorie restriction, such as 800 calories or less per day, has only short-term benefits and can actually make maintaining a lower weight more difficult. Research shows that the vast majority of overweight people who lose weight on very restricted diets regain the weight they lost plus additional pounds. In addition, this method of weight reduction is associated with the development of gallstones in some people.

Success is not usually achieved with very restricted diets for a variety of complex physiological and psychological reasons. The physiological reasons include reduced breakdown of body fat, increased fat storage in the body, decreased mobilization of stored fat to be used as fuel, and lowering of the resting metabolic rate (see pages 85–86). The psychological reasons involve the belief that "dieting would work if only I had more willpower" and the constant feeling of deprivation experienced by many dieters. Most people who are following a severely restricted diet lose several pounds during the first few weeks, leading to an elevated mood and increased energy. This initial success gives the feeling that severely restricted diets do work. Prolonged rigid caloric restriction, however, often leads to uncontrolled food cravings and binge eating, which cause dieters to feel out of control and experience guilt and self-loathing because of their self-perceived gluttony. This experience often makes people reluctant to continue following the diet.

The Living Heart Diet's "nondieting" approach to weight control has four components:

1. Develop support with a health professional and some of your friends and/or family members.

2. Normalize your eating pattern by eating three meals each day (do not skip meals or add snacks between meals). Some people may be able to lose weight eating six small meals per day; however, for many people the "small" meals expand to six "regular" meals, increasing calorie intake and possibly even resulting in weight gain.

3. Gradually reduce your fat intake (which will decrease calorie intake).

4. Gradually increase your level of physical activity. Be realistic. Set short-term goals that you can achieve. Many people working to lose excess weight set a goal based on their "ideal body weight" (see pages 358–59 in the Appendix), which may be unrealistically low. It is important to remember that each person is different and that "ideal body weight" as defined for the average person may not in fact be the best weight

for you. Discuss your desirable weight with your physician. When you decide to lose weight, set realistic, short-term goals, such as a loss of ½ to 1 pound per week. *Remember, losing 1 pound per week adds up to 52 pounds in a year.*

You can set appropriate individual goals within each component of the nondieting approach, such as:

1. Develop support. For example:

   - Visit a registered dietitian or other qualified health professional on a regular basis.

   - Find a "health partner" and support each other's efforts.

2. Normalize your eating pattern. For example:

   - Eat three meals per day.

   - Do not eat between meals.

   - Do not skip meals.

3. Gradually decrease your intake of fat. For example:

   - Select leaner meat.

   - Switch from whole milk to ½% low-fat milk.

   - Limit meat, poultry, and fish to 6 ounces cooked per day.

   - Order grilled or baked fish when eating in restaurants.

4. Gradually increase your physical activity (after receiving an okay from your physician). See page 82 for additional information about starting a program of physical activity. For example:

   - Walk 10 minutes three times during the next week.

   - Investigate where you can walk when it is too wet, cold, or hot to be out of doors.

   - Gradually increase the number of times you walk.

   - Gradually increase the length of time you walk.

   - Join a group of "mall-walkers."

Start with those goals that will have the greatest impact on how you feel, as well as on your weight. For example, you may feel tired most of the time, or frustrated because of uncontrolled food binges. Perhaps you skip breakfast and drink coffee all morning, eat a light lunch, have a large evening meal, snack on high-fat foods throughout the evening, drink too much alcohol, crave sweets, and sleep poorly. If so, your first concern is probably simply to start feeling better. In this situation a normalized eating pattern is one of the best ways for you to improve your overall sense of well-being. Eating three meals a day should help decrease food cravings and binges. Reducing or cutting out snacking should decrease calories and fat intake; not snacking at night will save calories and make it easier to eat breakfast the next morning. Reducing caffeine and alcohol may improve your sleep, thereby increasing your energy, so you will feel like exercising regularly. All of these changes will help you lose weight.

An important goal of the "nondieting" approach of the Living Heart Diet is learning to tell the difference between the two types of hunger: physiological and psychological. Physiological hunger, or true hunger, is the feeling of physical emptiness in the body. On the other hand, psychological hunger (cravings) is the urge to eat something in response to the environment or emotions. Examples of psychological hunger are eating at a particular time of day, whether or not you are hungry, and responding to the sight of food, such as snacking in response to a television commercial.

METHODS

Three methods are often helpful in losing weight:

1. Selecting lower-fat foods (which are also lower in calories)

2. Counting calories

3. Choosing servings of food from each food group

Each method is very effective—there is not a "best" that applies to everyone. The best choice for you depends on which method you prefer and the amount of structure you want. Selecting lower-fat foods is the least structured of these three methods, and counting servings of food from each food group is the most structured. Keeping a food diary and a weight chart can be helpful in using any of these methods.

All the recipes in this book are moderately low in calories; the exact number of calories is provided with each recipe. You can use the Living Heart Diet menus, which begin on page 186, to help you implement any of the methods described below.

SELECTING LOWER-FAT FOODS – The "selecting lower-fat foods" method works well for most people. It involves selecting foods that contain less fat than is typically consumed and emphasizes eating more vegetables and fruits and eating moderate amounts of starches (such as bread, cereals, pasta, and rice), low-fat or fat-free dairy products, and lean meat, poultry, and fish. Lower-fat foods are lower in calories than their higher-fat counterparts. However, some fat-free foods are actually higher in calories than similar foods labeled "low fat." This is especially true for commercially prepared fat-free desserts because of the extra sugar and other sweeteners added when fat is left out (see page 138 for a discussion of fat replacers). *Remember, "fat free" does not mean "calorie free."*

Five types of changes make the "selecting lower-fat foods" method easy to use:

1. Selecting lower-fat foods in place of their higher-fat counterparts. For example, choose:

   • ½% low-fat milk in place of whole milk

   • Lean meat with the fat trimmed off in place of fatty meat

- Low-fat cheese in place of Cheddar or American cheese

- Fat-free frozen desserts in place of ice cream

- Fat-free cookies in place of regular cookies

2. Choosing smaller servings of foods that contain fat. For example:

   - Limit meat, fish, and poultry to no more than 6 ounces cooked per day.

3. Selecting lower-fat foods of a different type to replace higher-fat foods. For example:

   - Substitute grilled fish for steak.

4. Selecting low-fat preparation methods for foods eaten at home and away from home. For example:

   - Grill instead of fry.

   - Steam instead of sauté.

5. Increasing consumption of fat-free and low-fat foods. For example:

   - Include three servings of fat-free (skim) or low-fat dairy products daily.

   - Include five or more servings of fruits and vegetables each day.

   - Increase the use of "free" foods shown on pages 354–55 in the Appendix.

For an extensive list of foods that are lower in fat and calories, please see the food groups starting on page 345 in the Appendix. The lists indicate foods to choose and foods to decrease. For additional information on the selection of foods in supermarkets, see Chapter 7, and for guidelines on selecting foods when eating away from home, see Chapter 8. All the menus (which start on page 186) and the recipes (which start on page 207) in this book are moderately low in calories.

If you are having trouble reaching your weight-loss goals, you may find it helpful to keep a food diary for several days and to ask a registered dietitian or other qualified health professional to review it with you. You may also find it helpful to use the "counting calories" method described below or to add up the grams of fat in the foods you eat (see pages 42–44). By counting calories you can see exactly how many calories each food provides to help you determine where you need to make changes. Of course, it is also important to review your program of physical activity. How often are you exercising and how much? It may be time to increase your exercise.

COUNTING CALORIES – The "counting calories" method is very effective for people who want a little more detail and structure in their weight-loss program than the "selecting lower-fat foods" method provides. Counting calories involves writing down everything you eat or drink and adding up the calories provided by those foods. You can find the calories in foods in the Nutrition Facts portion of food labels and in the food table in the Appendix, starting on page 372. Information on calories is provided for each menu and recipe in this book.

The method of "compensating" works well with calorie counting. It consists of selecting a wide variety of foods, including a few high-calorie choices. By selecting primarily foods that are low in calories, you can compensate for the high-calorie foods. Pages 356–59 in the Appendix provide two methods for helping you estimate the number of calories you need daily.

CHOOSING SERVINGS OF FOOD FROM EACH FOOD GROUP – The "choosing servings of food from each food group" method is ideal for individuals who prefer a structured meal plan and who want to eat about the same number of calories and similar amounts of carbohydrate, protein, and fat each day. The first step is to estimate the number of calories you need (see pages 356–59 in the Appendix). The next step is to find your calorie level in the following table and determine the *number of servings* from each of the nine food groups for your calorie level. Information on each food group and the amount equal to a serving is in the Appendix, starting on page 345. A variety of foods can be used within each food group; for example, the dairy products group includes milk, cheese, and yogurt, and the bread group contains rice, pasta, cereal, crackers, potatoes, and popcorn.

SERVINGS OF FOOD ACCORDING TO DAILY CALORIE LEVEL

Food Group	Daily Servings Allowed						
	1,200 Cal	1,400 Cal	1,600 Cal	1,800 Cal	2,000 Cal	2,200 Cal	2,500 Cal
Meat, poultry, fish	6 oz	6 oz	6 oz	6 oz	6 oz	6 oz	6 oz
Egg yolks	3/wk	3/wk	3/wk	3/wk	3/wk	3/wk	3/wk
Dairy products	2	2	3	3	3	4	4
Fats, oils	3	3	4	5	6	7	8
Bread, cereal, pasta, starchy vegetables	3	4	4	6	7	7	10
Vegetables*	4+	4+	4+	4+	4+	4+	4+
Fruits	3	3	3	3	3	5	5
Sweets, alcohol†	0	100 cal	200 cal	200 cal	200 cal	200 cal	200 cal
Free foods	✔	✔	✔	✔	✔	✔	✔

*More nonstarchy vegetables may be included if desired.
†This food group is not usually included in a diabetic meal plan.
✔ = Not limited at any calorie level.

The Daily Eating Pattern on page 75 can be used to list the number of servings from each food group for the total day. These totals can then be divided among the meals and snacks eaten each day.

In addition, a food diary, as shown on page 76, can be used with this method. Write the name of the food group for each food you eat in the column on the right. Servings of food you eat can then be tallied in the space at the top, as shown in the example on page 77.

DAILY EATING PATTERN

Calories _____   Date _____

Daily Totals

_____ Ounces of meat, poultry, fish
          (pages 345–46)
_____ Egg yolks per week (page 347)
_____ Servings of dairy products
_____ (pages 347–48)
_____ Servings of fats, oils (pages 348–49)
          Servings of bread, cereal, pasta, starchy
_____ vegetables (pages 349–51)
          Servings of nonstarchy vegetables
_____ (pages 351–52)
_____ Servings of fruit (pages 352–53)
          Calories from sweets/alcohol
_____ (pages 353–54)
  ✔ Free foods (pages 354–55)

Breakfast

_____ Serving(s) of fruit
_____ Serving(s) of bread or cereal
_____ Serving(s) of fats, oils
_____ Serving(s) of dairy products
  ✔ Free foods

Midmorning Snack

_____ Serving(s) of _____
_____ Serving(s) of _____
  ✔ Free foods

Lunch

_____ Ounce(s) of meat, poultry, fish
_____ Serving(s) of bread, pasta, starchy
          vegetables
_____ Serving(s) of vegetables
_____ Serving(s) of fats, oils
_____ Serving(s) of fruit
_____ Serving(s) of dairy products
_____ Calories from sweets/alcohol
  ✔ Free foods

Afternoon Snack

_____ Serving(s) of _____
_____ Serving(s) of _____
  ✔ Free foods

Dinner

_____ Ounce(s) of meat, poultry, fish
_____ Serving(s) of bread, pasta, starchy
          vegetables
_____ Serving(s) of nonstarchy vegetables
_____ Serving(s) of fats, oils
_____ Serving(s) of fruit
_____ Serving(s) of dairy products
_____ Calories from sweets/alcohol
  ✔ Free foods

Evening Snack

_____ Serving(s) of _____
_____ Serving(s) of _____
  ✔ Free foods

✔ = As desired

FOOD DIARY

Food Groups*

Name_____

Day_____ Date_____

Exercise_____

	Goals		Servings Eaten
	_____	Meat	_____
	_____	Dairy	_____
	_____	Fat	_____
	_____	Bread	_____
	_____	Veg	_____
	_____	Fruit	_____
	_____	Sweets/ Alcohol	_____

Write ONE food item on each line.

Time & Place	Amount	Food—How Prepared	Food Group*

*M = meat; D = dairy; B = bread, cereal, pasta, starchy vegetables; V = vegetables; F = fruit; S/A = sweets and alcohol.

FOOD DIARY   Food Groups*

	Goals		Servings Eaten
Name Pat Doe	6	Meat	///
Day Thursday Date 9/8	3	Dairy	//
Exercise walked 2 miles in 35 minutes	5	Fat	///
	6	Bread	///
	4	Veg	//
	3	Fruit	/
	2	Sweets/ Alcohol	/

Write ONE food item on each line.

Time & Place	Amount	Food—How Prepared	Food Group*
7 am	2 slices	wheat bread, toasted	2 B
home	2 tsp	margarine, diet	1 Fat
	½ cup	orange juice, unsweetened	1 F
	1 cup	½% low-fat milk	1 D
12 noon	2 cups	tossed salad w/ tomato	1 V
café	2 tbsp	low-cal dressing	1 Fat
	6	saltine crackers	1 B
	3 oz	chicken breast, skinless, baked	3 M
	½ cup	green beans, seasoned	1 V & 1 Fat
3 pm	1 cup	½% low-fat milk	1 D
	2	fat-free fig bars	1 S/A

M = meat; D = dairy; B = bread, cereal, pasta, starchy vegetables; V = vegetable; F = fruit; S/A = sweets/alcohol.

FOLLOW-UP AND MAINTENANCE

It is important to have regular follow-up during the process of losing weight and even more important afterward. Many people find it beneficial to have someone with whom they can "check in" on a regular basis. For example, it is fairly common for people who have lost weight to make an appointment every few months with a registered dietitian to help them keep on track. Regular follow-up while losing weight and after weight has been lost allows you to have someone to

- Record your weight on a regular basis

- Evaluate your progress toward reaching your goal weight, or evaluate how you are maintaining your goal weight

- Help you set new goals regarding food selection

- Evaluate your level of physical activity

The only way to keep from regaining weight you have lost is to make some permanent lifestyle changes and to remain aware of your food intake and level of physical activity. The best way to predict whether you will be able to keep weight off after losing it is to assess your physical activity: individuals who take part in regular physical activity are more likely to keep weight off after losing it.

Once you have identified a method for losing weight that works for you, you will need to continue it after you have lost weight. Of course, after you reach your goal weight, you will be able to increase your intake of fat-free and low-fat foods. Be careful not to add too many calories or you may begin to regain the weight you lost. It will take fewer calories to maintain your new, lower weight because it takes fewer calories for you to do the same amount of physical activity (for example, to walk across a room) than it did before you lost weight. *Remember, people who go back to old eating habits after losing weight will regain the weight they lost, and usually gain a few more pounds.*

Many people who have successfully lost weight find it helpful to weigh themselves on a regular basis and periodically to record their food intake. These measures will help you increase your awareness and avoid slipping back into old habits.

Physical Activity in Weight Control

The tendency toward physical inactivity—being a "couch potato"—has become a major health risk for Americans. It is estimated that only 22% of American adults exercise regularly and intensely enough to reach current fitness guidelines; another 54% exercise once in a while at a level of intensity too low to result in health and fitness gains, and 24% do not exercise at all. Regular physical activity is essential to a successful weight control program. Losing weight and keeping it off requires both a well-balanced diet and regular physical activity.

There are several reasons that the recommendations for physical activity were expanded in the mid-1990s. The long-accepted exercise prescription has been to perform from 30 to 60 minutes of moderate- to high-intensity exercise (such as briskly walking uphill, jogging, or mowing the lawn with a hand mower) three or more times per week; however, less than one-fourth of Americans followed this recommendation to exercise regularly. Recent research studies show that many of the health benefits associated with exercise can be obtained by performing moderate-intensity physical activities. Moderate-intensity activities are effective even when they are done over several short periods of time; that is, the time spent doing these activities is cumulative. Therefore, the current recommendation is to engage in moderate-intensity activity (defined as enough to expend about 200 calories per day) almost every day. You can burn 200 calories walking briskly enough to travel two miles in about 30 minutes. Or you can accumulate your 200 calories by a combination of exercises such as brisk walking, gardening, and playing table tennis. The health benefits of physical activity are directly proportional to the total amount of activity performed. However, increased longevity is associated with approximately 4 hours per week of vigorous exercise, which confers a reduction in mortality rate of approximately 20%.

The four steps used in making dietary changes can also be used to help you establish a habit of regular physical activity:

1. **Assessment.** Assess your present situation in relation to exercise (planned physical activity). Be sure to check with your physician before beginning any program of physical activity; your physician may recommend that you be tested on an exercise treadmill to evaluate your level of physical fitness. Assess your personal goals for a physical activity program and your reasons for wanting to begin exercising now. Do you have reasonable expectations for what exercise can do for you? It is also helpful to identify the factors in your life that have prevented you from exercising regularly in the past and develop a plan for exercising in spite of these barriers. For example, if you live in an area where it rains frequently, you can identify a place, such as a shopping mall, where you can walk indoors, or get a stationary bicycle or treadmill to use at home.

2. **Goal Setting.** Goal setting is a very important part of establishing a lasting program of physical activity. Set reasonable, short-term goals for yourself. For example, if you are sedentary, you may wish to begin walking 10 to 15 minutes three times per week and then gradually increase the number of days you walk, the length of time you walk, and your speed. There is no ideal level of exercise for everyone—even a small amount of physical activity is better than no activity. Research shows that individuals at a moderate level of fitness have a greatly reduced risk for death, including death from heart disease or cancer, compared with sedentary people.

3. **Methods.** Many options are available to help you select the method of exercise that is best for you. You may decide to exercise indoors or outdoors; at home or in a gymnasium; alone, in a group, or with a personal trainer; by walking, jogging, or using various types of exercise equipment. Experiment until you find the activities you enjoy. Most people find walking to be the most convenient form of physical activity; it has low risk for injury and requires only good walking shoes. If you are a beginning exerciser, you may benefit from varying the type of activity in developing your program. For example, in a week's time you might walk outdoors or on a treadmill and ride an indoor or outdoor bicycle; you might also do some upper body muscular endurance training by lifting some light hand weights.

4. **Follow-up and Maintenance.** Follow-up consists of keeping track to make sure you have reached your goals for regular physical activity. The important thing is that you establish a habit of being physically active that becomes as automatic as eating or brushing your teeth. Some people find that keeping a diary of their physical activity (such as the one below) helps them make permanent lifestyle changes; a blank exercise diary is provided that you can copy and use.

EXERCISE DIARY

Name __Pat Doe__   Beginning Date __9/18__
Target Exercise Heart Rate __140__   Beats per Minute _____

Day/Date	Warm-up	Exercise	Cool-down	Total Minutes
Sun 9/18	stretched, strolled —8 min.	walked 1 mile in 18 min.	strolled, stretched —7 min.	33
Mon 9/19	stretched, biked slowly—8 min.	rode exercise bike 20 mph—16 min.	biked slowly, stretched—7 min.	31
Wed 9/21	stretched, strolled —9 minutes	walked 1¼ miles in 21 min.	strolled, stretched —7 min.	37

EXERCISE DIARY

Name _____   Beginning Date _____

Target Exercise Heart Rate _____   Beats per Minute _____

Day/Date	Warm-up	Exercise	Cool-down	Total Minutes

BEGINNING YOUR PROGRAM OF PHYSICAL ACTIVITY

Most people are motivated to start exercise programs because of the health-related benefits they hope to gain. However, continuing a program of physical activity depends on its providing enjoyment, convenience, and social support. You are also more likely to continue doing an exercise that is performed at a moderate intensity, as opposed to one that is more strenuous.

There are several points to consider before you begin any exercise program. First and foremost, it is *very* important that you check with your physician before beginning any program of physical activity. People who are apparently healthy can usually begin a moderate exercise program without supervision after receiving their physician's approval. However, people who are at high risk for coronary heart disease or who have coronary heart disease should have an exercise electrocardiogram (ECG) to establish a suitable level of exercise, as should people with certain other medical conditions or risks.

TYPES OF PHYSICAL ACTIVITY – Exercise can be separated into endurance, strength (resistance activities), and flexibility activities. For all these types of exercise, the goal in each workout is to work your muscles at a level that requires just a little more effort than is comfortable. When an exercise becomes so easy that it takes no real effort, it is time to increase the number of times you exercise per week, exercise for a longer period each time, or increase the intensity of the exercise. But *never* push yourself to the point of joint pain or chest pain. Although minimal to moderate muscle soreness is normal for a couple of days after a strength-training workout, "no pain, no gain" is just not true for endurance and flexibility exercises.

- Endurance exercises build stamina and burn calories, both during the exercise and for a period of time after exercise is completed.

- Strength training strengthens and builds muscle.

- Flexibility exercises increase the ability of your joints to move through a wider range of motion.

Endurance exercises use the large muscles, such as those in the hips and legs, continuously at a moderate intensity for 20 to 60 minutes. These activities include walking briskly outdoors or on a treadmill, hiking, jogging, outdoor and indoor bicycling, swimming, rowing, climbing stairs or using a stair-climbing machine, aerobic dancing, and cross-country skiing. When performed at a moderate intensity, endurance activities are aerobic ("with oxygen"); this means that the muscle being worked burns both oxygen and fuel (from the food you have eaten in the last 3 to 8 hours and/or from body fat) to produce energy for prolonged muscle contraction. If endurance activities are performed at a high enough intensity to make you breathless, not enough oxygen is able to get to the muscle, and the exercises are no longer aerobic. Aerobic endurance exercises are especially useful in cardiovascular conditioning, that is, increasing the strength and efficiency of the heart.

Strength training includes activities such as weight lifting, sit-ups, push-ups, and other body-lifting exercises. In these exercises, specific muscles are worked more intensely for a brief period of time. Strength-training activities are typically anaerobic ("without oxygen"), since the muscle is worked at a moderate to high intensity for too brief a time to allow oxygen to be used in the production of energy. Strength training is done differently depending on whether your primary goal is to strengthen muscle or to increase muscle endurance. Muscle size is increased by using heavy weights and performing few repetitions of an exercise; exercises to increase muscular endurance have more repetitions using lighter weights. For example, a muscle endurance workout could consist of several sets of each exercise with each set being 5, 10, 20, or more repetitions.

The aim of flexibility exercises is to make your body more supple. They include activities such as bending, stretching, and yoga. In flexibility exercises, you extend the muscle until it develops light to moderate tension and then hold it for about 10 counts or 10 seconds. Flexibility exercises should be done slowly and evenly; do not bounce or push too hard when the muscle is in its stretched position, or you could cause small tears in muscles and ligaments.

WARM-UP AND COOL-DOWN – Two essential—but often neglected—parts of any good program of physical activity are the warm-up and cool-down periods. Warm-up exercises are of two types: general stretches and total body movements or low-intensity movements that are similar to the exercise you plan to perform. For example, joggers and runners might walk briskly for several minutes before beginning to jog or run. As the name suggests, warm-up exercises gradually increase physical activity, which allows the entire body to adjust properly to get ready for physical effort.

Cool-down exercises allow your body's circulation and metabolism to gradually return to nonexercising levels. You cool down by walking around or doing light stretching or calisthenics.

DESIGNING YOUR PERSONAL PROGRAM OF PHYSICAL ACTIVITY

Most health experts suggest developing a program of physical activity that is based on aerobic endurance exercises to improve cardiovascular fitness. A good basic program might consist of 5 to 10 minutes of warm-up exercises, 20 to 30 minutes of endurance exercises, 20 minutes of strengthening activities, and 5 to 10 minutes of cool-down and flexibility activities. Of course, you will need to start with an exercise period that is shorter than 20 minutes and increase the time as your level of fitness increases.

Your exercise "dosage" is a combination of (1) frequency, or how often you exercise, (2) duration, or how long you exercise at one time, and (3) intensity, or how much effort you exert during exercise. The level of intensity of endurance exercises is typically measured by comparing your heart rate (pulse count) during exercise with a target exercise heart rate. If you plan to use heart rate to measure the intensity of your exercise, *talk with your physician about your recommended target heart rate during exercise.* Your target exercise heart rate is based on your age and physical condition. A simple way to estimate your target exercise heart rate is to (1) subtract your age from 220 to get your maximum heart rate and then (2) multiply your maximum heart rate by an appropriate percent, based on your level of fitness. *Never try to exercise at your maximum heart rate.* For most people who are just beginning to exercise, maximum heart rate is multiplied by about 60% to get the target exercise heart rate. The following table lists suggested target exercise heart rates at different ages and levels of activity.

TARGET EXERCISE HEART RATE

Age	60% Maximum Heart Rate	70% Maximum Heart Rate	80% Maximum Heart Rate
20	120	140	160
25	117	137	156
30	114	133	152
35	111	130	148
40	108	126	144
45	105	123	140
50	102	119	136
55	99	116	132
60	96	112	128
65	93	109	124
70	90	105	120

For example, a man age 45 who is starting an exercise program has a target exercise heart rate of 105 per minute (220 − 45 = 175; 175 × 0.60 = 105). A 45-year-old man who is physically fit might calculate his target exercise heart rate at 80% of his maximum heart rate, or 140 (175 × 0.80 = 140).

The heart rate can be measured by gently pressing the first two fingers of your hand on the inside of the opposite wrist. At first you may have to try several times to find the best spot to count your heart rate; practice doing this before you begin to exercise. To measure the heart rate per minute, stop exercising and immediately count heartbeats with your first count as zero (to ensure accuracy of your estimate), either for 6 seconds (and multiply by 10) or for 10 seconds (and multiply by 6). Do not pause between stopping exercise and taking your heart rate or the count will not be accurate. You may prefer to purchase an accurate heart rate monitor.

Once you have a regular program of aerobic endurance exercise in place, you may wish to add some moderate-intensity strength training, such as doing some sit-ups, push-ups, or other exercises that isolate individual areas of muscle. You may want to seek the help of a qualified personal trainer to guide you toward your strength goals in a safe manner.

AVOIDING INJURY

Exercising in a way that avoids injury is one of the best ways to ensure that you continue your physical activity program. Many people set unrealistic goals for their exercise program, trying to go from complete inactivity to a very ambitious daily workout. To be of long-term value, any program of physical activity needs to be a permanent change; there is no benefit—and there is increased risk for injury—from trying to do too much too soon. Here are some tips on avoiding injury:

- Always warm up for 5 to 10 minutes before you exercise and cool down for 5 to 10 minutes after exercising (see page 83 for information on warm-up and cool-down periods).

- Do not keep exercising if you feel very tired; avoid excessive fatigue.

- Stop exercising if you feel pain.

- Stop exercising immediately if you feel sick, dizzy, nauseated, or weak, or have chest pressure or pain or shortness of breath (contact your physician if you experience these symptoms).

- Check your heart rate at regular intervals to make sure you are not exceeding your target exercise heart rate (see pages 83–84).

Physical activity is relatively safe for most overweight individuals who have not been exercising as long as they begin their program slowly. It is important to learn how to perform different exercises properly, both to maximize results and to minimize risk for injuries. Careful supervision is especially vital for children, adolescents, and the elderly who are taking part in strength training. There is a small, temporary increase in risk for heart failure during exercise, especially for people who have been inactive for long periods of time. Although small, this increase in risk emphasizes the importance of checking with your physician before beginning to exercise.

HEALTH BENEFITS OF PHYSICAL ACTIVITY

Many health benefits are associated with performing regular moderate physical activity. There is a strong link between being physically active and controlling your weight. In fact, a program of regular exercise is the most reliable predictor of success in keeping weight off after you lose it. As was mentioned earlier, regular aerobic endurance exercise both burns calories during exercise and increases the rate at which your body burns calories for a period after you stop exercising. For example, if you burned an extra 300 calories per day, 6 days per week, this could result in a loss of 27 pounds in a year (300 calories × 6 days = 1,800 calories/week × 52 weeks = 93,600 ÷ 3,500 calories per pound = 27 pounds). Regular aerobic endurance exercise also favors burning fat as a fuel, whereas brief, strenuous activities tend to burn carbohydrate in the form of glucose from glycogen (carbohydrate stored in muscle and liver).

Strength training can also play a part in weight control. For all but the most physically active, about two-thirds of the calories burned each day are used to maintain vital bodily functions, such as heart and lung activity, when at complete physical and mental rest; this is called the resting (or basal) metabolic rate. The remaining one-third are burned in physical activity and as the result of eating and digesting food. Your resting metabolic rate depends on the amount of lean body mass you have. Although "lean body mass" literally means everything that is not fat (primarily water, muscle, and bone), the term lean body mass as used in this section refers to muscle. Physical activity that increases muscle, such as some strength training, raises the resting metabolic rate and increases the calories being burned when you are not active. Since, in equal volumes, muscle weighs more than fat, individuals who do enough strength training to appreciably increase their muscle mass may not lose much weight; however, they will change their body composition and reduce excess body fat. As part of a weight control program, regular exercise indirectly contributes to controlling blood pressure (see Chapter 4 on high blood pressure, beginning on page 89) and helping prevent the development of non-insulin-dependent diabetes mellitus (see Chapter 5 on managing diabetes, beginning on page 110). Research has shown other important health benefits to be linked to regular exercise. Performing regular moderate aerobic endurance exercise has been shown to

- Reduce death rates from all causes

- Reduce risk for heart attack and stroke

- Increase blood levels of HDL-cholesterol ("good" cholesterol) and, in some people, decrease LDL-cholesterol ("bad" cholesterol)

- Decrease blood pressure

- Decrease triglyceride level

- Help in weight reduction

- Improve glucose tolerance

- Strengthen bones, muscles, heart, and lungs

- Increase strength and energy

- Help in stress management

- Improve sleep

- Improve body image and enhance self-esteem

Performing regular strength training has been shown to

- Increase strength and flexibility

- Enhance self-concept and sense of adequacy and worth

- Help preserve lean body mass during weight loss

- Reduce muscle weakness in the frail elderly

- Increase bone density, muscle mass, muscle strength, and balance in postmenopausal women

In addition, strength training may increase bone mass, improve the ratio of HDL-cholesterol to LDL-cholesterol, reduce risk for broken bones, and help individuals return to normal physical activity after a heart attack.

Drug Therapy for Obesity

Obese patients often find it difficult to lose weight and to maintain any weight loss that is achieved. This frustration with the inability to control weight has led to increasing interest in drug therapy for weight control.

Obesity typically has not been treated as a disease. However, viewing obesity as a chronic disease could make treatment with drug therapy more acceptable for physicians and patients. As is the case with chronic diseases such as high blood pressure and diabetes, it is possible that long-term drug therapy might be helpful in controlling, but not curing, obesity.

Research has shown that drugs are effective in producing short-term weight loss and, in some individuals, maintenance of lowered weight for extended periods of time. The drugs currently approved for use in the United States act in one of two ways:

1. Adrenergic agents (for example, phentermine) speed up metabolism and increase the number of calories burned.

2. Serotoninergic agents (for example, fenfluramine, fluoxetine) increase the availability of serotonin in the brain.

Effects of Drug Therapy for Obesity

One of the concerns in using drugs to treat obesity is that most existing drugs are recommended only for short-term treatment (usually 12 weeks) of a long-term disorder. There is growing interest in developing drug therapy that can be used for longer periods. A recent study using a combination of fenfluramine and phentermine reported significant weight loss, which some individuals maintained for more than three years. However, the lost pounds returned when the drugs were withdrawn. Side effects of the treatment included dry mouth, fatigue, diarrhea, and modest central nervous system complaints, almost all of which disappeared after a few weeks. The study participants experienced improvements in blood pressure, cholesterol and triglyceride levels, and glucose tolerance.

Drugs should be considered as only one part of a comprehensive weight management program that includes a low-fat diet and regular physical activity. The rationale for using adrenergic or serotoninergic agents in combination with behavior modification is that these drugs reduce hunger, making it easier for individuals to develop healthy eating habits. More research is needed, with careful long-term follow-up to determine which drugs work in which groups of patients. A better understanding of the biochemical mechanisms involved in the development of obesity may help in the long-term management of body weight.

Chapter 4

The Living Heart Diet in Preventing and Treating High Blood Pressure

High blood pressure (hypertension) affects about one in four adults in the United States. The heart is especially susceptible to damage by high blood pressure, as are the brain, kidneys, and eyes. Uncontrolled high blood pressure can lead to stroke, kidney failure, or loss of eyesight, and it can contribute to heart attack, congestive heart failure, and peripheral vascular disease (narrowing of blood vessels in the legs and sometimes the arms due to the formation of plaque and/or changes in the blood vessels themselves). Most cases of high blood pressure cannot be cured; however, high blood pressure associated with certain kidney diseases (such as pheochromocytoma, hyperaldosteronism, and renovascular disease) are curable. Many cases of high blood pressure can be prevented through exercise and control of weight, sodium intake, and alcohol intake.

High blood pressure often has no symptoms, and it is possible to have elevated blood pressure for years without knowing it. Dietary changes and other lifestyle modifications to help prevent high blood pressure are especially important because many people sustain heart, brain, kidney, or eye damage before their high blood pressure is discovered. For this reason high blood pressure is known as a "silent crippler" or "silent killer." Yet the only thing required to diagnose this condition is routine blood pressure measurements, which are quick, simple, painless, and often free of charge.

Fortunately, there are excellent methods for controlling high blood pressure, including lifestyle changes and medications. Control of the incurable type of high blood pressure usually requires a lifetime commitment to therapy. When blood pressure is only mildly elevated, lifestyle changes can sometimes lower it enough that drugs are not required. It is very important that people maintain lifestyle changes and, if taking medications to lower blood pressure, stay on their medications, since lifestyle changes and medications control but do not cure high blood pressure.

What Is blood pressure?

Blood pressure is a measure of the pressure that blood exerts against the inside of the artery wall. It consists of two numbers: Systolic blood pressure, which is listed first, is the pressure of the blood flow when the heart beats. Diastolic blood pressure, which is listed second, is taken between heartbeats. The values are given in millimeters of mercury, abbreviated as mm Hg.

A typical blood pressure reading for a healthy adult might be 125/75 mm Hg (systolic/diastolic). Levels vary according to age and other factors and can temporarily be increased by influences such as fear, stress, recent exercise, eating a heavy meal, and some illnesses and medications. A systolic reading of 139 mm Hg together with a diastolic reading of 89 mm Hg is usually considered the upper limit for normal blood pressure for adults, although a value of, for example, 120/80 mm Hg may carry less risk for cardiovascular disease. Blood pressure is defined as high when systolic pressure is higher than 139 mm Hg or diastolic pressure is higher than 89 mm Hg for an extended period of time. However, there is no exact threshold for average or high risk: risk exists across a range of values. The higher the blood pressure over an extended period, the greater the risk for damage to body organs, such as the heart, kidneys, and brain.

CLASSIFICATION OF BLOOD PRESSURE IN ADULTS

Category	Systolic mm Hg	Diastolic mm Hg
Optimal*	Below 120	Below 80
Normal	Below 130	Below 85
High normal	130–139	85–89
High blood pressure		
Mild	140–159	90–99
Moderate	160–179	100–109
Severe	180–209	110–119
Very severe	210 or higher	120 or higher

*Unusually low readings should be evaluated for clinical significance. Definitions from the Fifth Report of the Joint National Committee on Detection, Evaluation, and Treatment of High Blood Pressure, Bethesda: NHLBI, 1992.

What causes high blood pressure?

There are two categories of high blood pressure in terms of cause: essential and secondary. In 90% to 95% of all cases of high blood pressure, the cause is unknown. These cases are called essential hypertension. Secondary hypertension results from another disease or condition, such as kidney disease (including pheochromocytoma, hyperaldosteronism, and renovascular disease) or pregnancy. When the cause of secondary hypertension is resolved or corrected, the high blood pressure usually disappears. The discussion of high blood pressure in this book deals with essential hypertension.

Blood pressure rises with age. From young adulthood to early middle age, high blood pressure is more common in men than in women; after this stage of life, the reverse is true. There are certain conditions under which a woman may be more likely to develop high blood pressure. Some women who have normal blood pressure develop high blood pressure during pregnancy. A woman who takes oral contraceptives may be more likely to develop high blood pressure if she (1) is overweight, (2) has mild kidney disease, (3) has a family history of high blood pressure, or (4) developed high blood pressure when she was pregnant.

High blood pressure seems to run in some families; a person who has a parent with high blood pressure is more likely to develop it than someone whose parents have normal blood pressure. High blood pressure is much more common in blacks than in whites.

Age, family history of disease, and race cannot be changed. However, lifestyle factors, which can be changed, also play important roles in the development of high blood pressure. The main lifestyle contributors to high blood pressure are (1) excessive calorie intake and overweight, (2) high sodium intake, and (3) heavy consumption of alcohol (in excess of three drinks per day; see page 93 for definition of one drink). Other modifiable lifestyle factors that have been implicated include a sedentary lifestyle, stress, and low intakes of potassium, calcium, magnesium, and fiber.

KEY LIFESTYLE CHANGES FOR PREVENTING AND TREATING HIGH BLOOD PRESSURE

The lifestyle changes listed below are proven effective in lowering blood pressure. They help in both the *prevention* and the *treatment* of high blood pressure.

LIFESTYLE CHANGES THAT HELP PREVENT AND TREAT HIGH BLOOD PRESSURE

- **Reach and maintain a desirable body weight (see pages 356–59 in the Appendix).**
- **Take part in regular physical activity (see page 78).**
- **Limit alcohol intake to no more than 1 ounce of pure alcohol, which is about 2 regular drinks, per day (see page 93).**
- **Reduce sodium to 2,400 mg or less per day; this amount of sodium is equivalent to about 1⅛ teaspoons of salt (see page 93).**

In prevention, these changes are particularly important for people who have a family history of high blood pressure. For people who have already developed high blood pressure, making these lifestyle changes is crucial even when medication to lower blood pressure is being taken. As noted above, some patients with only mildly elevated blood pressure who make appropriate lifestyle changes may avoid the use of drugs. These lifestyle changes have many other health benefits as well. They are especially helpful for the many people with high blood pressure who have other risk factors for heart disease, such as high blood cholesterol or diabetes. Lowering blood pressure in a person who has diabetes also helps prevent damage to the small blood vessels of the eyes and kidneys.

Weight Control

Weight control is one of the most important factors in preventing and treating high blood pressure. Being overweight is closely correlated with increased blood pressure, and blood pressure decreases in proportion to weight loss. Most people who have high blood pressure and are more than 10% above ideal weight are able to lower their blood pressure with weight loss. In many cases moderate sustained weight loss (about 10 pounds or more) returns mild or moderate high blood pressure to normal. A decrease in blood pressure usually occurs early in a weight reduction program. Weight loss has the additional advantage of enhancing the effectiveness of medications to lower blood pressure.

Anyone who has high blood pressure and is overweight should strive to lose weight. The weight loss program should be individualized and monitored by a health professional, and it should include regular planned physical activity. Ways to accomplish weight loss are discussed in Chapter 3, which begins on page 67.

Physical Activity

Sedentary people are as much as 50% more likely than active, fit people to develop high blood pressure. Regular aerobic physical activity can lower systolic blood pressure by about 10 mm Hg in people with high blood pressure. How physical activity helps control blood pressure is not well understood. It is known that physical activity has beneficial effects on blood pressure independent of weight loss.

To lower blood pressure, it is more effective to take part in physical activity every day than just three times per week. Low- to moderate-intensity aerobic (endurance) exercise is as effective as high-intensity exercise in reducing mild to moderate high blood pressure. It is recommended that everyone develop a regular program of dynamic, moderate-intensity, low-resistance physical activity, such as walking, cycling, dancing, or swimming. You should check with your physician before starting an exercise program.

Alcohol

It has been estimated that as many as 7% of cases of high blood pressure can be traced to alcohol intake of three or more drinks per day. Reducing high alcohol intake lowers blood pressure in individuals who have blood pressure in the normal range as well as in those who have high blood pressure; it may help prevent the development of high blood pressure. Excessive alcohol intake can cause resistance to medications used to treat high blood pressure.

People with high blood pressure who drink alcoholic beverages should do so in moderation; women who are pregnant should not drink because of the risk of birth defects. Moderate alcohol intake is defined as a maximum of 1 ounce of pure alcohol (ethanol) per day. One ounce of pure alcohol is often equated to two drinks, because each drink typically contains ½ ounce of alcohol. The following alcoholic beverages contain ½ ounce of alcohol, and each is considered one drink:

ONE ALCOHOLIC DRINK*

- **12 fluid ounces of regular or light beer**

- **5 fluid ounces of table wine**

- **3 fluid ounces of fortified wine, such as sherry, port, marsala, or Madeira**

- **1½ fluid ounces (a "jigger") of 80-proof liquor or 1 fluid ounce of 100-proof liquor, such as rum, bourbon, Scotch, vodka, tequila, or gin**

*Limit intake to no more than 2 drinks per day.

In addition to its effects on blood pressure, alcohol provides calories with no nutritional benefit and can increase appetite in some people, making weight control more difficult. Further, in recent studies alcohol consumption reduced the body's ability to clear fat (particularly saturated fat) from the blood after a meal. Therefore, for people who consume alcoholic beverages, it is especially important to decrease intake of saturated fat to the level recommended on the Step I Diet (8% to 10% of calories) or the Step II Diet (less than 7% of calories). The calorie content of common alcoholic beverages is shown in the Appendix, starting on page 370.

Sodium

Sodium is a necessary element in the diet and is chiefly obtained in sodium chloride, that is, common salt. It is needed to maintain fluid balance in the body and for other physiological functions. However, the amount of sodium adults need daily is only 500 milligrams (mg), many times less than the 4,000 to 5,800 mg typically consumed by Americans. If no salt were added to food during processing or cooking, there would still be an adequate amount of sodium in the diet.

There is a strong association between the amount of sodium consumed and blood pressure. A low-sodium diet reduces blood pressure in people with blood pressure in the normal range as well as in those with high blood pressure.

Following a low-sodium diet can be a challenge because salt and sodium-containing compounds are added to most commercially prepared foods. The National High Blood Pressure Education Program recommends a daily intake for everyone of no more than 2,400 mg of sodium (the amount in 1⅛ teaspoons of salt). The American Heart Association's recommendation for the general public is similar: no more than 3,000 mg. These lower levels of sodium are recommended both to help prevent high blood pressure and to treat it. A high-sodium diet decreases the effectiveness of blood pressure medications. Techniques for lowering sodium intake are discussed on page 100.

People who reduce their sodium intake find that it usually takes several weeks to get accustomed to the taste of lower-sodium foods. People are not born with a taste for salt: it is learned.

There are several sources of sodium in the diet, as shown below.

MAJOR SOURCES OF SODIUM IN THE DIET

- **Sodium added to food during processing and manufacturing**
- **Sodium added to food during preparation, both at home and in restaurants, and at the table**
- **Sodium that occurs naturally in water and food**

SODIUM ADDED IN FOOD PROCESSING

The greatest source of sodium in the American diet—accounting for up to 80%—is the salt and other sodium compounds added to food during processing. Food manufacturers add sodium not only for taste but also because it acts as a preservative. "Salt" and "sodium" are related, but they do not mean the same thing. Salt (sodium chloride) contains about 40% sodium and 60% chloride. One-fourth teaspoon of salt contains 533 mg of sodium.

SODIUM-CONTAINING COMPOUNDS ADDED TO FOOD DURING PROCESSING

Baking powder	Sodium caseinate
Baking soda (sodium bicarbonate)	Sodium citrate
Disodium phosphate	Sodium dioxide
Monosodium glutamate (MSG)	Sodium hydroxide
Saccharin (sodium saccharide)	Sodium metabisulfite
Salt (sodium chloride)	Sodium nitrate
Sodium alginate	Sodium nitrite
Sodium benzoate	Sodium propionate
Sodium bisulfite	Sodium sulfite

Examples of processed foods that are high in sodium are cured meats; pickled foods; cheese; many convenience foods, including most canned, frozen, and shelf-stable entrees and dinners; ready-to-eat cereals; and baked goods leavened with baking soda and/or baking powder. Bread (a processed food) is a primary contributor of sodium to the diet. Even though a slice of bread contains only about 150 mg of sodium, the amount of bread typically eaten each day causes the total sodium to add up. Ready-to-eat cereal is another large contributor of sodium. The following list includes commonly eaten foods that are typically high in sodium; lower-sodium varieties of some of these foods are available. Amounts of sodium in commonly eaten foods are shown in the Appendix, starting on page 372.

COMMON FOODS HIGH IN SODIUM

Anchovies	Nuts, salted
Bacon	Olives
Barbecue sauce	Pastrami
Bologna	Pepperoni
Bread and rolls (several servings a day)	Pickles
Buttermilk	Pizza
Cereal, ready-to-eat	Pretzels
Cheese	Salad dressing (regular and fat free)
Chips, potato, corn, and other snack	Salami
Corned beef	Sauerkraut
Crackers with salted tops	Sausage
Frankfurters	Seeds, salted
Frozen entrees and dinners (check label)	Soup (all types)
Ham	Soy sauce
Jerky	Steak sauce
Meat, canned or frozen in sauce	Wieners (beef, pork, chicken, turkey)
Meat, cured	Worcestershire sauce
Meat, kosher	

LABELING SODIUM IN FOOD – In 1993 the Food and Drug Administration (FDA) established guidelines for "nutrient content claims" concerning certain nutrients. Nutrient content claims for sodium establish the maximum level of sodium that can be found in a standard serving of a food labeled "sodium free," "very low sodium," "low sodium," or "reduced sodium." The FDA has established standard servings for the foods commonly found in the American diet. The following table shows the nutrient content claims for sodium for single foods and for main dishes and meal products, such as frozen entrées and dinners. Nutrient content claims for calories, fat, saturated fat, and cholesterol and claims specifically applied to meat, poultry, and fish (lean and extra lean) are on pages 134–36.

DEFINITIONS OF NUTRIENT CONTENT CLAIMS FOR SODIUM

Nutrient Content Claim	Definition of Sodium Level
Sodium free	Less than 5 mg per serving of an individual food or per labeled serving of a main dish or meal product
Very low sodium	35 mg or less per serving of an individual food or per 100 grams (about 3½ ounces) of a main dish or meal product
Low sodium	140 mg or less per serving of an individual food or per 100 grams of a main dish or meal product
Reduced sodium	Contains at least 25% less sodium per serving of an individual food or per 100 grams of a main dish or meal product than reference food (see page 133 for definition of a reference food)
Salt free	Food must fit the definition of sodium free
Unsalted	No salt added during processing to a food to which sodium is usually added (unsalted foods that are not sodium free must have this fact stated on the label)
Light	"Light" may be used without qualification if the sodium is reduced by at least 50% in a food providing 3 grams or less of fat and 40 calories or less per serving compared with a reference food
Light in sodium	Sodium is reduced by 50% or more in an individual food when compared with a reference food that contains more than 3 grams of fat or more than 40 calories per serving; may be used in labeling a meal product that meets the definition for low sodium
Lightly salted	50% less sodium has been added than is normally added to a reference food ("lightly salted" foods that are not low sodium must have this fact stated on the label)
Healthy*	In an individual food, 3 grams or less of fat, 1 gram or less of saturated fat, 60 mg or less of cholesterol, and 480 mg or less of sodium* and must contain at least 10% of Daily Value of vitamin A, vitamin C, iron, calcium, protein, or fiber per serving

(continued)

Nutrient Content Claim	Definition of Sodium Level
	In a main dish or meal product, 3 grams or less of fat and 1 gram or less of saturated fat per 100 grams and per serving, and 90 mg or less of cholesterol and 600 mg or less of sodium per serving

Sodium level to be lowered in individual foods to 360 mg or less and in main dishes and meal products to 480 mg or less by 1998.

SODIUM ADDED DURING COOKING AND AT THE TABLE

About 15% of the sodium in the American diet is in the form of salt added to food during cooking and at the table. Salt and seasonings containing salt are added to most restaurant and fast foods. Remember, ¼ teaspoon of salt contains 533 mg of sodium.

SODIUM IN LEAVENING AGENTS AND SEASONINGS

Leavening Agent or Seasoning (¼ tsp except where noted)	Sodium mg
Baking powder	122
Baking soda	242
Celery salt	376
Garlic salt	315
Lemon pepper	86
"Lite" salt	244
Monosodium glutamate (MSG)	154
Onion salt	397
Seasoned salt	342
Soy sauce (1 tbsp)	1,029
Soy sauce, reduced-sodium (1 tbsp)	600

As the table above shows, it is possible to add a lot of sodium to food in the form of salt without actually using a saltshaker. One way to limit your sodium intake is to choose ingredients that contain less sodium for the dishes you make. These foods are often labeled "low sodium" or "reduced sodium." Remember, not all "reduced-sodium" ingredients are as low in sodium as the term suggests. For example, although reduced-sodium soy sauce is 40% lower in sodium than regular soy sauce, 1 tablespoon still provides 600 mg of sodium, or one-fourth of the maximum daily recommended intake of sodium (2,400 mg). Adding seasonings that do not contain sodium to foods will give them a distinct flavor without the use of salt or salty seasonings. It is important to read the Nutrition Facts portion of food labels for the sodium content of the foods and recipe ingredients you buy.

The recipes in this book are either moderately low in sodium or accompanied by a low-sodium variation. Some of the recipes call for the addition of a small amount of salt and are still fairly low in sodium; however, you can reduce the sodium in these recipes even further by omitting the salt. The sodium content is listed with the nutrient information for each recipe in this book.

TIPS FOR REDUCING SODIUM IN FOODS PREPARED AT HOME

- Add lemon juice, garlic, onion, and/or pepper to foods for flavor.
- Substitute herbs and spices for salt in recipes and at the table.
- Use more fresh food and less processed food.
- Use a small amount of a salt substitute in place of salt. To avoid the bitter taste of a salt substitute, add it to foods after they have been cooked. The use of "lite" salt is not recommended because it still contains sodium.
- Use garlic powder, celery powder, and onion powder instead of garlic salt, celery salt, and onion salt.

The following table lists some simple substitutions that you can make in preparing recipes to lower the sodium in the finished products.

RECIPE SUBSTITUTIONS TO LOWER SODIUM

Regular Product	Amount	Use Product Labeled	Sodium Reduced Approximately mg*
Baking powder	1 tsp	Low-sodium baking powder (3 tsp)	485
Beans, pinto, canned	1 cup	Cooked from dried beans without salt	410
Broth or meat stock, salted, beef or chicken	1 cup	Low-sodium bouillon† Beef Chicken	580 720
Buttermilk	1 cup	Skim, ½%, or 1% low-fat milk (1 cup minus 1 tbsp) plus lemon juice or vinegar (1 tbsp)	130
Cheese, American processed	1 oz	Low-sodium Low-fat & low-sodium	230 320
Cheese, Cheddar	1 oz	Low-sodium Low-fat & low-sodium	60 90

(continued)

Regular Product	Amount	Use Product Labeled	Sodium Reduced Approximately mg*
Cottage cheese	½ cup	No salt added	435
		Dry curd	450
Garlic salt	¼ tsp	Garlic powder	240
Tomatoes, canned	1 cup	No salt added	360
Tomato juice	1 cup	Salt-free	850
Tomato paste	½ cup	No salt added	950
Tomato sauce	½ cup	No salt added	705
Tuna, canned in water	2 oz	Unsalted	165
		Low-sodium	75
Vegetables, canned	1 cup	No salt added	225–520

*Values rounded to nearest 5.

†Refers only to "low-sodium" broth or bouillon; "light in salt" or other reduced-sodium broth or bouillon is higher in sodium.

NATURALLY OCCURRING SODIUM

Sodium that occurs naturally in water and food accounts for about 10% of the sodium consumed each day. Sodium is found in all plant and animal foods; examples are shown in the table below.

NATURALLY OCCURRING SODIUM IN FOODS

Food	Amount	Sodium mg
Meat, poultry, or fish	3 oz	75
Skim or low-fat milk	1 cup	120
Rice or pasta, cooked	1 cup	Less than 5
Fresh vegetables	½ cup	5–25
Fresh fruit	1 medium piece	2

All natural water supplies contain sodium, although the concentration varies depending on the source. Water from brackish or saline wells may contain several thousand milligrams of sodium per quart. Even rainwater contains a very small amount of sodium (1 mg per quart). Local water supplies differ widely in sodium content, which may be as low as 1 mg per quart or as high as 1,500 mg per quart. Someone drinking 8 cups of water containing 1,500 mg of sodium per quart gets 3,000 mg of sodium from that water alone. To find out the sodium content of your water supply, call your local health department or water department, or ask your physician to send a sample of your water to the laboratory that does your blood analysis. If your local water supply is high in sodium, you may wish to use distilled water or a bottled water without sodium for preparing foods and beverages and for drinking. Also, some water softeners increase the sodium content of water by exchanging sodium for calcium.

TECHNIQUES FOR LOWERING SODIUM INTAKE

Changing your eating habits to lower your intake of sodium is not a simple process. It involves being aware of the sodium in all the food you eat at home and especially away from home. To help ensure success in lowering your sodium intake, you can use the same techniques for changing dietary habits that registered dietitians teach their patients: assessment, goal setting, methods, and follow-up. These techniques are described on pages 41–50 and pages 69–78.

First, assess your current eating habits. Which foods are providing most of your sodium? It is helpful (and often surprising) to write down all the foods you eat for several days and add up the sodium they contain. Remember, the recommended intake of sodium is no more than 2,400 mg per day or the level recommended by your physician.

Second, based on your assessment of your current eating habits, set realistic goals for substituting lower-sodium foods for those that are high in sodium. For example, one simple change you could make would be to replace a ready-to-eat breakfast cereal that is high in sodium with one that contains little or no sodium, such as shredded wheat. Another important change you could make would be to choose a cooked-to-order entree in a restaurant and ask that it be prepared without salt.

Counting the milligrams of sodium in the foods you eat is an excellent method for decreasing your sodium intake. You can find information on the sodium content of food in the Nutrition Facts portion of food labels and in the food table beginning on page 372 of the Appendix. Sodium content is provided for each of the Living Heart Diet menus (which begin on page 186) and for the Living Heart Diet recipes (which begin on page 207).

Another method for decreasing sodium intake is called compensating. Compensating is a user-friendly way of living comfortably with a low-sodium diet. It consists of eating a few high-sodium foods that you really like and compensating for them by selecting other foods that are very low in sodium. First, identify your favorite high-sodium foods and prioritize them; then, identify the foods you like that are very low in sodium. Next, look at the sodium content of foods eaten for the total day rather than just the sodium in one food or even a single meal. The Appendix can be used to determine the sodium content of foods you eat frequently. For example, you can compensate for the 1,200 mg of sodium in a ham sandwich that contains 2 ounces of ham by making the sandwich with unsalted bread, eating cereal that is unsalted (shredded wheat instead of raisin bran) for breakfast, and using flavored vinegar as dressing on your tossed salad instead of French dressing. These changes alone save about 1,000 mg of sodium.

CONTROLLING SODIUM WHEN EATING AWAY FROM HOME

Controlling sodium intake when eating away from home can be a challenge. Most restaurants do not have information available on the sodium content of the foods they serve. The amount of sodium can vary widely in the same dish when it is prepared by different chefs. Most restaurant food has salt added to it, and many dishes contain monosodium glutamate (MSG), which is a high-sodium flavor enhancer often added to food. A restaurant meal can easily contain 1,000 to 5,000 mg of sodium. Beginning on page 372 of the Appendix, the sodium content is listed for many American, Mexican, Italian, and Chinese restaurant foods. *Remember: you can always request that salt be left out of food that is cooked to order, but sodium cannot be decreased in foods prepared ahead of time, such as casseroles, soups, and sauces.*

The tips below will help you select lower-sodium foods in restaurants that serve typical "American" foods and in those that serve ethnic cuisines. Another book in our series, *The Living Heart Guide to Eating Out,* contains extensive information on selecting lower-sodium, lower-fat American and ethnic foods when eating away from home (see back of book for order form).

AMERICAN CUISINE – The following practical tips will help you avoid excess sodium when you eat out in American restaurants and fast-food establishments that serve typical American foods.

Breakfast and Brunch

- Choose fruit or fruit juice instead of tomato or vegetable juice.

- Have a meat-free breakfast or brunch, since most breakfast meats (bacon, sausage, ham, Canadian bacon) are high in sodium.

- If you order an egg (as part of your egg allowance for one week), specify that it be poached or boiled.

- If you order an omelet (as part of your egg allowance), ask that cheese and salt be omitted.

- Select an unsalted cereal, such as shredded wheat, puffed wheat, or puffed rice.

Lunch and Dinner

- Order salad or fruit as an appetizer instead of soup.

- Select salads that do not contain cheese or cottage cheese.

- Choose fruit or fresh vegetables as a salad instead of ordering higher-sodium prepared salads, such as tuna, chicken, pasta, or potato salad or pickled vegetables.

- Use oil and vinegar (from separate bottles, so that you can control the amount of oil), flavored vinegar, or lemon juice as a dressing for salad instead of a prepared dressing.

- Choose cooked-to-order dishes, such as grilled, broiled, or baked meat or fish, and ask that salt, MSG, and soy sauce be omitted during preparation. In dishes prepared ahead of time, such as casseroles, soups, and foods with gravies or sauces, the salt cannot be reduced.

- If an entrée is served with breading, topping, or sauce, remove it before eating the entrée.

- Condiments—including salt, pickles, olives, soy sauce, meat sauces, salad dressings, catsup, and mustard—are high in salt.

- Use lemon juice with fish instead of tartar sauce, cocktail sauce, or catsup.

- On your baked potato, use toppings such as green onion, chives, lemon juice, or a small amount of margarine.

- Ask that your vegetables be served without sauce or cheese.

- Choose yeast breads, such as hard rolls or sliced bread, instead of higher-sodium breads made with baking powder, such as biscuits, cornbread, or muffins.

- For dessert, choose fruit, gelatin, frozen yogurt, or sherbet, because these foods are lower in sodium than most baked desserts.

- If fruit pie is selected, decrease sodium and fat by eating only the filling and leaving the crust.

Fast Foods and Sandwiches

- Request "fresh" cooked turkey or roast beef instead of meats processed with sodium, such as deli-type turkey or roast beef. Grilled chicken is also a good choice; request that salt not be added to it.

- Ask that a salad or carrot sticks be substituted for chips if they come with a sandwich.

- Order lettuce, tomato, and/or onion for your sandwich instead of pickles, cheese, catsup, and/or steak sauce.

- Ask for sweet pickles with your sandwich instead of dill or sour pickles, which are higher in sodium.

- Order a small hamburger without cheese instead of a cheeseburger or a quarter-pound or other large hamburger.

Pizza

- Specify little or no cheese on your pizza.

- Order vegetable toppings (except olives) instead of meat toppings, which are high in sodium and fat.

- Order your pizza without anchovies.

ETHNIC CUISINES – In Chapter 8, "The Living Heart Diet Guide to Selecting Food When Eating Out," there are tables comparing the fat, saturated fat, and sodium in Chinese (see page 161), Italian (see page 164), and Mexican (see page 166) restaurant meals to the Daily Values (at 2,000-calorie level) for these nutrients.

Cajun

- Boiled seafood makes a good appetizer.

- Choose grilled seafood, chicken, or steak, and request that salt not be used in preparation. Cajun favorites such as jambalaya, creole dishes, gumbo, and étouffée are made ahead of time, and the sodium cannot be reduced.

Chinese

- Ask that MSG, salt, and soy sauce not be used in the preparation of your food; most foods prepared ahead of time and many of the sauces used in preparation already have these ingredients in them. It is best to choose a restaurant that states on the menu that no MSG is used in the food.

- Choose steamed foods, such as fish or dumplings.

- Sweet-and-sour, plum, and duck sauces are much lower in sodium than soy, oyster, and bean sauces.

- Check the sodium content for selected Chinese foods on page 380 of the Appendix.

French

- Choose cooked-to-order dishes, such as grilled fish and vegetables; ask that salt be omitted and that sauce be served on the side so that you can control the amount you eat.

- Order fruit or sorbet for dessert.

Greek and Middle Eastern

- Choose baked fish or chicken and ask that salt be omitted during cooking. Selections such as moussaka, spanakopita, dips, and sauces are made ahead of time, and the sodium in them cannot be reduced.

- Feta cheese is high in sodium.

Indian

- Choose tandoori or tikka meat instead of an entrée prepared with a sauce, such as curry sauce.

Italian

- Choose dishes that are cooked to order, and ask that salt be omitted during food preparation. Lasagna, ravioli, and cannelloni, which are made ahead of time, contain cheese and salt.

- Use vinegar or lemon juice on salad instead of Italian dressing.

- Choose granita without whipped cream for dessert.

- See sodium content for selected Italian foods on page 387 of the Appendix.

Japanese

- Japanese food is typically high in sodium because of the salt, MSG, and soy sauce used in soups and cooking broths, sauces, marinades, and salad dressings.

- Order plain steamed rice and use very little, if any, dipping sauce.

- Although sashimi is low in sodium, eating raw fish can be hazardous.

Mexican

- Ask that cheese not be added to your food.

- Choose grilled chicken, fish, or fajitas, and ask that salt not be added during cooking. Avoid dishes made ahead of time, such as burritos, enchiladas, and tacos, in which sodium cannot be reduced.

- Use salsa as a salad dressing on fajita salad instead of chile con queso, which is high in sodium and fat.

- See sodium content for selected Mexican foods on page 389 of the Appendix.

Thai and Vietnamese

- Order one less entrée than the number of people dining together and share.

- Avoid peanut sauce, which is high in sodium and fat.

- Select steamed rice instead of fried rice.

Other Dietary Considerations

Research into the causes and treatment of high blood pressure has led scientists to study the effects of various other nutrients and foods on blood pressure. Some nutrients—such as potassium and calcium—have a positive effect on blood pressure, while other nutrients—such as protein, carbohydrate, and fiber—have not yielded consistent research results.

POTASSIUM

Studies have shown an inverse relation between blood pressure and dietary intake of potassium—that is, low potassium intake is associated with higher blood pressure and vice versa. It has been suggested that lower intake of potassium accounts for the higher prevalence of high blood pressure in blacks than in whites in the United States. High intake of potassium may help protect against developing high blood pressure, and low intake may increase blood pressure. In addition, potassium seems to enhance the beneficial effect of restricting sodium in the diet.

Adequate potassium intake is especially important for people with high blood pressure. Low levels of potassium in the blood may result from the diuretic therapy often used for patients with high blood pressure. It may be necessary for these patients to add potassium in the form of a potassium supplement or potassium-containing salt substitute, or to switch to a potassium-sparing diuretic.

Potassium supplementation is probably not as important as controlling body weight and reducing sodium intake in most people. Potassium supplementation may be important in *preventing* high blood pressure in people with a low dietary intake of potassium.

There is not a Recommended Dietary Allowance (RDA) for potassium. However, the recommended daily minimum intake used in food labeling is 3,500 mg, an amount that can easily be obtained by increasing consumption of fruits, vegetables, and beans. As a rule, processing decreases potassium and increases sodium in foods. Good sources of potassium are listed from high to low in the table below.

POTASSIUM CONTENT OF SELECTED FOODS

Food	Potassium mg*
White beans, cooked (¾ cup)	750
Salt substitute containing potassium (¼ tsp)	715
Potato, baked (1 medium)	610
Pinto beans, cooked (¾ cup)	600
Yogurt, low-fat, plain (1 cup)	575
Baked beans, vegetarian, canned (¾ cup)	565
Lentils, cooked (¾ cup)	550
Lima beans, cooked (¾ cup)	545
Kidney beans, cooked (¾ cup)	535
Tomato juice, salt-free (1 cup)	535
Cantaloupe, cubed (1 cup)	495
Orange juice, frozen, reconstituted (1 cup)	475
Yogurt, low-fat, w/ fruit (1 cup)	475
Black beans, cooked (¾ cup)	460
Honeydew melon, cubed (1 cup)	460
Tomatoes, unsalted, canned (¾ cup)	460
Apricots, dried, uncooked (9 halves or ¼ cup)	450

(continued)

POTASSIUM CONTENT OF SELECTED FOODS (CONT.)

Food	Potassium mg*
Banana (1 large)	450
Milk, low-fat, protein-fortified (1 cup)	445
Spinach, frozen, cooked (¾ cup)	425
100% bran ready-to-eat cereal (¾ cup)	410
Brussels sprouts, frozen, cooked (¾ cup)	380
Grapefruit juice (1 cup)	380
Milk, low-fat (1 cup)	380
Pork, tenderloin, cooked (3 ounces)	370
Watermelon, cubed (2 cups)	370
Carrot juice (½ cup)	360
Prune juice (½ cup)	355
Prunes, dried (5 medium)	315
Avocado (¼ medium)	300
Apple juice (1 cup)	295
Flounder, cooked (3 oz)	290
Nectarine (1 medium)	290
Beef, round, cooked (3 oz)	285
Blackberries (1 cup)	280
Pink salmon, unsalted, canned (3 oz)	275
Beets, sliced, canned (¾ cup)	260
Tomato, fresh (1 medium)	255
Strawberries, sliced (1 cup)	250
Carrot, raw (1 medium)	235
Orange (1 medium)	235
Cherries, sweet, raw (15)	230
Turkey, unprocessed, roasted (3 oz)	225
Chicken, roasted (3 oz)	205
Tuna, water-packed, unsalted (½ cup)	200
Grapefruit (½ medium)	165

Adapted from USDA, Composition of Foods, Agriculture Handbook series no. 8 (Washington, D.C.: USDA, 1976–1992).
*Values rounded to nearest 5.

CALCIUM

In most population studies there is an inverse relation between dietary calcium and blood pressure—that is, a high intake of dietary calcium is associated with lower blood pressure and vice versa. Calcium deficiency is associated with an increased prevalence of high blood pressure, and an increase in dietary calcium may help lower blood pressure. Calcium has a greater blood pressure–lowering effect in some patients, but there is no way to predict which patients will benefit. Even though an increase in dietary calcium may help lower blood pressure, the results from research studies using large doses of calcium as supplements have not been convincing.

The RDA for calcium is 1,200 mg for both sexes ages 11 to 24 years, and 800 mg for younger children and for adults age 25 years and above. For the purposes of food labeling, a single recommendation of 1,000 mg of calcium is used. Dairy products are the best source of calcium; other sources include dark-green leafy vegetables and some fish and shellfish. For a list of foods high in calcium, see page 183.

MAGNESIUM

There is evidence to suggest that low intake of magnesium is associated with higher blood pressure. However, the evidence is not strong enough to justify recommending magnesium supplementation for the purpose of lowering blood pressure. In a study using magnesium tablets, some of the patients had gastrointestinal complaints, such as loose stools or diarrhea. What is recommended is maintaining an adequate dietary intake of magnesium.

The RDA for magnesium depends on age and sex. For males, it is 270 mg for ages 11 to 14 years, 400 mg for ages 15 to 18, and 350 mg for ages 19 and older. For females, it is 280 mg for ages 11 to 14 years, 300 mg for ages 15 to 18, and 280 mg for ages 19 and older. For the purposes of food labeling, a single level of 400 mg of magnesium is used. Magnesium is found in a wide variety of foods, as shown in the table below, which lists some of the best sources from high to low.

MAGNESIUM CONTENT OF SELECTED FOODS

Food	Magnesium mg*
Tofu, firm (½ cup)	120
Almonds (¼ cup)[†]	105
Halibut, cooked dry heat (3 oz)	90
Wheat germ, toasted (¼ cup)	90
Pumpkin and squash seed kernels, roasted (1 tbsp)[†]	75
Peanuts, dry-roasted (¼ cup)[†]	65
Sesame seeds, whole, dried (2 tbsp)[†]	65
Spinach, frozen, cooked (½ cup)	65

(continued)

MAGNESIUM CONTENT OF SELECTED FOODS

Food	Magnesium mg*
Black beans, cooked (½ cup)	60
Fortified oat flakes cereal (1 cup)	60
Baked potato with skin (1 medium)	55
Navy beans, cooked (½ cup)	55
Blackstrap molasses (1 tbsp)	45
Oatmeal, cooked (¾ cup)	40
Milk, 1% low-fat (1 cup)	35
Bread, whole-wheat (1 slice)	25
Chicken breast, skinned, roasted (3 oz)	25
Green peas, frozen, cooked (½ cup)	25
Beef, top round, trimmed, braised (3 oz)	20
Fruits	10–25

Adapted from USDA, Composition of Foods, *Agriculture Handbook series no 8 (Washington, DC: USDA, 1976–1992).*
Values rounded to the nearest 5.
†*These foods are high in fat.*

CAFFEINE

Caffeine can raise blood pressure, especially in people who do not normally consume it; however, regular consumption of caffeine appears to decrease this tendency. Although there is presently no general recommendation to limit caffeine as a way of lowering blood pressure, reducing caffeine intake may be appropriate for individuals who are sensitive to it. Primary sources of caffeine in the diet are coffee, tea, chocolate, and some soft drinks (regular and sugar free). Caffeine content for selected foods appears on page 62.

DIETARY FATS

It has been shown that a diet lower in saturated fat and higher in polyunsaturated fat decreases both systolic and diastolic blood pressure. Studies have also shown that large quantities of omega-3 fatty acids, which are found primarily in fish-oil supplements and high-fat fish, lower blood pressure in some people. However, the use of fish-oil supplements is not recommended for the treatment or prevention of high blood pressure because of potential side effects with a high intake of fish oil.

PROTEIN AND CARBOHYDRATE

In clinical studies, varying the levels of protein and carbohydrate in the diet has not had consistent effects on blood pressure.

FIBER

Several studies have shown that dietary fiber helps lower blood pressure, while other studies have not shown this effect. However, including good sources of fiber in the diet is recommended for other health benefits, such as a reduction in risk for gastrointestinal cancer.

GARLIC AND ONION

Studies conducted to evaluate the effect of increased consumption of garlic or onion on blood pressure have not obtained consistent results. However, several studies suggest that an intake of 600 to 900 mg of garlic powder (about ⅓ teaspoon) per day lowers systolic and diastolic blood pressure both in people with normal blood pressure and in those with high blood pressure.

Other Lifestyle Considerations

Scientists have tried to identify other aspects of lifestyle that may play a direct or indirect role in the development and control of high blood pressure. Two lifestyle changes often recommended to people with high blood pressure are stopping smoking and decreasing stress.

SMOKING

Although smoking cessation is not directly related to high blood pressure, it is essential for good health. Cigarette smoking is a major risk factor for heart disease and is the leading cause of preventable premature death in the United States.

STRESS

There is some evidence that chronic life stress, including job strain and a lack of decision-making ability, can contribute to the development of high blood pressure. However, even though handling stress well is an important part of general well-being, it is not clear that stress management techniques can either prevent or control high blood pressure. Stress management is not currently endorsed by medical authorities as an effective therapy for high blood pressure.

Controlling High Blood Pressure with Medication

Very effective medications are available for controlling high blood pressure. Medications are used in addition to weight control, regular planned physical activity, sodium restriction, moderating alcohol intake, and other changes in lifestyle, not in place of these measures. Weight loss in overweight patients with high blood pressure causes blood pressure medications to work more effectively. Medications to lower blood pressure are also more effective when patients are following a low-sodium diet. Adherence to lifestyle recommendations may allow the number and doses of medications to be decreased. As noted in this chapter's introduction, if you are taking blood pressure medication, it is very important to continue taking it, since medication controls rather than cures high blood pressure.

Chapter 5

The Living Heart Diet in Managing Diabetes

Diabetes management consists of a combination of diet, exercise, weight control, and, if necessary, medication (oral medication or insulin). Diet is the cornerstone of diabetes treatment. Medical nutrition therapy for diabetes includes specific recommendations for fat, saturated fat, and cholesterol intake, as well as for carbohydrate (starch and sugar) intake, since people with diabetes frequently have elevated blood triglyceride and low HDL-cholesterol levels; they may also have elevated total cholesterol or LDL-cholesterol. Sodium restriction to help prevent or control high blood pressure is also recommended for people with diabetes. Diabetes mellitus is a major independent risk factor for cardiovascular disease; people with diabetes are three to four times more likely to develop cardiovascular disease than people without diabetes.

Medical Nutrition Therapy for Diabetes

The American Diabetes Association has established the following goals for medical nutrition therapy for diabetes:

- To assist people with diabetes in making changes in nutrition and exercise habits that lead to improved diabetic control

- To maintain blood glucose levels as near normal as possible by balancing food intake with oral medications or insulin and levels of physical activity

- To achieve desirable blood levels of triglyceride and cholesterol

- To provide adequate nutrition for achieving and maintaining a reasonable body weight (including the special needs of growing children and adolescents, pregnant and lactating women, and people recovering from illness)

- To prevent and treat serious complications of diabetes, including hypoglycemia, kidney disease, neuropathy (diseases of the nervous system), high blood pressure, and cardiovascular disease

- To improve overall health through optimal nutrition

Diabetic patients are advised to follow the recommendations for fat and cholesterol intake made for the general public, that is, a daily intake providing

- 30% or less of calories from fat

- 8% to 10% of calories from saturated fat

- Less than 300 milligrams (mg) of cholesterol per day

Diabetic patients with known atherosclerotic disease, like other people with atherosclerotic disease, should follow the Step II Diet. In the Step II Diet, as discussed in Chapter 2, saturated fat is reduced to less than 7% of calories and cholesterol is reduced to less than 200 mg per day.

EXCHANGE LISTS

Exchange Lists are often used in developing meal plans for individuals with diabetes. In this book the Exchange Lists are called Food Groups and Serving Sizes and appear in the Appendix on pages 345–55. A description of how to use the Food Groups and Serving Sizes to control calories, carbohydrate, and fat is provided on page 74 of Chapter 3, on weight control, and is called "Choosing Servings of Food from Each Food Group."

The recipes in this book (which begin on page 207) include exchanges when applicable. For example, one serving of Black-Eyed Pea and Chicken Soup on page 234 can be counted as 1 starch/bread and 2 meat exchanges. For recipes that are too high in refined sugars, "not applicable" appears in the space usually used for exchanges.

WEIGHT CONTROL

Obesity, especially centered in the waist or abdomen, is often associated with type II diabetes, also called non-insulin-dependent diabetes mellitus (NIDDM) or late-onset diabetes. More than 80% of patients with type II diabetes are overweight at the time their diabetes is diagnosed. Reaching and maintaining a reasonable weight, which reduces blood glucose levels, is a priority in medical nutrition therapy for diabetes. For overweight patients, mild to moderate weight loss can improve control of blood glucose levels even if the traditional "ideal" body weight is not achieved. (See pages 358–59 in the Appendix for information on desirable weights for men and women.) For some patients with diabetes, the physician may recommend a weight greater than the "desirable" weights shown in the tables as a more reasonable goal for weight loss.

Moderate calorie restriction (250 to 500 calories less than the average daily intake) and initiation of regular exercise are important to a healthy weight control plan for people with diabetes. It is important to remember that consuming large amounts of foods labeled "low calorie," "sugar free," or "fat free" can provide too many calories. See Chapter 3, on weight control, for additional information about losing weight and keeping it off.

Fat Intake and Levels of Blood Cholesterol and Triglyceride

When elevated blood cholesterol levels do not decrease to goal levels after following a diet that contains 8% to 10% of calories from saturated fat and less than 300 mg of cholesterol per day, an eating plan with less than 7% of calories from saturated fat and dietary cholesterol of less than 200 mg daily may be necessary. As noted above, all patients with atherosclerotic disease *begin* dietary therapy with this intensified diet.

Diabetic patients with very high triglyceride levels (greater than 1,000 mg/dL) may need to decrease their intake of all types of fat. For additional information on fat intake and lowering cholesterol and triglyceride levels, see Chapter 2, beginning on page 31.

Sugars and Other Nutritive Sweeteners

Recent research has suggested that first priority be given to the total amount of carbohydrate consumed rather than the source of carbohydrate. However, some physicians specializing in diabetes management believe that restriction of all refined sugars and the naturally occurring sugars in fruits and fruit juices is essential to good blood glucose control. The degree to which sugars are allowed or restricted in a diabetic meal plan will depend on the approach to treatment recommended by the individual physician and the response of the individual patient. If limited amounts of refined sugars such as sucrose and sucrose-containing foods are allowed in a diabetic meal plan, these foods should be *substituted* for other carbohydrate-containing foods instead of simply added to the meal plan. The nutrient content of foods high in refined sugars, which are frequently high in calories and fat, needs to be taken into consideration.

All nutritive sweeteners (that is, sweeteners providing calories) in a food must be included in the list of ingredients on the food label. To identify the nutritive sweeteners in a food, look for the following terms in the list of ingredients on the label:

COMMON NUTRITIVE SWEETENERS

Corn syrup	Maple syrup
Dextrose (glucose)	Molasses
Fructose	Sorbitol*
Fruit juice or fruit juice concentrate	Sucrose (table sugar)
High-fructose corn syrup	Sugar
Honey	Turbinado (partially refined cane sugar)
Maltose	Xylitol*
Mannitol*	

Sugar alcohols

Since 1994 the Nutrition Facts portion of food labels has included the grams of sugars present in a standard serving of a food. The term "sugars" encompasses sucrose and most other nutritive sweeteners. It also includes the naturally occurring sugars in milk, fruits, and fruit juices. Sugar alcohols (sorbitol, mannitol, and xylitol) are not included in the "sugars" listed on the Nutrition Facts portion of a food label. Manufacturers have the option of listing grams of sugar alcohols separate from other sugars on the label. Sugar alcohols raise blood sugar less than sucrose and other carbohydrates, although the American Diabetes Association does not consider them to have an advantage over other nutritive sweeteners.

The inclusion of more complete information on sugar content in labeling foods makes it easier for diabetic patients restricting their intake of sugars to identify appropriate food choices. As a help to diabetic patients, the third edition of *The Living Heart Brand Name Shopper's Guide* (see last page for order form) not only indicates foods low in fat, saturated fat, and cholesterol, but also includes the amount of carbohydrate in each food.

The Food and Drug Administration allows the following nutrient content claims to be made regarding sugars:

- "Sugar free"—less than 0.5 gram of sugars per serving and with no ingredient that is sugar

- "Reduced/less sugar"—at least 25% less sugars per serving than reference food

- "No added sugar"—no sugar or ingredient containing sugar is added during processing

SUGAR SUBSTITUTES

Nonnutritive sweeteners, or sugar substitutes, provide few or no calories. Saccharin, the oldest sugar substitute, is marketed under several brands. Aspartame is marketed as Equal for table use and as

NutraSweet when used as an ingredient. Acesulfame K is marketed under the brand names Sunette and Sweet One. People with diabetes can safely consume all approved nonnutritive sweeteners.

FIBER

The American Diabetes Association recommends that people with diabetes consume from 20 to 35 grams of dietary fiber per day from a wide variety of foods—the same recommendation that has been made for the general public. Although increased fiber intake may be beneficial in treating or preventing some gastrointestinal disorders, it is considered to have an insignificant effect on control of blood glucose levels.

ALCOHOL

Diabetic patients should follow their physician's recommendations about alcohol use. Hypoglycemia is a major concern because alcohol may increase the risk for hypoglycemia in diabetic patients treated with sulfonylureas or insulin. Diabetic individuals who are pregnant or who have a history of alcohol abuse should totally abstain from alcohol, and there are other special situations in which alcohol should not be consumed. Patients with high triglyceride levels should abstain from alcohol.

SODIUM AND HIGH BLOOD PRESSURE

Approximately 50% of diabetic adults also have high blood pressure. Physicians often prescribe a reduced sodium intake to help lower blood pressure in people with high blood pressure. Recommendations for sodium intake vary: some health authorities recommend a daily intake of no more than 3,000 mg of sodium for the general population, while other health authorities recommend a slightly lower level of 2,400 mg. Sodium and high blood pressure are discussed in more detail in Chapter 4, beginning on page 89.

VITAMINS AND MINERALS

Generally, a diabetic patient following a balanced diet should not need a vitamin–mineral supplement. At present there is insufficient evidence to support taking supplements of the antioxidants vitamin C, vitamin E, and beta-carotene. Supplementation with chromium or with magnesium is not recommended except in cases of a deficiency of these minerals. Potassium supplementation may be necessary in cases of loss through use of diuretics. Individuals with diabetes should follow their physician's recommendations about taking supplements.

Detecting Diabetes

It is estimated that 6% of the U.S. population has diabetes. Although more than half of these people have been diagnosed as having diabetes, the remainder are unaware that they have the disease.

A number of factors are typical of people who are more likely to develop diabetes. Overweight is one factor over which you may have control. You are more likely to develop diabetes if you

- Are overweight

- Have a family history of diabetes

- Are age 40 or older

- Are black, Hispanic, or Native American

The following are warning symptoms of diabetes. See your physician if you are experiencing two or more of these symptoms:

- Blurred vision

- Dry skin or dry mouth

- Frequent urination

- Excessive thirst

- Extreme hunger

- Unexplained weight loss

- Irritability

- Weakness or fatigue

- Drowsiness

- Itching

- Tingling or numbness in hands or feet

- Recurring or hard-to-heal infections of the skin, gums, or bladder

- Nausea or vomiting

At present there is no cure for diabetes; however, this disease can be controlled. Vigorous efforts—diet, exercise, weight control, glucose monitoring, and, when necessary, medication—can be used to control blood glucose levels and may prevent or delay the complications of diabetes.

Chapter 6

The Living Heart Diet for Vegetarians

Vegetarianism is becoming an increasingly popular way to eat healthfully. Vegetarian diets are nutritionally adequate when carefully planned, and they can help reduce risk for coronary heart disease (CHD), obesity, high blood pressure, diabetes mellitus, and certain types of cancer. Vegetarian diets are consistent with the Dietary Guidelines for Americans and the Food Pyramid, both of which emphasize consuming larger amounts of plant foods and smaller amounts of animal foods.

There is no single definition for a vegetarian diet. All vegetarians avoid red meat; however, some vegetarians include fowl, fish, eggs, and dairy products in addition to fruits, vegetables, grains, legumes, seeds, and nuts.

GENERAL TYPES OF VEGETARIANISM		
Type	Does Not Eat	Does Eat
Semi-vegetarian	Meat	Plant foods, fish, fowl, dairy products, and eggs
Pesco-vegetarian	Meat and fowl	Plant foods, fish, dairy products, and eggs

(continued)

Type	Does Not Eat	Does Eat
Lacto-ovo-vegetarian	Meat, fowl, and fish	Plant foods, dairy products, and eggs
Lacto-vegetarian	Meat, fowl, fish, and eggs	Plant foods and dairy products
Ovo-vegetarian	Meat, fowl, fish, and dairy products	Plant foods and eggs
Vegan	All animal products	Plant foods

People from all age groups and all walks of life turn to a vegetarian lifestyle for a variety of reasons. The most common reasons cited for following a vegetarian diet are

- Religious beliefs

- Desire to spare natural resources by eating lower on the food chain

- Issues of world hunger

- Kindness to animals

- Belief that a vegetarian diet is healthier

- Financial concerns (plant foods cost less)

- Preference for plant foods

Only one of the issues listed above will be addressed in this book: the healthfulness of a vegetarian diet.

Health Benefits of Vegetarianism

Many research studies have shown lower rates of several chronic degenerative diseases and conditions in people who follow a vegetarian diet. It is not easy to separate the effects of vegetarian eating from those of the lifestyle factors that often accompany it, such as having a desirable weight, taking part in regular physical activity, and abstaining from alcohol, caffeine, smoking, and illicit drugs. Nevertheless, it is clear that vegetarianism is associated with health benefits.

VEGETARIANISM AND HEART DISEASE

Vegetarians are less likely than nonvegetarians to die of CHD. Vegans as well as those vegetarians who eat dairy products and eggs in addition to plant foods tend to have lower blood levels of total cholesterol and LDL-cholesterol than nonvegetarians. HDL-cholesterol and triglyceride levels vary, depending on the type of vegetarian diet being followed.

Dietary cholesterol is found only in animal foods, such as meat, fish, poultry, eggs, and dairy products. A great deal of the saturated fat in the U.S. diet comes from meat, poultry, and high-fat dairy products. A vegetarian diet is not always lower in total fat than a nonvegetarian diet; however, a vegetarian diet is typically lower in saturated fat and higher in polyunsaturated fat.

Dean Ornish, M.D., conducted a study in which the participants were patients with severe CHD. Improvement in coronary artery plaque was seen among the participants who followed a program combining a very low fat vegetarian diet (less than 10% of calories from fat) with smoking cessation, moderate exercise, and stress management. Information on a very low fat diet is on page 40.

VEGETARIANISM AND HIGH BLOOD PRESSURE

Population studies suggest that on average vegans have lower blood pressure than people eating both animal and plant foods. This difference in blood pressure may be due to several differences in diet. The vegan diet is higher in fiber, lower in animal protein, and usually lower in calories and fat, especially saturated fat, compared with a nonvegetarian diet. The lower blood pressure could also be the result of other lifestyle characteristics shared by many vegetarians, such as taking part in regular physical activity and abstaining from smoking. In addition, vegetarians tend to be leaner than nonvegetarians, and obesity is associated with high blood pressure.

VEGETARIANISM AND CANCER

The National Cancer Institute (NCI) estimates that diet may be related to one-third of cancer deaths. The NCI has stated that (1) cruciferous vegetables (those in the cabbage family) may reduce risk for cancer, (2) diets low in fat and high in fiber may reduce risk for colon cancer, and (3) diets rich in foods containing vitamin C and beta-carotene may reduce risk for some cancers.

Seventh-Day Adventists who are vegetarians are one group who have lower rates of colon cancer than the general population. This decreased incidence may be due to lower intake of total fat, saturated fat, cholesterol, and/or caffeine; increased intake of fruits and vegetables; increased intake of calcium (in lacto-vegetarians); increased fiber intake; or some combination of these factors. Eating less meat and animal protein has been associated with lower rates of colon cancer in some, but not all, studies.

Research studies have suggested an association between a low-fat diet that is high in plant foods and fiber and a reduced risk for some other kinds of cancer as well. There is some evidence for a link between vegetarian eating and reduced risk for breast cancer.

VEGETARIANISM AND DIABETES

Because they tend to be leaner, vegetarians are at lower risk than nonvegetarians for developing type II diabetes mellitus, also called non-insulin-dependent or adult-onset diabetes mellitus.

VEGETARIANISM AND OTHER DISEASES

Vegetarian eating is associated with decreased risk for constipation. It is also linked to lower rates of alcoholism, perhaps reflecting the limited consumption of alcohol that is often a part of the vegetarian lifestyle. There is preliminary evidence that a vegetarian diet contributes to lower risk for developing several other disorders, including osteoporosis, gallstones, kidney stones, and diverticular disease. Whether the reduced risks are due to the diet or to other lifestyle characteristics shared by many vegetarians is not known.

VEGETARIANISM AND CALORIE INTAKE

Vegetarians, especially vegans, usually have body weight closer to desirable than nonvegetarians. The lower rates of CHD, high blood pressure, diabetes mellitus, and some types of cancer among vegetarians are possibly linked to their lower rates of obesity; obesity contributes to all these disorders.

Some vegetarians may have difficulty consuming enough plant foods to maintain a desirable weight. For these individuals it may be necessary to use a larger amount of oils low in saturated fat (see table on page 53) in food preparation and to increase consumption of higher-fat plant foods, such as nuts. Sufficient calorie intake is especially important for women who are pregnant.

Guidelines for Vegetarian Diets

It is important that a vegetarian diet be carefully planned to ensure adequate intake of all nutrients. The possibility of inadequate intake of nutrients increases as the range of food choices becomes narrower. For example, ovo-vegetarians and vegans need to take extra care in planning their diets and may need supplementation with vitamin B_{12}. Vitamin B_{12} is further discussed on pages 121–22.

Semi-vegetarian, pesco-vegetarian, lacto-ovo-vegetarian, and lacto-vegetarian diets can be adequate in vitamin B_{12} without supplementation. However, the amounts of fowl, fish, eggs, and dairy products eaten and the frequency of consumption need to be carefully evaluated. It may be helpful to have a registered dietitian who is familiar with vegetarian diets review the adequacy of the diet. The table on pages 125–26 provides vegetarians with a guide for selecting foods. People following a vegetarian diet need to pay special attention to the nutrients discussed below.

PROTEIN

Plant sources can provide adequate protein if two conditions are met: a wide variety of high-quality protein plant foods are selected, and adequate calories are consumed to meet the body's needs. Amino acids are the building blocks of proteins. There are two types of amino acids in relation to diet: essential (those that are not made in the body) and nonessential (those that are made in the body). Soybeans and animal products (meat, fowl, fish, dairy products, and eggs) are called "complete" protein sources because each contains all the essential amino acids; each food can be eaten as the sole source of protein. Whole grains, vegetables, seeds, nuts, and legumes (other than soybeans) are "incomplete" protein sources because each of these foods does not contain all the essential amino acids.

It is not necessary to eat particular combinations of incomplete plant proteins at each meal to obtain all the essential amino acids necessary for growth and repair of body tissue, as was previously recommended. Vegetarians who consume an adequate amount of protein overall from a variety of sources get a sufficient supply of essential amino acids. However, some people may still wish to combine at a meal plant proteins that complement one another through supplying all the essential amino acids when eaten together. Those individuals may combine legumes (lentils, black-eyed peas, chickpeas, peanuts, or lima, broad, kidney, pinto, navy, mung, or black beans) with grains (wheat, corn, rice, bulgur, oats, barley, millet, or buckwheat). A number of vegetarian food products made to look like meats are available; they usually contain soybeans, which, as noted above, are a complete protein source.

Protein recommendations vary for different age groups:

RECOMMENDED DIETARY ALLOWANCES FOR PROTEIN

Category	Age in Years	Grams of Protein per Day per Pound of Body Weight
Infants	0–½	1.00
	½–1*	0.73
Children	1–3	0.55
	4–6	0.50
	7–10	0.45
Adolescents and adults		
Males	11–14	0.45
	15–18	0.41
	19 and above	0.36
Females (nonpregnant)	11–14	0.45
	15 and above	0.36

Adapted from National Research Council, Recommended Dietary Allowances, *10th ed. (Washington, D.C.: National Academy Press, 1989).*
*First birthday.

For example, a 35-year-old man who weighs 150 pounds needs 54 grams of protein per day (150 × 0.36 = 54); if he weighed 180 pounds, his recommended protein level would be 65 grams per day. Note that protein needs per pound are higher in infancy, childhood, and adolescence than in adulthood; these higher levels are to support growth.

The Recommended Dietary Allowance (RDA) for protein for pregnant women averages 60 grams daily. For lactating women, the RDA is 65 grams of protein daily for the first 6 months and 62 grams of protein daily for the second 6 months.

Vegetarian diets are usually lower in total protein than nonvegetarian diets; however, most non-vegetarian Americans consume much more protein than they need. Some studies have shown health benefits from eating less protein than is present in the typical American diet. For example, lower protein levels are associated with better calcium retention in vegetarians. Lower protein may also mean a lower intake of total fat, saturated fat, and cholesterol, which reduces risk for CHD and certain types of cancer. Special care must be taken to ensure that children receive adequate protein for optimal growth and development. The table below shows how much protein and fat and how many calories are found in selected animal and plant sources of protein.

SELECTED PLANT AND ANIMAL SOURCES OF PROTEIN

Food	Protein g	Fat g	Calories
Chicken breast, skinless, roasted (3 oz)	27	3	142
Eye of round roast, braised (3 oz)	25	5	149
Beef tenderloin, trimmed, broiled (3 oz)	24	8	170
Flounder, broiled (3 oz)	21	1	99
Red beans & rice (1 cup)	15	1	316
Macaroni & cheese (1 cup)	12	19	402
Peanut butter, regular (2 tbsp)	8	16	190
Oatmeal, cooked (1 cup)	6	2	145
Potato, baked, w/ skin (1 medium)	5	<1	220
Corn, cooked (1 cup)	4	2	132
Whole-wheat bread (1 slice)	3	1	70
Cornflakes (1 cup)	2	<1	110

Adapted from USDA, Composition of Foods, *Agriculture Handbook series no. 8 (Washington, D.C.: USDA, 1976–1992).*

Vegetarians need to be careful not to consume too many calories in an effort to meet their protein needs. For example, to obtain the 31 grams of protein in 3 ounces of braised lean top round steak (160 calories), it takes almost 2½ cups of cooked pinto beans at a cost of 525 calories.

VITAMIN B$_{12}$

The RDA for vitamin B$_{12}$ is very small, only 2 micrograms per day for adults, slightly lower for young children, and a little higher for women who are pregnant or lactating. However, vitamin B$_{12}$ is an essential dietary component, necessary for normal function in the metabolism of all cells in the body. Since this vitamin does not occur in plant foods, there is a real possibility of a deficiency in vegetarians who eat no animal foods. Those vegetarians who consume dairy products, which contain small amounts of vitamin B_{12}, are less likely to develop a deficiency. The following sources of vitamin B_{12} are from high to low.

VITAMIN B_{12} CONTENT OF SELECTED FOODS

Food	Vitamin B_{12} mcg
Clams, cooked in moist heat (3 oz)	84.1
Beef liver, braised (3 oz)	60.4
Oysters, eastern, cooked in dry heat (3 oz)	23.6
Beef tenderloin, trimmed, broiled (3 oz)	2.1
Ground beef, extra-lean, broiled medium (3 oz)	1.8
Yogurt, fat-free, plain (8 oz)	1.4
Halibut, baked (3 oz)	1.2
Tuna, white, canned in water, drained (3 oz)	1.0
Yogurt, low-fat, fruit-flavored (8 oz)	1.0
Milk, skim (1 cup)	0.9
Cottage cheese, 1% low-fat (4 oz)	0.7
Pork chop, loin, broiled (3 oz)	0.7
Egg, cooked (1 medium)	0.6
Ice milk (½ cup)	0.4
Chicken breast w/o skin, roasted (3 oz)	0.3
Cheese, mozzarella, part-skim (1 oz)	0.2

Adapted from USDA, Composition of Foods, *Agriculture Handbook series no. 8 (Washington, D.C.: USDA, 1976–1992).*

Vegans need to incorporate reliable vitamin B_{12} supplementation into their diet to avoid developing a deficiency. The best source is cyanocobalamin, which is available in supplements and can be found in foods fortified with vitamin B_{12}, such as soy beverages, some brands of breakfast cereal, and selected brands of nutritional yeast. From 80% to 94% of the vitamin B_{12} described as present in seaweed, spirulina, and tempeh (and other fermented foods) is in fact inactive and is not a reliable source of vitamin B_{12}.

IRON

Vegetarians and nonvegetarians are at equal risk for not reaching the RDA for iron. Dietary iron is classified as nonheme or heme. Nonheme iron, which is present in plant foods, is not as well absorbed as the heme iron found in animal foods. Plant sources of iron include whole grains, dark-green leafy vegetables, and iron-fortified bread and cereal products. The absorption of nonheme iron is increased by the consumption of certain foods and decreased by others. It is increased by consumption of vitamin C (see pages 176–77) and is decreased by consumption of fiber, phytates (indigestible compounds in the outer husks of cereal grains), and tea (because of the tannin content). In vegetarian diets that incorporate a variety of foods, consumption of foods that increase absorption of nonheme iron usually balances the effect of foods that decrease absorption. More information on iron appears on pages 178–79, including the RDA and selected food sources.

CALCIUM

Dairy products are the primary source of calcium; some plant foods contain calcium but at much lower levels. However, calcium deficiency is rare in vegetarians even when intake is below the recommended level. Vegetarians probably need less calcium because they have lower intakes of animal protein and absorb more calcium from the food they eat than nonvegetarians. More information on calcium appears on pages 182–83, including the RDA for different age groups and selected food sources.

VITAMIN D

The body requires vitamin D to utilize the calcium and phosphorus needed to form bone. Vitamin D is formed by the body in the presence of sunlight; the most concentrated food source is fish liver oil. Milk is fortified with vitamin D to ensure an intake sufficient for the proper utilization of calcium.

A vitamin D supplement may be necessary for vegetarians who do not consume vitamin D–fortified dairy products and who cannot get sufficient vitamin D from sunshine. These groups include dark-skinned individuals, infants whose only source of vitamin D after age 4 to 6 months is breast milk, and children with limited exposure to sunlight, either through choice or because of living in a northern climate or a culture in which children wear clothing shielding their skin from the sun.

ZINC

Zinc plays an important role in most metabolic pathways. Vegetarians who eat a wide variety of foods and meet calorie needs usually have an adequate intake of zinc. Good plant sources of zinc include legumes, grains, and nuts; the best source, however, is animal foods, including meat, fowl, fish, and shellfish (especially oysters). If zinc supplements are taken, they should not exceed 15 mg per day, since a zinc intake only slightly above the RDA has been shown to impair copper status in the body. More information on zinc, including the RDA and selected food sources, is found on pages 185–86.

FIBER

Vegetarians usually have a higher intake of fiber than nonvegetarians. Animal foods do not contain fiber; plant foods are the only source. An adequate intake of fiber is important to good health. See page 59 for additional information on fiber and good sources of fiber.

KEY PLANT SOURCES OF NUTRIENTS

The following table lists good plant sources of those nutrients discussed above that are most likely to be low in a vegetarian diet:

PLANT SOURCES OF SELECTED NUTRIENTS

Nutrient	Plant Sources
Vitamin B$_{12}$	Some cereals, fortified soy milk, some brands of nutritional yeast, some soy products
Iron	Dried beans, tofu, legumes, dark-green leafy vegetables (spinach, beet greens, and chard), whole grains, dried fruits, prune juice, bulgur wheat, blackstrap molasses, iron-fortified cereals and breads such as whole-wheat bread Absorption of iron is increased by vitamin C, found in citrus fruits and juices, tomatoes, strawberries, broccoli, peppers, dark-green leafy vegetables, potatoes with skins
Calcium	Tofu (prepared with calcium), broccoli, seeds, nuts, spinach, kale, turnip and collard greens, bok choy, legumes (beans and peas), fortified soy milk, calcium-enriched grain products, tortillas processed with lime
Vitamin D	Fortified margarine
Zinc	Whole grains (especially the germ and bran portions), whole-wheat bread, legumes, nuts, tofu

RECOMMENDATIONS FOR VEGETARIANS

The American Dietetic Association made the following recommendations in its 1993 position paper on vegetarian diets:

- Choose a wide variety of foods and ensure that the caloric intake is adequate to meet energy needs.

- Keep intake of sweets and fatty foods, which have a low nutrient density, to a minimum.

- Choose whole-grain or unrefined grain products instead of refined grain products whenever possible, or use fortified or enriched cereal products.

- Consume a variety of fruits and vegetables, including good sources of vitamin C.

- If dairy products are consumed, use low-fat or nonfat varieties.

- Limit egg yolks to three or four per week.

- Vegans should have a reliable source of vitamin B_{12}, such as some fortified breakfast cereals, fortified soy beverages, or cyanocobalamin supplementation.

- If exposure to sunlight is limited, a vitamin D supplement may be necessary.

- Vegetarian and nonvegetarian infants who are solely breast-fed beyond 4 to 6 months of age should receive supplements of iron and, if exposure to sunlight is limited, vitamin D.

Vegetarian and nonvegetarian women who are pregnant usually need iron and folic acid supplements. Vegetarians usually have higher intakes of these nutrients than nonvegetarians.

The following food guide for vegetarians was published by the American Dietetic Association.

DAILY FOOD GUIDE FOR VEGETARIANS

Food Group	Daily Servings	Serving Sizes
Breads, cereals, rice, & pasta	6 or more	1 slice bread
		½ bun, bagel, or English muffin
		½ cup cooked cereal, rice, or pasta
		1 oz ready-to-eat cereal
Vegetables	4 or more	½ cup cooked or 1 cup raw
Legumes & other meat substitutes	2–3	½ cup cooked beans
		4 oz tofu or tempeh
		1 cup soy milk
		2 tbsp nuts or seeds (high in fat; use sparingly in a low-fat diet)
Fruits	3 or more	1 piece fresh fruit
		½ cup canned or cooked fruit
		¾ cup fruit juice
Dairy products	Optional— up to 3	1 cup skim, ½%, or 1% low-fat milk
		1 cup fat-free or low-fat yogurt
		1½ oz low-fat cheese
Eggs	Optional— limit to 3–4 yolks per week	1 whole egg or 2 egg whites

(continued)

Food Group	Daily Servings	Serving Sizes
Fats, sweets, & alcohol	Go easy on these foods and beverages	Oil, margarine, & mayonnaise
		Cakes, cookies, pies, pastries, & candies
		Beer, wine, & distilled spirits

Adapted from Eating Well—the Vegetarian Way *(Chicago: American Dietetic Association, 1992).*

Eating the Vegetarian Way

Becoming a vegetarian is more complicated than simply dropping meat from the diet. You may wish to start slowly, first reducing meat portions and eating more meals without meat, instead of making an abrupt change in lifelong eating habits. Educate yourself about vegetarian cuisine. To avoid monotony, invest in some vegetarian cookbooks, which may also include menu ideas.

As with a nonvegetarian diet, the secret of a healthy vegetarian diet is to eat a wide variety of foods, including whole-grain food products, legumes, fruits, vegetables, nuts, seeds, low-fat dairy products (if allowed) or a fortified soy milk substitute, and a limited number of eggs (if allowed). Tofu is an excellent source of protein and is a good substitute for meat.

There are some practical considerations in implementing a vegetarian diet. Many people find it easier to begin including higher-fiber foods gradually in order to decrease the risk of gastrointestinal discomfort, such as bloating, cramping, and excess gas. In addition, there are products on the market for minimizing gas production when eating gas-forming high-fiber foods.

The following tips may help you in low-fat vegetarian eating:

BREAKFAST

- Serve fresh or dried fruit with cooked or ready-to-eat whole-grain cereal and use skim, ½%, or 1% low-fat milk.

- Try eggs, within your recommended intake, or egg substitute either cooked in very little oil or with nonstick cooking spray. Egg or egg substitute can be used as an ingredient in French toast, pancakes, or waffles.

- Enjoy a variety of tasty whole-grain breads, such as English muffins, bagels, and low-fat or fat-free muffins. Use little margarine or simply fruit spread or preserves.

LUNCH

- Combine whole-grain breads with a variety of interesting fillings, such as low-fat or fat-free cream cheese and raisins or chopped nuts, low-fat or fat-free cheese with tomato and other vegetables, or peanut butter and jelly.

- Low-fat or fat-free yogurt can be combined with fresh fruits or vegetables.

- Serve whole-grain crackers or bread with a hearty soup made of lentils, beans, or vegetables.

- Try a pasta salad with vegetables and use a low-fat or fat-free dressing.

- Order a vegetarian pizza with a thin crust instead of a thick crust.

- Salad bars are great for vegetarian eating; try tossed greens, pasta salads, bean salads, tabouli salad, garbanzo beans, tomatoes, broccoli, cauliflower, and other raw and cooked vegetables. Remember that olives, avocado, and regular salad dressings contain fat, which will increase your calories. Ask if a low-fat or fat-free dressing is available.

DINNER

- Prepare macaroni and cheese with low-fat or fat-free cheese.

- Top a baked potato with low-fat cottage cheese, plain low-fat or fat-free yogurt, vegetables, and/or low-fat or fat-free cheese.

- Combine pasta, vegetables, and beans as a casserole or salad (see page 204 for directions for cooking dried beans).

- Serve ratatouille with pasta or rice (see recipe on page 252).

- Enjoy spicy red beans and rice, a favorite in the southern and southwestern United States (see recipe on page 254).

- Make spinach lasagna with low-fat or fat-free ricotta or cottage cheese and part-skim mozzarella cheese (see recipe on page 251).

- Try delicious vegetarian chili, available in the supermarket or made from the recipe on page 236.

- Prepare a quick meal of healthy nachos by covering baked tortilla chips with fat-free canned refried beans, low-fat or fat-free cheese, and chopped tomato and jalapeño peppers, and then heating.

- Experiment with tofu or soybean-based meat substitutes in stir-fried dishes and casseroles; tofu is very bland and takes on the flavor of the foods with which it is combined (see pages 205–6 for preparation of tofu).

Chapter 7

The Living Heart Diet Guide to Selecting Food in Supermarkets

Since 1994 federal law has required food manufacturers to provide detailed information on labels about the nutrients in most supermarket foods (see sample food label on page 129). The Nutrition Facts portion of the label makes it easier to select foods that are lower in calories, total fat, saturated fat, cholesterol, and sodium and that are good sources of vitamins, minerals, and fiber.

Nutrition Labeling

The Food Safety and Inspection Service, which is part of the U.S. Department of Agriculture (USDA), is responsible for labeling meat and poultry. The labeling of all other foods is under the jurisdiction of the Food and Drug Administration (FDA), which is part of the Department of Health and Human Services.

Some information in the Nutrition Facts portion of a food label is mandatory, and some is voluntary. Mandatory items include serving size, servings per container, and the amounts of specific nutrients provided by one serving (see below). The introduction of mandatory standard serving sizes in 1994 made it easier to read and interpret the nutrition information found on food labels.

STANDARD SERVING

A standard serving is the amount of food used by all manufacturers to calculate the calories and nutrients stated in the Nutrition Facts portion of the label. For example, a standard serving of frozen yogurt is ½ cup (4 fluid ounces); manufacturers must provide nutrition information based on this serving and can no longer use 3 fluid ounces or some other amount as a serving. Each type of food has a different standard serving. For example, the serving size is 1¾ ounces for bread, 1 ounce for cheese, 1 ounce for cookies, 1 cup for milk, 8 ounces for refrigerated yogurt, and 4.4 ounces for spaghetti sauce. Use of standard servings makes it possible to compare the calories and specific nutrients in a product with those in similar products.

THE FOOD LABEL AT A GLANCE

Serving sizes are stated in both household and metric measures. The serving sizes, which reflect the amounts people actually eat, are consistent across product lines.

The **list of nutrients** includes those of most importance to the health of consumers, most of whom need to avoid getting *too much* of certain nutrients (such as fat, saturated fat, and cholesterol) and *too little* of other nutrients (such as fiber and certain vitamins and minerals).

The label lists the number of calories per gram of fat, carbohydrate, and protein.

Nutrition Facts

Serving Size ½ cup (114g)
Servings Per Container 4

Amount Per Serving

Calories 90   Calories from Fat 30

% Daily Value*

Total Fat 3g	5%
Saturated Fat 0g	0%
Cholesterol 0 mg	0%
Sodium 300 mg	13%
Total Carbohydrate 13g	4%
Dietary Fiber 3g	12%
Sugars 3g	
Protein 3g	

Vitamin A 80% • Vitamin C 60%
Calcium   4% • Iron   4%

*Percent Daily values are based on a 2,000 calorie diet. Your daily values may be higher or lower depending on your calorie needs:

		Calories:	2,000	2,500
Total Fat	Less than		65g	80g
Sat Fat	Less than		20g	25g
Cholesterol	Less than		300mg	300mg
Sodium	Less than		2,400mg	2,400mg
Total Carbohydrate			300g	375g
Dietary Fiber			25g	30g

Calories per gram:

Fat 9 • Carbohydrate 4 • Protein 4

Calories from fat are shown on the label to help consumers meet dietary guidelines that recommend that no more than 30% of calories come from fat.

% Daily Value shows how a food fits into an overall daily diet at the 2,000-calorie level (see page 131).

Most labels provide the grams of fat, saturated fat, carbohydrate, and fiber and the milligrams of cholesterol and sodium that represent the Daily Value at 2,000 calories; some labels also provide the Daily Values at the 2,500-calorie level.

NUTRIENTS ON FOOD LABELS

The nutrition information that is included in the Nutrition Facts portion of the food label is shown below. All the nutrition information given on a food label is for a standard serving.

NUTRIENTS INCLUDED ON FOOD LABELS

✔ Calories

✔ Calories from fat

Calories from saturated fat

✔ Total fat—in grams—and percent of Daily Value

✔ Saturated fat—in grams—and percent of Daily Value

Stearic acid—in grams

Polyunsaturated fat—in grams

Monounsaturated fat—in grams

✔ Cholesterol—in milligrams—and percent of Daily Value

✔ Sodium—in milligrams—and percent of Daily Value

Potassium—in milligrams

✔ Total carbohydrate—in grams—and percent of Daily Value

✔ Dietary fiber—in grams—and percent of Daily Value

Soluble fiber—in grams

Insoluble fiber—in grams

✔ Sugars—in grams

Sugar alcohols (including sorbitol, mannitol, and xylitol)—in grams

Other carbohydrate, consisting of the difference between total carbohydrate and the sum of dietary fiber, sugars, and (if declared) sugar alcohols—in grams

✔ Protein—in grams

✔ Vitamin A—as percent of Daily Value

✔ Vitamin C—as percent of Daily Value

✔ Calcium—as percent of Daily Value

✔ Iron—as percent of Daily Value

Other essential vitamins and minerals

✔ = *mandatory information*

DAILY VALUES

Some of the nutrition information listed above is given as a percent of the Daily Value. The percent of the Daily Value shows what part of a whole day's recommended intake is provided by a standard serving of that food. Some Daily Values are maximum amounts and some are minimum amounts of a nutrient recommended in a day's intake. Examples of Daily Values that indicate maximum amounts are fat, saturated fat, and cholesterol; examples of Daily Values that indicate minimum amounts are carbohydrate, fiber, vitamins A and C, calcium, and iron. Some Daily Values, such as those for cholesterol and sodium, are the same at all calorie levels, while those for fat, saturated fat, protein, carbohydrate, and fiber vary according to the calorie level.

RECOMMENDED DAILY VALUES

Change by Calorie Level

Total fat	Maximum of 30% of calories
Saturated fat	Less than 10% of calories
Protein	10% of calories
Carbohydrate	At least 60% of calories
Fiber	At least 11.5 grams per 1,000 calories

Remain the Same at All Calorie Levels

Cholesterol	Maximum of 300 mg
Sodium	Maximum of 2,400 mg
Vitamin A	5,000 international units
Vitamin C	60 mg
Calcium	1,000 mg
Iron	18 mg

An intake of 2,000 calories is used to calculate the percent of Daily Value appearing on the label for the nutrients that change with the calorie level. The actual percent of Daily Value for these nutrients will differ for people eating more or less than 2,000 calories. Although the FDA chose the 2,000-calorie level as "average," many individuals will have a calorie intake that is either higher or lower than 2,000 calories. The Daily Values used on food labels apply to all people 4 years of age or older except women who are pregnant or lactating. The following table shows the variable Daily Values for four calorie levels.

RECOMMENDED DAILY VALUES* ACCORDING TO SAMPLE CALORIE LEVELS

	1,500 Calories	1,800 Calories	2,000 Calories	2,500 Calories
Total fat	Max 50 g	Max 60 g	Max 65 g	Max 85 g
Saturated fat	Max 15 g	Max 20 g	Max 20 g	Max 30 g
Protein	About 40 g	About 45 g	About 50 g	About 65 g
Carbohydrate	Min 225 g	Min 270 g	Min 300 g	Min 375 g
Fiber	Min 15 g	Min 20 g	Min 25 g	Min 30 g

g = grams; max = maximum; min = minimum.
*Values rounded to nearest 5.

Suppose you purchase ice cream that provides 12 grams of fat in a ½-cup standard serving. The label will list the 12 grams as 18% of the Daily Value for total fat, since 12 is 18% of the maximum 65 grams of fat allowed at 2,000 calories per day (12 ÷ 65 = 0.18, or 18%).

However, if you consume 1,800 calories per day, your maximum fat intake is 60 rather than 65 grams, so a serving of the ice cream accounts for 20% of your Daily Value for fat (12 ÷ 60 = 0.20, or 20%). If you consume only 1,200 calories per day, your maximum fat intake is 40 grams, so a serving of the ice cream contributes 30% of your total day's fat allowance (12 ÷ 40 = 0.30, or 30%).

On the other hand, if you consume more than 2,000 calories per day, the ice cream accounts for a smaller percent of your Daily Value for fat. For example, at 2,500 calories, your maximum fat allowance is 83 grams (rounded to 85 grams), so one serving of the ice cream accounts for 14% of your fat allowance for the day (12 ÷ 85 = 0.14, or 14%).

In the same way you can use the information on the label to calculate the percent Daily Value for saturated fat, protein, carbohydrate, and fiber for different calorie levels. To determine how many calories you should be eating each day, see pages 356–59.

FOODS NOT SUBJECT TO MANDATORY LABELING

At the time of the publication of this book, nutrition labeling is required for most, but not all, foods. Exceptions include

- Single-ingredient raw meat and poultry
- Restaurant food
- Food produced by small businesses
- Food produced for immediate consumption, such as that served in a cafeteria or on an airplane or sold by sidewalk vendors
- Food shipped in bulk, not for sale in that form to consumers

- Medical foods, such as that used in enteral nutrition (tube feedings)

- Plain coffee and tea, some spices, and other foods without significant amounts of any nutrients

The FDA has established a voluntary point-of-purchase nutrition information program for raw fruit, vegetables, and fish. Supermarkets providing point-of-purchase nutrition information can choose to use stickers on individual foods, such as bananas; furnish information on large posters or signs; or list information in pamphlets, brochures, leaflets, or notebooks available for consumers to take home. Point-of-purchase nutrition information must include the name of the fruit, vegetable, or fish; the serving size; and nutrient information similar to that which appears on other nutrition labels.

The USDA allows voluntary nutrition labeling of single-ingredient raw meat and poultry products and requires mandatory nutrition labeling for almost all other meat and poultry products, including processed meat and poultry. Processed meats include luncheon meats and ham.

NUTRIENT CONTENT CLAIMS FOR INDIVIDUAL FOODS

The FDA and USDA have guidelines for nutrient content claims appearing on food labels. Nutrient content claims, such as "low fat" and "cholesterol free," have very specific definitions. "Low fat," for example, means that a standard serving of a single food contains no more than 3 grams of fat (main dishes and meal products have different guidelines and are discussed below). Relative nutrient content claims, such as "reduced," "less," "more," or "light," are used when one food is compared with a "reference food." The following foods can be used as reference foods:

REFERENCE FOODS

- **Market leader's product**
- **Average of the top three regional or national brands**
- **Representative product data base**
- **Manufacturer's own product**
- **Competitor's product**

NUTRIENT CONTENT CLAIMS FOR MAIN DISHES AND MEAL PRODUCTS

Specific definitions have been established for main dishes and meal products (for example, frozen dinners). A main dish must weigh at least 6 ounces and contain at least two foods representing at least two of four food groups. The four food groups used by the FDA for this purpose are (1) bread, cereal, rice, and pasta; (2) fruits and vegetables; (3) milk, yogurt, and cheese; and (4) meat, poultry, fish, dried beans, eggs, and nuts. A meal product, which is represented as a breakfast, lunch, dinner, or meal, must weigh at least 10 ounces and contain at least three foods representing at least two of the four food groups. Unlike individual food products, the sizes of main dishes and meal products vary and no one level of calories, fat, saturated fat, cholesterol, or sodium can be specified for making nutrient content claims. For example, the maximum amount of fat allowed in a main dish labeled "low fat" depends on its weight; the more the main dish weighs, the more fat it may contain and still be labeled "low fat." The table on page 145 shows the maximum calories and grams of fat allowed for main dishes and meal products of different weights that are labeled "low calorie" or "low fat."

DEFINITIONS OF NUTRIENT CONTENT CLAIMS

The following table includes the nutrient content claims for calories, fat, saturated fat, and cholesterol and the definitions for "light" and "healthy" for food products except meat, poultry, and fish (see pages 96–97 for nutrient content claims for sodium). To simplify the tables, the word "serving" is used to mean "standard serving."

DEFINITIONS OF NUTRIENT CONTENT CLAIMS FOR FOODS EXCEPT MEAT, POULTRY, AND FISH

Nutrient Content Claim	Individual Food Products	Main Dishes and Meal Products
Calorie free	Less than 5 calories per serving	No definition
Low calorie	Less than 40 calories per serving	Maximum of 120 calories per 100 grams (see table on page 145)
Reduced calorie	At least 25% fewer calories per serving compared with reference food	At least 25% fewer calories per 100 grams compared with reference food
Fat free	Less than 0.5 gram of fat per serving	Less than 0.5 gram of fat per serving
Low fat	3 grams or less of fat per serving	3 grams or less of fat per 100 grams; must provide 30% or less of calories from fat (see table on page 145)
Reduced fat	At least 25% less fat per serving compared with reference food	At least 25% less fat per 100 grams compared with reference food
Saturated fat free	Less than 0.5 gram of saturated fat; less than 0.5 gram of *trans* fatty acids per serving	Less than 0.5 gram of saturated fat per serving; *trans* fatty acids 1% or less of total fat
Low saturated fat	1 gram or less of saturated fat per serving; 15% or less of calories from saturated fat	1 gram or less of saturated fat per 100 grams; 10% or less of calories from saturated fat
Reduced saturated fat	At least 25% less saturated fat per serving compared with reference food	At least 25% less saturated fat per 100 grams compared with reference food

(continued)

Nutrient Content Claim	Individual Food Products	Main Dishes and Meal Products
Cholesterol free	Less than 2 mg of cholesterol and 2 grams or less of saturated fat per serving	Less than 2 mg of cholesterol and 2 grams or less of saturated fat per serving
Low cholesterol	20 mg or less of cholesterol and 2 grams or less of saturated fat per serving	20 mg or less of cholesterol and 2 grams or less of saturated fat per 100 grams
Reduced cholesterol	At least 25% less cholesterol per serving compared with reference food	At least 25% less cholesterol per 100 grams compared with reference food
Sodium	See definitions on pages 96–97	
Light or lite	In a food normally providing 50% or more of calories from fat, fat is reduced by 50% or more per serving compared with reference food In a food normally providing less than 50% of calories from fat, calories are reduced by at least one-third (33⅓%) or fat is reduced by 50% per serving compared with reference food "Light" can be used without qualification if a food contains 40 calories or less and 3 grams or less of fat per serving and the sodium is reduced by 50% or more compared with reference food "Light" can describe a physical property, for example, "light in color" or "light in texture"	Meets definitions of "low calorie," "low fat," or both; label must clearly state whether "light" means low calorie, low fat, or both
Healthy	3 grams or less of fat, 1 gram or less of saturated fat, 60 mg or less of cholesterol, and 480 mg or less* of sodium per serving; must contain at least 10% of Daily Value of vitamin A, vitamin C, iron, calcium, protein, or fiber per serving	3 grams or less of fat and 1 gram or less of saturated fat per 100 grams and per serving; 90 mg or less of cholesterol and 600 mg or less of sodium* per serving; must contain at least 10% of Daily Value of vitamin A, vitamin C, iron, calcium, protein, or fiber per serving

*Sodium level to be lowered in individual foods to 360 mg or less and in main dishes and meal products to 480 mg or less by 1998.

Meat, poultry, fish, and game may be labeled "lean" or "extra lean," and meat and poultry products may be labeled "healthy" as described in the following table.

NUTRIENT CONTENT CLAIM DEFINITIONS FOR MEAT, POULTRY, FISH, AND GAME PRODUCTS

Nutrient Content Claim	Individual Food Products	Main Dishes and Meal Products Containing Meat or Poultry
Lean	Less than 10 grams of fat, less than 4.5 grams of saturated fat, and less than 95 mg of cholesterol per 100 grams and per serving	Less than 10 grams of fat, less than 4.5 grams of saturated fat, and less than 95 mg of cholesterol per 100 grams and per serving
Extra Lean	Less than 5 grams of fat, less than 2 grams of saturated fat, and less than 95 mg of cholesterol per 100 grams and per serving	Less than 5 grams of fat, less than 2 grams of saturated fat, and less than 95 mg of cholesterol per 100 grams and per serving
Healthy (applies to meat and poultry)	Single-ingredient raw meat and poultry, such as steak or chicken breasts, contain less than 5 grams of fat, less than 2 grams of saturated fat, and less than 95 mg of cholesterol per 100 grams and per serving (single-ingredient raw seafood or game must also contain 480 mg or less sodium*); must also contain 10% or more of the Daily Value for vitamin A, vitamin C, iron, calcium, protein, or fiber per serving All other meat, poultry, fish, and game products, such as canned fish and luncheon meats, must contain 3 grams or less of fat, 1 gram or less of saturated fat, 60 mg or less of cholesterol, and 480 mg or less of sodium* per serving; must also contain 10% or more of the Daily Value for vitamin A, vitamin C, iron, calcium, protein, or fiber per serving	3 grams or less of fat and 1 gram or less of saturated fat per 100 grams and per serving, and 90 mg or less of cholesterol and 600 mg or less of sodium* per serving; must also contain 10% or more of the Daily Value for vitamin A, vitamin C, iron, calcium, protein, or fiber per serving

*Sodium level to be lowered in individual foods to 360 mg or less and in main dishes and meal products to 480 mg or less by 1998.

HEALTH CLAIMS

Health claims for food are statements concerning links between specific elements in the diet and risk for certain diseases. At the time of the printing of this book, the FDA has approved eight health claims as shown below.

APPROVED HEALTH CLAIMS FOR FOOD

Nutrient	Health Claim
Increased Intake Can Be Beneficial	
Calcium	Reduced risk for osteoporosis (condition consisting of decreased bone mass)
Fruits, vegetables, and grain products that contain fiber	Reduced risk for cancer
Fruits, vegetables, and grain products that contain fiber, particularly soluble fiber	Reduced risk for coronary heart disease
Fruits and vegetables	Reduced risk for cancer
Foods naturally high in folic acid and folic acid supplements	Reduced risk for neural tube defects (a class of birth defects)
Decreased Intake Can Be Beneficial	
Saturated fat and cholesterol	Reduced risk for coronary heart disease
Fat	Reduced risk for cancer
Sodium	Reduced risk for high blood pressure

Selecting Foods Lower in Calories, Fat, Saturated Fat, and Cholesterol

Some foods, such as fruits, vegetables, many starchy foods, lean meats, and fat-free dairy products, are naturally fairly low in calories, fat, and sugar. However, most people enjoy eating cookies, candy, cakes, chips, cheese, salad dressing, margarine, and other foods that are higher in calories from the fat and/or sugar they contain. Increased public interest in limiting calories has led food manufacturers to develop thousands of new products that are formulated to be lower in calories, fat, and/or sugar.

NEW FOOD PRODUCTS

The availability of "special" low-calorie food products helps some people reduce the feeling of being deprived—one reason commonly given for not staying on a "diet." For decades food scientists have attempted to reduce calories in food without changing its flavor, texture, and acceptability. Chief interest has been in using sugar substitutes and/or fat replacers to replace all or some of the sugar and/or fat in foods.

SUGAR SUBSTITUTES – Sugar substitutes are substances that can be used to reduce the calories from sugar in a food. Caloric sugar substitutes provide fewer calories than the sugar they are replacing; noncaloric sugar substitutes provide no calories.

Caloric sugar substitutes such as fructose and corn syrup contain the same calories as sucrose when used in the same amount; however, because they are sweeter, they can be used in smaller amounts to achieve the same level of sweetness. Aspartame (sold under Equal®, NutraSweet®, and other brand names) is listed as a caloric sugar substitute even though it is so low in calories that it is almost calorie free; the tiny amount needed to equal the sweetness of 1 teaspoon of sugar (providing 16 calories) provides only ⅒ of a calorie. An example of a noncaloric sugar substitute is saccharin, which can be used in very small amounts to sweeten foods. The relative sweetening power of sugar substitutes is measured against that of sucrose (table sugar) (see page 369 of the Appendix).

Saccharin, the first artificial sugar substitute, is about 300 times sweeter than sucrose and has long been used in foods for individuals with diabetes. In the early 1970s the government imposed a ban on cyclamate, a sweetener approximately 30 times sweeter than sucrose. The manufacturer of cyclamate may petition the FDA for reapproval of its product because the research leading to the ban on cyclamate has been shown to have been seriously flawed. A number of caloric and noncaloric sugar substitutes are now available and others are being developed or are awaiting FDA approval.

FAT REPLACERS – The emphasis on lowering fat intake has led to a wider use of substances to replace all or part of the fat in foods. Some fat replacers come from substances that are already present in nature. For example, Simplesse® is a microparticulated protein that is made from protein from egg white and milk; it provides 1 to 2 calories per gram, compared with 9 calories per gram for fat. It is difficult for manufacturers to gain FDA approval for fat replacers that are synthetic, that is, that do not exist in nature. The best-known example of a synthetic fat replacer is olestra, which has not yet received FDA approval.

The challenge in using fat replacers in foods has been to duplicate the desirable qualities of fat while reducing the actual fat and calories present. Fat adds flavor, texture ("mouth feel"), and aroma to foods and has a high satiety value; that is, consumption of fat leads to a feeling of having hunger satisfied or feeling full.

Fat replacers are usually separated into three categories: carbohydrate based, protein based, and fat based. By far, the carbohydrate-based fat replacers represent the largest and most widely used type of fat replacer. Some of these products, such as carrageenan, have been in use for many years and do not require further FDA approval when they are used to replace fat. See pages 367–69 in the Appendix for information about specific fat replacers.

EFFECTS OF SUGAR SUBSTITUTES AND FAT REPLACERS – Studies conducted to see if use of caloric or noncaloric sugar substitutes or fat replacers results in weight loss have come to mixed conclusions. Although some research suggests that using sugar substitutes does not decrease overall intake of sugar and may increase appetite, most studies support a reduction in total calories with the use of sugar substitutes.

It is difficult to conduct research studies in humans that show the effects of the fat replacers used in reduced-fat and fat-free foods on weight and fat intake. Although low-fat foods can help an individual reduce fat intake to the recommended level of less than 30% of calories, use of these foods may or may not result in a reduction in total caloric intake. In some studies people consuming lower-fat foods compensated by eating a larger amount. Some low-fat foods are almost as high in calories as the regular-fat foods they are designed to replace, and some fat-free foods are no lower in calories than their low-fat counterparts, especially dessert-type foods such as cakes and cookies. It is important to notice the fat and calories listed on food labels.

Sugar substitutes, fat replacers, and the foods containing them can, if used properly, help individuals enjoy favorite foods while following an eating pattern that is lower in sugar and/or fat and that provides fewer calories than typically consumed. For substances that replace fat or sugar to aid in weight reduction, the calories "saved" by using them should not be replaced by increasing the intake of other foods.

Tips on Selecting Heart-Healthy Foods and Cooking Ingredients

For many foods in the following list, a cutoff point for fat is included, that is, the maximum amount of fat allowed in a serving for the food to be considered low fat. A cutoff is usually given only for total fat, rather than for saturated fat and cholesterol, to make your grocery shopping easier; foods low in total fat are usually low in saturated fat and are often low in cholesterol. You can find the grams of fat in the Nutrition Facts portion of the food label. *The Living Heart Brand Name Shopper's Guide,* another book in our series for heart health, lists more than 5,000 foods by brand name that are low in fat, saturated fat, and cholesterol (see order form on last page). Foods and ingredients that are low in fat are recommended for preparation of the recipes in this book.

Rules of Thumb for Selecting Food

Food except meat: No more than 3 grams of fat per serving

Meat: No more than 9 grams of fat per 3 ounces cooked

Processed meat: No more than 3 grams of fat per ounce

GUIDELINES FOR SELECTING FOODS LOW IN CALORIES, FAT, SATURATED FAT, AND CHOLESTEROL

Alcoholic beverages: Plain alcoholic beverages, such as bourbon and Scotch, provide calories but no fat. Irish cream contains fat in its purchased form; some mixed drinks (for example, grasshopper, White Russian, and brandy Alexander) contain fat in the form of cream added during preparation. If you drink alcoholic beverages, select one that is fat free.

Avocados: Unlike most fruits, avocados are high in fat and calories; however, they are a good source of monounsaturated fat, which is recommended in moderate amounts in eating plans to lower blood cholesterol.

Bacon: Bacon, whether made from pork, beef, or turkey, is too high in fat to be recommended in the Living Heart Diet.

Bacon bits, imitation: Imitation bacon bits and chips are usually made of soy flour and oil and are fairly low in calories and fat; they primarily contribute sodium.

Bagels: Bagels are low in calories and fat. Select varieties with no more than 3 grams of fat per serving.

Barbecue sauce: Barbecue sauce is fairly low in calories and contains a small amount of fat; it primarily contributes sodium. Select a brand that contains no more than 3 grams of fat per serving.

Beans: All beans (black, butter, garbanzo, great Northern, green snap, kidney, lima, navy, pink, pinto, red, soybeans, white, and yellow); black-eyed, green, and split peas; and lentils are naturally low in fat. Some baked beans have fat added. Choose plain beans that contain less than 0.5 gram of fat per serving and beans in sauce that contain no more than 3 grams of fat per serving.

Beef: Beef can be high or low in fat depending on the amount of fat marbled through it and the amount of fat on the outside of a cut. Choose "Choice" or "Select" grade beef with very little marbling and trim off all visible fat. Look for cuts with "loin" or "round" in the name. Select beef with no more than 9 grams of fat per 3 ounces cooked.

Biscuits and biscuit mixes: Most biscuits are high in fat from the shortening or other fat used to make them. There are two types of biscuit mixes: complete and incomplete. Complete mixes, which usually contain shortening, only require the addition of water; incomplete mixes require the addition of several ingredients. Biscuits made from an incomplete mix can be lower in fat than those made from a complete mix if you substitute water or skim milk for whole milk, use egg white or egg substitute instead of whole egg, and use less fat than suggested in the package directions. Reducing the fat added to an incomplete mix may change the texture of the finished product. Select prepared biscuits and biscuit mixes with no more than 3 grams of fat per serving.

Bread: Most breads, such as white and whole wheat, are low in calories and fat; exceptions are egg bread and cheese bread. Select breads with no more than 3 grams of fat per 50-gram serving (about 1¾ ounces). See also *Buns, Cornbread, French bread,* and *Rolls.*

Bread crumbs: See *Crumbs, bread.*

Bread, fruit and nut: Fruit and nut breads typically are high in calories and fat because they are made with eggs, whole milk, nuts, and/or butter, margarine, oil, or shortening. When using a mix, select one that will result in a prepared product containing no more than 3 grams of fat per serving.

Breading: See *Coating mixes.*

Breadsticks: Hard breadsticks are usually lower in calories and fat than soft breadsticks, which are often brushed with fat. Select breadsticks with no more than 3 grams of fat per serving.

Brownies: Brownies are usually high in fat from the butter, shortening, margarine, or oil used to make them. Some brownie mixes include directions for reducing the fat added during preparation. Choose a brownie mix that, when prepared, contains no more than 3 grams of fat per serving; this same limit applies to brownies that are ready to eat.

Buns: Sandwich buns (hamburger, hot dog, hoagie, hero, and submarine) are low in calories and fat. Select buns containing no more than 3 grams of fat per 1¾ ounces (approximately); because buns differ in weight, be sure to check the amount of fat in one whole bun.

Butter: Butter is high in saturated fat; its use is not recommended in an eating plan to lower blood cholesterol.

Buttermilk: Buttermilk with no more than 1% fat is recommended for a beverage and for cooking. Buttermilk contains about twice as much sodium as 1% low-fat milk.

Cakes and cupcakes: Cakes range in fat content from high to low. For example, cakes made with butter, shortening, margarine, oil, sour cream, cream cheese, coconut, and/or nuts are high in fat. Angel food cake is always fat free. Many cake mixes now provide directions for preparing a lower-fat cake by using skim, ½%, or 1% low-fat milk, egg substitute, and a reduced amount of oil or margarine. Several brands of prepared cakes are "low fat" or "fat free"; however, they are not calorie free. Select prepared cakes or cake mixes that, when prepared, provide no more than 3 grams of fat per serving.

Candy: Candies that are primarily sugar, such as hard candy, jelly beans, and gum drops, contain a negligible amount of fat. Higher-fat candies are those containing chocolate, caramel, nuts, or coconut. Choose candies that provide less than 0.5 gram of fat per serving; the serving size is ½ ounce for hard candies and 1⅖ ounces for other candies.

Carbonated beverages: Carbonated beverages contain no fat. The calories depend on the amount of sugar present; many lower calorie, artificially sweetened products are available.

Catsup: Catsup (ketchup) is low in calories and contains only a trace of fat; it primarily contributes sodium.

Cereals: Plain cooked cereals are low in fat and calories, while some flavored cooked cereals are higher in calories and fat. Ready-to-eat cereals vary widely in the calories and fat they provide. Choose cooked or ready-to-eat cereals containing no more than 3 grams of fat per serving. Notice the serving size for the ready-to-eat cereal you choose; some have a small serving size, such as ¼ cup, while other, lighter cereals have a larger serving size, such as 1¼ cups.

Cheese (including cream cheese): Regular cheeses are high in fat. For example, Cheddar cheese contains 9.4 grams of fat per ounce, and cream cheese contains 9.9 grams of fat per ounce. Since the fat in cheese is more than 60% saturated, high-fat cheeses are also high in saturated fat. The preferred types of cheeses are low fat (no more than 3 grams of fat per ounce) or fat free. Most low-fat and fat-free cheeses are good when eaten cold; however, a reduced-fat cheese gives a better texture in cooking than a fat-free cheese while still containing much less fat than regular cheese. The recipes in this book specify using cheese with no more than 5 grams of fat per ounce (such as part-skim mozzarella), as long as the completed dish is acceptably low in fat. In a few cases a recipe specifies using a small amount of regular grated Parmesan cheese; 1 ounce of grated Parmesan contains 8.5 grams of fat, but it takes almost 6 tablespoons of grated Parmesan to equal 1 ounce.

Chicken: See *Poultry.*

Chili sauce: Chili sauce is low in calories and contains little or no fat; it primarily contributes sodium.

Coating mixes: Check the label of the coating mix used when baking meat, fish, or poultry; select a brand with 3 grams or less of fat per serving.

Cocktail sauce: Cocktail sauce based on catsup and/or chili sauce is low in calories and contains little or no fat; it primarily contributes sodium.

Cocoa mixes: Cocoa mixes prepared with water or skim milk are usually low in fat. Sugar-free or diet cocoa mixes are lower in calories than regular cocoa mixes.

Coconut: Coconut meat, coconut milk, and coconut oil are very high in saturated fat and are not recommended in the Living Heart Diet.

Coffee: Plain coffee contains no calories or fat; however, some flavored coffee mixes include chocolate or creamers that contain fat and saturated fat. Select varieties that are fat free.

Coffeecakes: Coffeecakes are traditionally high in fat, often having 12 or more grams of fat per serving. Select coffeecake mixes and ready-to-eat coffeecakes with no more than 3 grams of fat per serving.

Cookies: Many cookies are traditionally high in fat. However, a growing number of fat-free and low-fat commercial cookies are available. Select cookies and cookie mixes containing no more than 3 grams of fat per serving. Notice the calories provided by one serving of cookies; cookies that are "low fat" or "fat free" are not calorie free and may not even be low in calories. The serving size for cookies is 1 ounce: in lighter or smaller cookies, this may represent several cookies; in heavier or larger ones, it may be only one cookie. Cookie mixes may contain fat or have directions for adding fat during preparation; decreasing the amount of fat used in preparation may affect the texture of the final product. The guidelines for cookies also apply to graham crackers.

Cooking ingredients: See *Ingredients.*

Cooking sprays: See *Nonstick cooking sprays.*

Cornbread: Cornbread is a high-fat bread because of the shortening or other fat it usually contains. There are two types of cornbread mixes: complete and incomplete. Complete mixes, which usually contain shortening and egg solids, require only the addition of water; incomplete mixes require the addition of several ingredients. Cornbread made from an incomplete mix can be lower in fat than that made from a complete mix if you substitute water or skim milk for whole milk, use egg white or egg substitute instead of whole egg, and use less oil than suggested in the package directions. Select cornbread mixes that, when prepared, provide no more than 3 grams of fat per serving.

Cottage cheese: Select cottage cheese with no more than 2% fat or containing no more than 3 grams of fat per serving.

Crackers: Crackers have two standard serving sizes: 1 ounce for those usually eaten as a snack, and ½ ounce for those not usually eaten as a snack. Crackers not usually eaten as a snack include saltines, soda crackers, oyster crackers, melba toast, hard breadsticks, and ice cream cones. Select a cracker with no more than 3 grams of fat per serving, and notice the number of crackers equal to a serving.

Crackers, graham: See *Cookies.*

Cream cheese: See *Cheese.*

Creamer, coffee: Coffee cream, half-and-half, and most nondairy creamers are high in fat and saturated fat. Nondairy creamers can be powdered or liquid. Select powdered creamers that have no more than 1 gram of saturated fat per teaspoon and liquid creamers with no more than 1 gram of saturated fat per tablespoon.

Cream pie fillings: See *Puddings and cream pie fillings.*

Cream, sour: See *Sour cream.*

Croissants: A croissant is a very high fat, crescent-shaped bread that is usually made with butter; it is not recommended in the Living Heart Diet.

Croutons: Many brands of croutons are sprayed with oil; select a brand with no more than 3 grams of fat per ¼-ounce serving.

Crumbs, bread: Choose bread crumbs with 3 grams or less of fat per 1-ounce serving.

Cupcakes: See *Cakes and cupcakes.*

Dinners: See *Main dishes and meal products.*

Dips: Select dips with no more than 3 grams of fat per 2-tablespoon serving. Dip mixes are low in fat but high in sodium and should be prepared with a dairy product that is nonfat or low fat, whether sour cream, yogurt, or cream cheese.

Doughnuts: Doughnuts are high in fat, from both the fat present in the dough and the fat used to deep-fry them; they are not recommended in the Living Heart Diet.

Eggs: The yolk of an average-size egg contains 213 milligrams of cholesterol, that is, two thirds of the recommended maximum daily intake of cholesterol for the Step I Diet (see page 36). It is recommended in the Living Heart Diet that egg yolks be limited to no more than three per week.

Egg substitutes: Most egg substitutes are primarily egg white combined with other ingredients. Select brands that contain no cholesterol and provide no more than 3 grams of fat per serving.

Enchilada sauce: Enchilada sauce is low in calories and contains little or no fat; it primarily contributes sodium.

English muffins: Most English muffins are low in calories and fat; choose an English muffin containing 3 grams or less of fat per serving.

Entrées: See *Main dishes and meal products.*

Fish and shellfish: Most finfish are low in fat and contain negligible saturated fat. The cholesterol content in 3 ounces of finfish ranges from 20 to 100 milligrams. Although most shellfish are very low in fat, some are high in cholesterol. For example, a 3-ounce serving of shrimp contains 165 milligrams of cholesterol, and the same amount of crayfish contains 150 milligrams.

French bread: Most French breads and rolls contain very little or no fat.

Frosting: Choose a frosting mix that, when prepared, contains less than 0.5 gram of fat per serving; the same fat limit applies to ready-to-eat frosting.

Frozen desserts: There are two types of frozen desserts: milk based and not milk based. Among the milk-based frozen desserts, ice milk, frozen yogurt, and sherbet are much lower in fat and saturated fat than ice cream. Select milk-based frozen desserts that contain no more than 3 grams of fat and 2 grams of saturated fat per ½-cup serving. Frozen desserts that are not milk based contain only a trace of fat. These products include sorbets, fruit ices, frozen fruit juice bars, and pops; select those that contain less than 0.5 gram of fat per serving. Remember that frozen desserts containing little or no fat still provide calories that can add up quickly when you eat several servings.

Frozen dinners: See *Main dishes and meal products.*

Frozen entrées: See *Main dishes and meal products.*

Frozen yogurt: See *Frozen desserts.*

Fruit and fruit juices: Fruit (except avocados and olives), fruit juices, and fruit nectars contain negligible fat.

Fruit and nut bread: See *Bread, fruit and nut.*

Fruit-flavored beverages: Select beverages that contain no fat.

Fruit ices: See *Frozen desserts.*

Fruit pie fillings: Select fruit pie fillings that contain no more than 3 grams of fat per serving. Although many fruit pie fillings contain no fat, some recipes call for the addition of butter or margarine, which can be omitted without affecting the flavor.

Game: Most game meat is low in fat. Wild duck and goose are lower in fat than domestic duck and goose. Choose game containing less than 9 grams of fat per 3 ounces cooked.

Gelatin: Select unflavored and flavored gelatins containing less than 0.5 gram of fat. The calories in flavored gelatin come primarily from sugar; sugar-free flavored gelatin is very low in calories.

Graham crackers: See *Cookies.*

Gravies: Select gravies—canned, in a jar, or dehydrated—that, when prepared, contain no more than 3 grams of fat per ¼ cup. Most commercial gravies are high in sodium.

Horseradish: Horseradish (an herb) is low in calories and contains little or no fat. Some horseradish sauces are combinations of horseradish with a mayonnaise-type dressing and are higher in calories and fat. Select brands that contain less than 0.5 gram of fat per serving.

Hot sauce: Hot sauce is very low in calories and contains no fat. Although hot sauce contributes sodium, the amount of hot sauce consumed is typically quite small, making it a good seasoning for low-sodium foods.

Ice cream: See *Frozen desserts.*

Ice cream cones: See *Crackers.*

Ice milk: See *Frozen desserts.*

Ice pops: See *Frozen desserts.*

Icing: See *Frosting.*

Ingredients: Many cooking ingredients, such as flour and sugar, contain no cholesterol and little or no fat or saturated fat. Commonly used cooking ingredients that do add fat to the finished product include butter, oils, shortening, margarine, mayonnaise, egg yolk, chocolate, nuts, coconut, cream cheese, sour cream, and whipped cream or other whipped topping. See page 362 in the Appendix for substitutions you can make to lower the fat, saturated fat, and/or cholesterol in the foods you prepare. The recipes in this book primarily use ingredients that are low in fat; small amounts of high-fat ingredients, such as oil, margarine, and nuts, are used in some recipes.

Instant breakfast mixes: Select products providing no more than 3 grams of fat per prepared serving. If the nutrition label gives information only for the dry mix, add the grams of fat in one serving of the mix to the amount of fat in the milk used (count skim milk as containing no fat).

Jam: See *Sweets.*

Jelly: See *Sweets.*

Juices: See *Fruit and fruit juices* and *Vegetables and vegetable juices.*

Lamb: Lamb can be high or low in fat depending on the amount of marbling and the amount of fat remaining on the outside of a cut. Choose lamb with very little marbling and trim the visible fat to provide a cut with no more than 9 grams of fat per 3 ounces.

Lentils: See *Beans.*

Luncheon meats: Traditional luncheon meats are made of pork, beef, or a combination of the two and are high in fat, calories, and sodium. Today's market offers many luncheon meats made from turkey, chicken, and/or lean beef and pork that are lower in calories and fat; some luncheon meats are also lower in sodium. Choose luncheon meats that contain no more than 3 grams of fat per ounce.

Main dishes and meal products: Main dishes and meal products are defined on pages 133–34, and the table below shows the maximum calories and fat allowed in "low-calorie" and "low-fat" products at various weights.

Weight of Package in Ounces	Maximum Calories	Maximum Grams of Fat
6	205	5
7	240	6
8	270	7
9	305	8
10	340	9
11	375	9
12	410	10
13	440	11

Calories rounded to nearest 5; fat rounded to nearest whole number.

For example, a meal product (frozen dinner) that weighs 10 ounces qualifies as low fat when it contains 9 grams or less of fat, whereas a dinner that weighs 13 ounces may contain up to 11 grams of fat and be considered low-fat, as discussed on pages 133–34.

Margarine: Margarine is made from vegetable oil that has been hydrogenated to make it more solid. The reduced-fat and fat-free margarines and spreads are lower in calories, fat, and saturated fat than regular margarine. Select margarines that contain no more than 2 grams of saturated fat per 1-tablespoon serving. (See discussion of *trans* fatty acids on pages 54–55.)

Marinara sauce: See *Spaghetti sauce.*

Marshmallows: See *Sweets.*

Mayonnaise and mayonnaise-type dressings: Regular mayonnaise and mayonnaise-type dressings are high in fat and calories; reduced-fat and fat-free mayonnaise and mayonnaise-type products are lower in fat and calories. Choose products that contain no more than 2 grams of saturated fat per tablespoon.

Meat: See *Beef; Fish and shellfish; Game; Lamb; Luncheon meats; Pork; Poultry; Turkey;* and *Veal.*

Meat substitutes: Most meat substitutes are made of soybeans, which are a good source of high-quality protein. Choose meat substitutes that provide no more than 3 grams of fat per serving.

Milk: Milk containing no more than 1% fat is recommended for cooking and as a beverage. Milk containing 2% fat contains almost 5 grams of fat per cup; the cutoff point for "low fat" is 3 grams or less of fat per serving. Skim milk or evaporated skim milk is used for Living Heart Diet recipes that call for milk.

Milkshakes: Milkshakes made with whole milk and ice cream are high in calories and fat; lower-fat milkshakes can be prepared using skim, ½%, or 1% low-fat milk and low-fat or nonfat frozen yogurt or other frozen desserts. Select commercial products that contain no more than 3 grams of fat per serving.

Mixers: Most drink mixers, such as carbonated beverages, contain little or no fat; the calories depend on the amount of sugar present. The mixer for piña coladas often contains fat. If using a mixer, select one that contains less than 0.5 gram of fat per serving.

Molasses: See *Sweets.*

Mousse mixes: See *Puddings and cream pie fillings.*

Muffins: Muffins are often high in calories and fat. Select low-fat or fat-free prepared muffins, and muffin mixes that contain no more than 3 grams of fat per 2-ounce prepared muffin.

Mustard: Plain mustard is low in calories and contains negligible fat; however, some flavored mustards contain added fat. Select mustards that contain less than 0.5 gram of fat per 1-teaspoon serving.

Nectar, fruit: See *Fruit and fruit juices.*

Nonstick cooking sprays: Cooking sprays provide a way of adding very small amounts of oil to "grease" pans for cooking. They may also be sprayed directly on foods, such as air-popped popcorn. Cooking sprays are not calorie free; the calories and fat consumed depend on the amount used.

Nut butters: Nut butters are high in calories and fat. Some nut butters are higher in saturated fat than the nuts from which they are made because of hydrogenation, which increases *trans* fatty acids. There are some reduced-fat peanut butters on the market; however, they may not be any lower in calories than regular peanut butter. Select nut butters that contain no more than 2 grams of saturated fat per 2 tablespoons.

Nuts: All nuts, except chestnuts and water chestnuts, are high in calories and fat; chestnuts and water chestnuts are very low in calories and fat. Choose nuts, such as almonds, that contain no more than 2 grams of saturated fat per 1-ounce serving.

Oils, vegetable: All oils are high in fat and calories. Use of the word "light" on a vegetable oil label does not mean that it is lower in fat and calories; it usually indicates a lighter color or flavor. Select an oil containing no more than 2 grams of saturated fat per 1-tablespoon serving. Canola oil is lower in saturated fat than other oils; other oils containing no more than 2 grams of saturated fat per tablespoon (from lowest to highest in saturated fat) include safflower, sunflower, corn, olive, sesame, soybean, and peanut oils.

Olives: Unlike most fruits, olives are high in fat and calories. Ripe, or black, olives contain more oil than green olives. Select olives with no more than 2 grams of saturated fat per ½-ounce serving.

Pancakes: There are two types of pancake mixes: complete and incomplete. Complete mixes, which usually contain shortening, require only the addition of water; incomplete mixes require the addition of several ingredients. Pancakes made from an incomplete mix can be lower in fat than those made from complete mixes if you substitute water or skim milk for whole milk, use egg white or egg substitute instead of whole egg, and use less fat than suggested in the package directions. Select pancake mixes that, when prepared, contain no more than 3 grams of fat per 3.9-ounce serving; the same fat limit applies to already-prepared pancakes.

Pasta: Choose pasta that contains less than 0.5 gram of fat per serving and no cholesterol; a serving is 2 ounces of dry pasta. Pasta dishes often have added margarine, oil, butter, cheese, or high-fat sauces or gravies. Choose prepared pasta dishes that contain no more than 3 grams of fat per serving.

Pasta sauce: See *Spaghetti sauce.*

Peanut butter: See *Nut butters.*

Peas, black-eyed, green, and split: See *Beans.*

Peppers: Fresh and pickled peppers are low in calories and contain little or no fat; many, but not all, canned peppers are high in sodium.

Pepper sauce: See *Hot sauce.*

Picante sauce: Picante sauce is low in calories and contains little or no fat; it primarily contributes sodium. Select brands that contain less than 0.5 gram of fat per serving.

Pickles: Pickles contain no fat; sweet and bread-and-butter pickles are higher in calories than dill pickles. Pickles primarily contribute sodium.

Pie fillings: See *Fruit pie fillings* and *Puddings and cream pie fillings.*

Pies: Most pies are high in fat because of the shortening, butter, lard, oil, or margarine used to make the crust; some pies also have fat added to the filling and/or topping. Select ready-to-eat pies and pie crusts that contain no more than 3 grams of fat per serving. In homemade pies fat can be reduced by making a "crustless" pie or by preparing pie or cobbler with no bottom crust but with strips of pastry on top.

Pita: Pita bread is low in calories and fat.

Pizza: Pizza is usually high in fat and calories from the cheese, sausage, pepperoni, and ground meat that it contains. Lower-fat pizza can be made using a low-fat or fat-free pizza or spaghetti sauce, part-skim mozzarella cheese, and vegetables. If meat is used, it should be lean or extra lean. Choose prepared pizza providing no more than 3 grams of fat per 5-ounce serving.

Pizza sauce: Pizza sauce is low in calories and contains little or no fat; it primarily contributes sodium. Select a pizza sauce that contains no more than 3 grams of fat per ½-cup serving.

Pork: Pork can be high or low in fat depending on the amount of marbling and the amount of fat remaining on the outside of a cut. Choose pork that has very little marbling, is trimmed of visible fat, and provides no more than 9 grams of fat per 3 ounces cooked. Cured pork, such as Canadian bacon and lean ham, is high in sodium.

Potato chips: See *Snacks.*

Poultry: Chicken and turkey meats are low in fat, but do not eat poultry skin, which is high in fat. Choose poultry that provides no more than 9 grams of fat per 3 ounces cooked. See also *Turkey.*

Processed meats: See *Luncheon meats* and *Sausage.*

Puddings and cream pie fillings: Most pudding mixes, cream pie filling mixes, and mousse mixes are low in fat; preparing them with skim, ½%, or 1% low-fat milk results in a finished product that is still low in fat. Using a sugar-free mix for pudding, cream pie filling, or mousse can further reduce calories. Select a mix that, when prepared, provides no more than 3 grams of fat per ½ cup of pudding or mousse or per 3 ounces of pie filling.

Relishes: Pickle relish and other pickled vegetables contain little or no fat. Relishes differ in calories depending on the amount of sugar present. Most relishes are high in sodium.

Rice: Plain rice, whether white, brown, or wild, contains negligible fat; the addition of margarine, oil, butter, cheese, and high-fat sauces or gravies increases both fat and calories. Choose rice dishes that contain no more than 3 grams of fat per serving.

Rice cakes: Plain rice cakes and popcorn cakes are low in fat and calories; most flavored or sweetened rice cakes are higher in calories.

Rolls, dinner: Hard rolls are low in calories and fat. Soft dinner rolls may contain fat, and their tops are often brushed with fat. Select dinner rolls that contain no more than 3 grams of fat per 1¾-ounce serving.

Rolls, sweet: See *Sweet rolls.*

Salad dressings: Regular salad dressings are high in fat and calories. There are many low-fat and fat-free salad dressings on the market. Choose a salad dressing containing no more than 2 grams of saturated fat per 2-tablespoon serving.

Salsa: Salsa is low in calories and contains little or no fat; it primarily contributes sodium.

Sauces: See individual sauce entries *(Barbecue, Catsup, Chili, Cocktail, Enchilada, Horseradish, Hot, Picante, Pizza, Salsa, Soy, Spaghetti, Steak,* and *Taco).*

Sausage: Sausage is usually high in fat; however, there are a variety of reduced-fat sausages on the market. Sausage products are high in sodium. Choose sausage that contains no more than 3 grams of fat per ounce.

Seasonings: Herbs and spices contain negligible fat and calories; they are usually low in sodium. However, seasonings vary in the amount of sodium they contain (see page 97).

Seeds: Most seeds are high in calories and fat. Select seeds that contain less than 2 grams of saturated fat per ounce; examples include roasted whole pumpkin, squash, and sesame seeds as well as dried, toasted, or dry-roasted safflower, sunflower, and sesame seed kernels.

Shellfish: See *Fish and shellfish.*

Sherbet: See *Frozen desserts.*

Snacks: The snacks category includes chips, popcorn, pretzels, fruit snacks, party mixes, trail mixes, and breakfast bars. Most regular chips are high in fat, calories, and sodium; baked chips and other reduced-fat chips, some of which are unsalted, are available. Plain popcorn contains negligible fat and sodium; light microwave popcorn provides appreciably less fat than regular microwave products. Hard pretzels are fat free but are high in sodium unless unsalted; some soft pretzels are brushed with fat. Most fruit snacks contain negligible fat; some products, such as banana chips, may be fried and therefore be higher in fat. Party mixes and trail mixes vary in their calories and fat, depending on their ingredients. Choose chips, popcorn, pretzels, fruit snacks, party mixes, and trail mixes that contain no more than 3 grams of fat per 1-ounce serving. Select breakfast bars, granola bars, and rice cereal bars that provide no more than 3 grams of fat in a 1.4-ounce serving. See also *Dips.*

Sodas: See *Carbonated beverages.*

Soft drinks: See *Carbonated beverages.*

Sorbet: See *Frozen desserts.*

Soups: Cream soups are usually higher in fat than broth-based soups. Most commercial canned, dehydrated, and frozen soups are high in sodium. Lower-fat, lower-sodium soups are available. Choose a soup that contains no more than 3 grams of fat per serving.

Sour cream: Select nonfat or low-fat sour cream that contains no more than 3 grams of fat per 1-ounce serving.

Soy sauce: Soy sauce is negligible in calories and fat. Regular soy sauce is very high in sodium. Even though the sodium in reduced-sodium soy sauce is decreased by 40%, the sodium content is still very high.

Spaghetti sauce: Most plain spaghetti, pasta, and marinara sauces are fairly low in calories and fat and high in sodium. Some low-fat, lower-sodium sauces are available. Commercial sauces that contain meat are usually higher in calories and fat. Select spaghetti sauce that contains no more than 3 grams of fat per ½-cup serving.

Sprays, cooking: See *Nonstick cooking sprays.*

Steak sauce: Steak sauce is low in calories and contains only a trace of fat; it primarily contributes sodium.

Stuffing: Choose brands of stuffing that contain no more than 3 grams of fat per serving. When making stuffing from scratch, reduce the fat in ingredients, such as cornbread and/or biscuits, defat broth used in the stuffing, and use less margarine or other fat in the recipe.

Sweet rolls: Sweet rolls are typically high in fat from the butter, margarine, oil, shortening, whole milk, cream cheese, and/or nuts used to make them. Select ready-to-eat low-fat and fat-free sweet rolls with no more than 3 grams of fat per 2-ounce serving.

Sweets: Sweet foods that contain negligible fat and consist primarily of sugar include honey, molasses, jam, jelly, syrups (corn, pancake and waffle, and fruit), preserves, marmalade, fat-free candy, and marshmallows. Higher-fat sweets include fudge and caramel sauce; choose sweets that contain no more than 3 grams of fat per serving. See also *Candy.*

Syrups: See *Sweets.*

Taco sauce: Taco sauce is low in calories and contains little or no fat; it primarily contributes sodium.

Tea: Plain tea contains no calories or fat; tea made from sugar-sweetened mixes provides calories. If milk is added to hot tea, choose skim, ½%, or 1% low-fat milk.

Tofu: Tofu (soybean curd or bean curd) contains fat but no cholesterol. It is a good source of protein and can be substituted for meat. (See pages 205–6 for preparation of tofu.)

Tortillas: Corn tortillas contain negligible fat unless they are fried; flour tortillas are higher in fat because they are made with lard or shortening. Choose tortillas that provide no more than 3 grams of fat per 1¾-ounce serving.

Turkey: Select a turkey that is not self-basting because extra fat has been injected into these birds. Turkey may be cooked with the skin on; however, the skin should be removed before the turkey is eaten. Turkey breast is especially low in fat. See also *Poultry.*

Veal: Most cuts of veal are low in fat and saturated fat. Veal is higher in cholesterol than beef because it comes from a young animal, in which cholesterol is concentrated in the tissues. Choose veal that provides no more than 9 grams of fat per 3 ounces cooked.

Vegetable oil: See *Oils, vegetable.*

Vegetables and vegetable juices: Vegetables naturally contain little or no fat. The addition of sauces, gravy, margarine, butter, sour cream, bacon, or cheese to vegetables increases fat and calories. Fresh and frozen vegetables typically contain little sodium; regular canned vegetables and vegetable juices are high in sodium, but unsalted and reduced-sodium products are available. Choose plain vegetables that contain less than 0.5 gram of fat per serving and vegetables in sauce that contain 3 grams or less of fat per serving.

Waffles: There are two types of waffle mixes: complete and incomplete. With complete mixes, which usually contain shortening, only water needs to be added; incomplete mixes require the addition of several ingredients. Waffles made with an incomplete mix can be lower in fat than those made with a complete mix if you substitute water or skim milk for whole milk, use egg white or egg substitute instead of whole egg, and use less fat than suggested in the package directions. Select frozen waffles and waffle mixes with no more than 3 grams of fat per serving.

Whipped toppings: Whipped toppings vary in the calories and fat they contain. Select whipped topping mixes that when prepared with skim milk contain no more than 3 grams of fat per 2 table-spoons; the same fat limit applies to frozen whipped toppings.

Yogurt: Sweetened, flavored yogurt is higher in calories than plain yogurt or artificially sweetened, flavored yogurt that contains the same amount of fat. Nonfat and low-fat yogurts are excellent sources of calcium. Choose yogurt that contains no more than 3 grams of fat per 8-ounce serving.

Yogurt, frozen: See *Frozen desserts.*

Chapter 8

The Living Heart Diet Guide to Selecting Food When Eating Out

Meals and snacks eaten away from home now represent a considerable portion of the average American's daily food intake. Surveys show that 42% of American adults eat at a family restaurant and 51% eat at a fast-food restaurant at least once a week. On average, Americans 8 years of age and older eat out 198 meals per year.

Learning how to choose low-calorie, low-fat foods when dining away from home is an important part of following the Living Heart Diet. In recent years an increasing number of restaurants have begun serving low-fat dishes and/or have expressed a willingness to prepare upon request dishes that are lower in fat. In a survey of restaurant owners, almost 70% said that a customer asking for a change in a menu item presented no problem. In this chapter you will find more than 100 practical tips on how to order lower-fat food in a restaurant and how to choose lower-fat food at a party; low-fat foods are usually lower in calories. Tips on choosing restaurant food that is low in both fat and sodium begin on page 154. For more detailed information on ordering low-fat restaurant food, you may wish to obtain *The Living*

Heart Guide to Eating Out, another book in our series (see order form on last page). It includes the calorie, fat, saturated fat, and cholesterol content in more than 1,500 American and ethnic restaurant foods. Tips on choosing lower-fat party food appear on page 168.

It is useful to do some extra planning to help guarantee that you get the type of food you want when you go out to eat. If you are not familiar with a restaurant's menu, telephone ahead and inquire about the menu selections. Call the chef in the afternoon when he or she is less busy and ask which menu selections are lowest in fat. Ask to have a menu sent to you by fax. Here are some sample questions you may wish to ask the chef or your waiter/waitress at the restaurant:

1. Which items on the menu can be prepared without fat?

2. Are low-fat salad dressings available?

3. Is the skin removed before chicken is cooked?

4. Is fat removed from beef, pork, lamb, or other meat before it is cooked?

5. Can meat, poultry, or fish be broiled or grilled without fat?

6. Can the sauce or gravy be served in a side dish rather than on the entrée?

7. Which vegetables are cooked at the time they are ordered so that fat can be decreased?

8. Is soft margarine available?

You will also want to read the menu carefully. The following common menu terms tell you that a food is high in fat:

MENU TERMS THAT MEAN HIGH FAT

à la king	casserole
Alfredo	cheese sauce
au beurre	creamy, creamed, or cream sauce
au gratin	crispy
basted	croquettes
batter-dipped	fried or deep fried
béarnaise	fritters
braised	fritto
breaded	gravy or in its own gravy
buttered or butter sauce	hash
carbonara	hollandaise

MENU TERMS THAT MEAN HIGH FAT (cont.)

meunière	prime (grade of meat that is highest in fat)
Newburg	sautéed
pan fried	scalloped
Parmesan or parmigiana	stuffed
potpie	tempura

As a rule, you will be safer ordering a menu item described as being baked, broiled dry (not basted with fat), grilled, poached, roasted, steamed, or in tomato sauce.

For many people, drinking alcoholic beverages is a part of eating away from home. Information on alcoholic beverages appears on pages 60 and 370–71.

American Cuisine

American cuisine is a mixture of dishes that originated in the United States and Americanized versions of popular ethnic foods, such as pizza, lasagna, croissants, French bread, and enchiladas. The following sections provide practical tips on selecting food lower in fat and saturated fat when eating out, whether at breakfast/brunch, lunch, or dinner, in restaurants that serve American cuisine. Tips on selecting food lower in sodium begin on page 101.

BREAKFAST/BRUNCH

Whether you are ordering breakfast or brunch from a menu or selecting dishes from a buffet, there are usually several low-calorie, low-fat choices available:

- Cooked cereals are low in fat; ask that butter or margarine not be added. Most ready-to-eat cereals, with the exception of some granolas, are low in fat.

- Request skim or low-fat milk as a beverage, to use on cereal, and as "cream" in your coffee.

- Ask for "dry" toast, English muffins, or bagels with margarine served on the side. Biscuits, muffins, sweet rolls, fruit and nut breads, and coffeecake are higher in fat.

- Ask that your waffles and pancakes be served without butter or margarine; instead, use syrup, fruit topping, or yogurt. If you want margarine, have it served on the side so that you can control the amount used.

- If selecting meat, choose Canadian bacon, lean ham, or a small lean breakfast steak. (Be sure to include meat eaten at breakfast in calculating your day's meat intake.) Bacon and sausage are too high in fat to be good choices.

- Choose one egg (within the recommended three yolks per week) that is poached, hard or soft cooked, or scrambled in little or no fat. If egg substitute is available, ask that it be prepared on a dry grill. Order a plain, vegetable, or Spanish omelet made with egg white and no cheese.

LUNCH

People eat a wide variety of foods for lunch: soup and salad, hamburger or sandwich, pizza, plate lunch, or ethnic cuisine. Several tips for finding lower-calorie, lower-fat foods are shown below. For suggestions on plate lunches (entrée, vegetables, bread, and dessert), see the Dinner section, which begins on page 156.

TYPES OF RESTAURANT

- Select an eating place that offers food cooked to order so that you can request that the amount of fat used in preparation be decreased.

- Choose a restaurant with a varied menu instead of one that serves a limited number of items that are all high in fat.

SOUP AND SALAD

- As a rule, broth-based soups are lower in fat than cream soups.

- Fresh fruit and vegetable salads are low in fat; have dressing served on the side so that you can control the amount you use. High-fat salads include tuna, chicken, meat, potato, macaroni, and pasta salads, as well as coleslaw and tabouli. Mayonnaise and oil dressings used on salads are typically high in fat but low in saturated fat.

- Ask if low-fat or fat-free salad dressings are available. Some restaurants provide separate containers of oil and vinegar to be used as salad dressing. Try using lemon juice, flavored vinegar, salsa, or marinated vegetables to dress your salad.

FAST FOOD AND SANDWICHES

- Choose a sandwich that will be prepared the way you prefer rather than one prepared ahead of time. Ask for less meat, no cheese or bacon, and generous amounts of lettuce, tomato, and onion.

- If the sandwich is on toast or a bun, ask that the bread not be brushed with fat.

- Request that margarine, mayonnaise, or oil-and-vinegar dressing be served on the side so that you can control the amount used. Mustard, catsup, barbecue sauce, steak sauce, and other meat sauces contain negligible fat.

- Choose a lower-fat sandwich filling such as sliced turkey or chicken, grilled or broiled chicken breast, or lean roast beef or ham instead of a higher-fat mixed filling (chicken, ham, tuna, or egg salad) or instead of a hamburger. If your sandwich contains a generous amount of meat, you may wish to order extra bread and share the sandwich with a companion.

- Select a small, plain hamburger without cheese and add lettuce, tomato, and onions; avoid high-fat selections such as cheeseburgers, hamburgers with large meat patties, and double-meat hamburgers. Request carrot sticks or a salad instead of French fries with your sandwich.

- Order a submarine or po-boy sandwich with turkey, lean roast beef, or lean ham instead of luncheon meats and omit the cheese; have the mayonnaise or oil-and-vinegar dressing served on the side so that you can control the amount used. Large sandwiches are best divided between two meals or split with a friend.

PIZZA

- Try eating a large salad before you begin eating your pizza to help curb your appetite.

- Choose a thin-crust pizza with mushrooms, onions, green peppers, and other vegetables and request less cheese. Thick-crust pizzas are usually higher in fat.

- Select a pizza without pepperoni, sausage, or hamburger meat; Canadian bacon is the only lean meat commonly available on pizza.

DINNER

At dinner, the most important tip is the same as for lunch choices and bears repeating: Choose a restaurant that offers cooked-to-order items so that you can request less fat in your food.

- If the restaurant serves large portions, consider splitting an entrée with a companion and adding soup or salad. Or ask for a "to-go" container and save leftover food for another meal. CLEANING YOUR PLATE IS AN OUTMODED IDEA—A LITTLE WASTE IS BETTER THAN A LARGE WAIST!

- Try ordering à la carte instead of a complete dinner so that you get only the items you want.

- At a cafeteria, look at all the food being offered and decide which low-fat dishes you will order before you start down the line, to avoid choosing too many items.

- When eating at a buffet, take reasonable-size servings of four or five lower-fat foods instead of filling your plate with some of everything.

APPETIZERS — See the section on lunch for tips on soups and salads.

- Choose an appetizer that is not fried.

- Select fresh fruit or vegetables as a good low-fat appetizer; avoid high-fat sauces or dips.

ENTRÉES

- You may wish to order two low-fat appetizers in place of an entrée.

- Select lean cuts of meat that have been roasted or baked, or have lean meat broiled or grilled without basting with fat; trim off any visible fat. Lean cuts of beef include sirloin, tenderloin, and filet mignon (cooked without bacon); lean cuts of pork are tenderloin, loin pork chops, center-cut baked ham, and ham steak; a lean cut of lamb is leg of lamb with the fat trimmed off. High-fat cuts of meat include brisket, ribs, rib-eye and T-bone steaks, and all prime cuts of meat.

- Request that the skin be removed before chicken is cooked.

- When ordering cooked-to-order entrées that are sautéed or stir-fried, request that little or no oil be used.

- Ask that gravies and sauces be served on the side so that you can control the amount used.

- Some fish may be dry if grilled or broiled without being basted with fat. Ask to have your fish poached or baked with a small amount of wine. The alcohol evaporates as food is cooked.

- Select grilled or broiled meat or fish instead of a casserole, which is usually high in fat because of the butter, oil, margarine, cream, sour cream, cheese, and/or ground meat used in preparation.

VEGETABLES AND STARCHES

- Choose a tomato-based sauce without meat, such as marinara, for pasta instead of a creamy sauce or cheese sauce.

- Select plain steamed or grilled vegetables instead of those served with butter or in cream sauce.

- Choose low-fat toppings for a baked potato, such as salsa, chives, scallions, green onions, lemon juice, hot peppers, catsup, or mustard, instead of butter, cheese, bacon, or sour cream. Potato toppings that contain some fat but that are low in saturated fat include reduced-fat salad dressings and a small amount of margarine. Examples of high-fat potato dishes are French fries, hash browns, and potatoes that are creamed, scalloped, au gratin, stuffed, or twice-baked.

BREADS

- Choose low-fat breads, such as hard rolls, hard breadsticks, or sliced bread, instead of croissants, muffins, biscuits, or cornbread. Most dinner rolls are prepared with fat and the tops are brushed with fat.

- Request soft margarine instead of butter on bread and rolls and use it sparingly.

DESSERTS

- Choose fresh fruit, sorbet, sherbet, low-fat or fat-free frozen yogurt, angel food cake, or gelatin without whipped cream, whipped topping, or sour cream.

- Decrease your fat intake by eating only the filling in fruit pie and cobbler (most of the fat is in the crust) and by removing frosting from cake. Most whipped toppings, even the nondairy types, are high in fat and saturated fat. Other high-fat desserts include ice cream, most cakes, mousse, cheesecake, and cookies.

BEVERAGES

For people who drink alcoholic beverages, the Living Heart Diet recommends no more than two drinks per day. Women who are pregnant should not drink alcoholic beverages because of the risk for birth defects. One drink is defined on page 60.

Calorie and alcohol levels of selected alcoholic beverages appear in the Appendix on pages 370–71. The amount of pure alcohol (ethanol) in one drink is about ½ ounce (14 grams). Many of the alcoholic drinks shown in the Appendix contain more alcohol than is considered one drink. For example, 4 fluid ounces (½ cup) of the following alcoholic beverages is equivalent to about two drinks: a daiquiri (not frozen), a Manhattan, and a martini. The following tips can help you choose beverages when you are eating away from home:

- If you drink alcoholic beverages, select one without fat instead of a brandy Alexander, White Russian, grasshopper, golden Cadillac, piña colada, eggnog with brandy, or hot buttered rum, all of which contain fat.

- Coffee, tea, sparkling water, soft drinks, fruit juice, and fruit-flavored drinks contain no fat.

- Request skim or 1% low-fat milk as a beverage and for coffee instead of whole milk or cream.

SNACKS

Many Americans are in the habit of snacking between meals, especially during the evening and when away from home. Foods that are popular for snacking include ice cream, chocolate candy, cookies, and popcorn. Some of these snacks are so high in fat, saturated fat, and sodium that they can provide more than 100% of the Daily Value for these nutrients at the 2,000-calorie level and an even higher percent of the Daily Value at lower calorie levels. (An explanation of Daily Value appears on pages 131–32.) The table below shows the grams of fat and saturated fat and the milligrams of sodium in some common snacks and the percent of the Daily Value these values represent at the 2,000-calorie level. For example, the medium container of "buttered" popcorn shown in the table contains 135 grams of fat, which is 210% of the maximum amount of fat (100% of the Daily Value is 65 grams). Remember, if you consume less than 2,000 calories, the percent Daily Value will be higher for each snack shown in the table.

COMPARISON OF SNACKS: FAT, SATURATED FAT, SODIUM, AND PERCENT DAILY VALUES* AT 2,000-CALORIE LEVEL

Snacks	Fat g (% Daily Value)	Saturated Fat g (% Daily Value)	Sodium mg (% Daily Value)
Banana split (3 scoops ice cream, 2 oz fudge sauce, 1 cup whipped topping)	40 (60%)	25 (125%)	255 (10%)
Cookies, chocolate chip (3 cookies w/ 3-in diameter)	25 (40%)	10 (50%)	165 (5%)
Corn chips (3 cups)	30 (45%)	5 (25%)	440 (20%)
Hot fudge sundae	20 (30%)	10 (50%)	140 (5%)
Milk chocolate candy bar, plain, king size (4 oz)	35 (55%)	20 (100%)	95 (5%)
Milk chocolate candy bar w/ peanuts, extra-large (7 oz)	65 (100%)	35 (175%)	65 (5%)
Popcorn, "buttered," medium container at movie theater (12–16 cups)	135 (210%)	25† (125%)	2,560 (105%)
Popcorn, microwave (1 bag, or about 9 cups)	20 (30%)	5 (25%)	605 (25%)
Trail mix (1 cup)	45 (70%)	10 (50%)	345 (15%)

Values rounded to nearest 5.
*% Daily Values appear in parentheses; based on 65 g fat, 20 g saturated fat, and 2,400 mg sodium (2,000-calorie level).
†Saturated fat will vary depending on the type of fat used for popping and "buttering" popcorn.
Values for other popular snacks are shown in the Appendix, starting on page 372.

Ethnic Cuisines

Ethnic restaurants are becoming increasingly popular in the United States. A survey by the National Restaurant Association found that 78% of people polled had eaten in a Chinese restaurant, 76% in an Italian restaurant, and 74% in a Mexican restaurant, making these three the most popular ethnic cuisines. The following section includes tables that compare meals from ethnic cuisines to the Daily Values for fat, saturated fat, and sodium at the 2,000-calorie level (see pages 132–32 for explanation of Daily Values).

The food served in ethnic restaurants often differs from dishes of the same name prepared in the country of origin. The Americanized versions of these native dishes are usually much higher in fat than the originals. Often, large amounts of meat, poultry, cheese, and/or fat are added to dishes that were primarily legumes, grains, and vegetables originally. These additions increase the total fat and saturated fat content.

It may be even more necessary to ask questions in an ethnic restaurant than in an eating establishment that serves American cuisine. When eating out, don't hesitate to inquire about the ingredients in a menu selection and to ask how it is prepared. *As a paying customer, you should not hesitate to ask for exactly what you want—and expect to get it!*

The tips listed below can help you select food lower in fat and saturated fat from 10 popular ethnic cuisines; tips on selecting lower-sodium food when eating out in ethnic restaurants begin on page 102.

CAJUN

- Choose seafood that is grilled or broiled instead of fried; although shrimp and crayfish are high in cholesterol, they are low in total fat when prepared with only a small amount of fat and can be eaten occasionally.

- Select plain or even "buttered" rice in preference to "dirty" rice, which is typically made with chicken or turkey livers, gizzards, and bacon fat.

- Request that "blackened" foods be prepared with very little fat.

- If possible, order red beans and rice prepared without sausage.

- The fat content of any dish, of course, will depend on how it is made; as a rule, creole and jambalaya dishes are lower in fat than étouffée and gumbo.

CHINESE

The food served in many Chinese restaurants in the United States is high in fat and sodium. The following table shows the fat, saturated fat, and sodium in some Chinese restaurant meals in light of the Daily Values at the 2,000-calorie level; higher-fat meals are listed first, and lower-fat ones are listed second. Remember, the lower your calorie level, the higher the percent of the Daily Value for fat each of these meals represents. Values for other Chinese foods are shown on page 380 of the Appendix.

COMPARISON OF CHINESE RESTAURANT MEALS: FAT, SATURATED FAT, SODIUM, AND PERCENT DAILY VALUES* (AT 2,000-CALORIE LEVEL)

Meals	Fat g (% Daily Value)	Saturated Fat g (% Daily Value)	Sodium mg (% Daily Value)
HIGHER-FAT CHINESE MEALS			
Beef & broccoli dinner: 6 fried chicken wings, hot/sour soup, & beef & broccoli stir-fry w/ fried rice	85 (130%)	20 (100%)	3,700 (155%)
Lemon chicken dinner: shrimp toast, won ton soup, lemon chicken, & fried rice	105 (160%)	20 (100%)	4,305 (180%)
Moo goo gai pan dinner: 6 fried won tons, moo goo gai pan, fried rice, & bean curd w/ soybean milk	85 (130%)	15 (75%)	5,550 (230%)
Sweet-and-sour pork dinner: 2 large egg rolls, sweet/sour pork, & fried rice	65 (100%)	15 (75%)	4,955 (205%)
LOWER-FAT CHINESE MEALS			
Chop suey dinner: won ton soup, 6 steamed vegetable dumplings, chicken & shrimp chop suey, & steamed rice	25 (40%)	5 (25%)	3,710 (155%)
Shredded pork w/ garlic sauce dinner: velvet corn soup, shredded pork w/ garlic sauce, steamed rice, & lychee (fruit) in syrup	20 (30%)	5 (25%)	2,150 (90%)
Shrimp and snow peas dinner: egg drop soup, shrimp & snow peas, steamed rice, & 1 fortune cookie	15 (25%)	5 (25%)	2,085 (85%)

Adapted from Michael E. DeBakey, Antonio M. Gotto, Jr., and Lynne W. Scott, The Living Heart Guide to Eating Out *(New York: MasterMedia, 1993), and from Nutrition Data System, University of Minnesota, Minneapolis.*
Values rounded to nearest 5.

*% Daily Values appear in parentheses; based on 65 g fat, 20 g saturated fat, and 2,400 mg sodium (2,000-calorie level).

The following tips will help you select lower-fat food when eating in a Chinese restaurant; tips for selecting lower-sodium Chinese food are found on page 103.

- Since most Chinese dishes are prepared at the time they are ordered, you can request that very little oil be used to stir-fry food.

- Since the portions served in Chinese restaurants are often large, order fewer servings than there are people and share.

- Select steamed dumplings as a low-fat appetizer instead of fried egg rolls, which are high in fat.

- Choose steamed rice instead of fried rice, which is high in fat.

- Request that water chestnuts, which are fat free, be substituted for cashews and peanuts in entrées. Nuts add calories and fat.

- Choose steamed foods instead of fried foods at dim sum meals (which consist of a variety of small appetizers and snacks).

FRENCH

- You may wish to call ahead to the restaurant to see if it serves "light" dishes.

- French cuisine is famous for its sauces, many of which are high in fat. Wine sauces, such as bordelaise, are usually lower in fat than creamy sauces, such as béarnaise, hollandaise, and Mornay sauces, which typically contain butter, milk, eggs, and/or cheese.

- Some French chefs add butter to sauces immediately before serving them; to decrease the fat in the dish, ask that extra butter or oil be omitted.

- Choose French bread, which is low in fat, instead of croissants.

- Select fresh fruit (without crème), sorbet, or fruit ice as a light dessert.

GREEK AND MIDDLE EASTERN

- Choose appetizers such as rice mixtures in grape leaves, cucumber and yogurt dip, and baked stuffed eggplant, which are lower in fat than calamari (squid, often served fried), hummus, and fish roe dip. Ask that the olive oil that is often added to dips right before they are served be omitted.

- Ask that the feta cheese and olives be served on the side of your Greek salad so that you can more easily control the amount eaten.

- Order baked chicken or grilled fish and ask that olive oil not be added before the entrée is served. The fat cannot be decreased in entrées that are prepared ahead of time, such as pastitsio, moussaka, and spanakopita.

- Ask that lean meat be used in shish kebab.

- The pita bread served with appetizers and entrées is low in fat.

- Order a chicken pita sandwich instead of a gyro, which typically contains a high-fat mixture of lamb and beef; have the yogurt sauce (made with whole milk) served on the side so that you can control the amount used.

- Choose rizogalo (rice pudding) as dessert instead of galaktoboureko (custard pie) or baklava, which is a high-fat pastry.

INDIAN

- Request that chapati, roti, and naan (Indian breads) not be brushed with ghee (clarified butter).

- Select a vegetable salad or raita (spiced yogurt with cucumbers).

- Order tandoori or tikka meats or a kebab instead of entrées with a sauce. Request that meat not be brushed with fat.

ITALIAN

Many popular meals served in Italian restaurants contain more than 100% of the Daily Value for fat, saturated fat, and/or sodium. Dishes that have been sautéed and baked with cheese and a sauce containing oil, such as veal parmigiana and eggplant parmigiana, are especially high in fat. Casserole dishes, such as lasagna, that contain meat, cheese, tomato sauce, and oil in addition to the pasta are high in fat and sodium. A serving of fettuccine Alfredo, which has butter, cream, and cheese in the sauce, is especially high in saturated fat; one average serving provides 115% of the Daily Value for saturated fat at the 2,000-calorie level. A dinner including fettuccine Alfredo, as shown in the table below, provides 175% of the Daily Value for saturated fat. The table below includes both meals that are higher in fat and meals that are lower in fat. Values for other Italian foods are in the Appendix on page 387.

COMPARISON OF ITALIAN RESTAURANT MEALS: FAT, SATURATED FAT, SODIUM, AND PERCENT DAILY VALUES* AT 2,000-CALORIE LEVEL

Meals	Fat g (% Daily Value)	Saturated Fat g (% Daily Value)	Sodium mg (% Daily Value)
HIGHER-FAT ITALIAN MEALS			
Beef lasagna dinner: caponata (sautéed eggplant & other vegetables), beef lasagna, 1 slice garlic bread, & tiramisu	80 (125%)	35 (175%)	3,600 (150%)
Eggplant Parmesan dinner: minestrone (soup), eggplant Parmesan, & 1 slice garlic bread	110 (170%)	25 (125%)	2,655 (110%)
Fettuccine Alfredo dinner: stuffed artichoke, fettuccine Alfredo, 1 slice garlic bread, & coffee granita with whipped cream	75 (115%)	35 (175%)	1,555 (65%)
Spaghetti dinner: fried calamari, spaghetti w/ meat sauce, 1 slice garlic bread, & zabaglione (made w/ cream)	75 (115%)	30 (150%)	2,780 (115%)
LOWER-FAT ITALIAN MEALS			
Linguine w/ clam sauce dinner: linguine w/ red clam sauce, Italian spinach (sautéed in oil), 1 slice garlic bread, & coffee granita (w/o whipped cream)	25 (40%)	5 (25%)	1,470 (60%)
Pasta primavera dinner: minestrone (soup), pasta prima-vera, 1 slice garlic bread, & cappuccino	30 (45%)	5 (25%)	2,245 (95%)
Veal marsala dinner: minestrone (soup), veal marsala, tossed salad w/ 1 tablespoon Italian dressing, & 1 slice garlic bread	30 (45%)	10 (50%)	1,025 (45%)

Adapted from Michael E. DeBakey, Antonio M. Gotto, Jr., and Lynne W. Scott, The Living Heart Guide to Eating Out *(New York: MasterMedia, 1993), and from Nutrition Data System, University of Minnesota, Minneapolis. Values rounded to nearest 5.*

*% Daily Values appear in parentheses; based on 65 g fat, 20 g saturated fat, and 2,400 mg sodium (2,000-calorie level).

The following tips will help you select lower-fat Italian foods; see pages 103–4 for tips on choosing foods that are lower in sodium in an Italian restaurant.

- Ask that cooked-to-order dishes consisting of sautéed meat, poultry, fish, or vegetables be prepared with very little oil. Lasagna, ravioli, and other foods that are prepared ahead of time usually contain high-fat ingredients such as butter, cheese, cream, ground meat, and/or sausage.

- Choose tomato-based sauces, such as pomodoro and marinara, instead of cream sauces, such as Alfredo sauce; ask that marinara sauce be substituted for Alfredo sauce when pasta is served as a side dish.

- Choose granita (frozen mixture of water, sugar, and flavoring) instead of zabaglione (made with egg yolk, wine, and sugar) or tiramisu (mixture of coffee, cookies, mascarpone or cream cheese, egg yolk, rum or brandy, and cocoa).

JAPANESE

- Start your meal with a clear soup that does not contain egg.

- Sushi (vinegar-flavored rice with raw seafood) and sashimi (sliced raw fish) are popular appetizers in Japanese cuisine; however, raw fish can contain viruses, bacteria, and parasites and is not recommended.

- Sukiyaki, teriyaki, shabu shabu, and yosenabe are entrées that are low in fat.

- Several Japanese entrées are high in cholesterol because they contain egg; these include oyako donburi (chicken omelet over rice), chawan mushi (chicken and shrimp in egg custard), and sushi when it contains an omelet.

MEXICAN

If you do not select carefully when dining in a Mexican restaurant, it is possible to exceed 100% of the Daily Value for fat, saturated fat, and/or sodium in just one meal. The table below looks at higher-fat and lower-fat Mexican meals in view of Daily Values at the 2,000-calorie level.

COMPARISON OF MEXICAN RESTAURANT MEALS: FAT, SATURATED FAT, SODIUM, AND PERCENT DAILY VALUES* AT 2,000-CALORIE LEVEL

Meals	Fat g (% Daily Value)	Saturated Fat g (% Daily Value)	Sodium mg (% Daily Value)
HIGHER-FAT MEXICAN MEALS			
Beef enchilada dinner: 2 beef enchiladas, 2 tamales, refried beans, & Spanish rice	95 (145%)	40 (200%)	2,825 (120%)
Beef taco dinner: 2 beef tacos, refried beans, Spanish rice, & 2 sopaipillas	70 (110%)	25 (125%)	2,365 (100%)
Nacho dinner: 10 nachos w/ ground beef, refried beans, & cheese; flan	90 (140%)	40 (200%)	1,665 (70%)
Taco salad dinner: 24 tortilla chips & salsa; taco salad w/ grilled beef, cheese, guacamole, & sour cream (tortilla bowl eaten)	80 (125%)	30 (150%)	2,785 (115%)
LOWER-FAT MEXICAN MEALS			
Chicken fajita dinner: 2 soft corn tortillas w/ salsa, 2 chicken fajitas w/ soft corn tortillas, & Spanish rice	15 (25%)	5 (25%)	2,200 (90%)
Chicken taco dinner: 2 soft chicken tacos, frijoles a la charra, & Spanish rice	25 (40%)	5 (25%)	3,210 (135%)
Chicken taco salad dinner: 2 steamed corn tortillas, salsa, chicken taco salad (w/o guaca-mole, sour cream, & cheese) (tortilla bowl not eaten), & sherbet	15 (25%)	5 (25%)	1,540 (65%)

Adapted from Michael E. DeBakey, Antonio M. Gotto, Jr., and Lynne W. Scott, The Living Heart Guide to Eating Out (New York: MasterMedia, 1993), and from Nutrition Data System, University of Minnesota, Minneapolis. Values rounded to nearest 5.
*% Daily Values appear in parentheses; based on 65 g fat, 20 g saturated fat, and 2,400 mg sodium (2000-calorie level).

In the table above, the beef enchilada dinner provides 95 grams of fat and 40 grams of saturated fat—145% of the Daily Value for fat and 200% of the Daily Value for saturated fat at the 2,000-calorie level. The percent of the Daily Value for these nutrients is even higher at lower calorie levels. Values for other Mexican foods appear on page 389 of the Appendix. The following tips will help you select lower-fat foods in a Mexican restaurant; see page 104 for tips on ordering Mexican food that is lower in sodium.

- As soon as you are seated, request steamed or baked corn tortillas. Use them (in place of chips) with salsa as an appetizer instead of nachos (fried tortilla chips topped with re-fried beans, ground beef, and cheese). Guacamole is high in fat but low in saturated fat.

- Order chicken or beef fajitas and ask that little or no fat be used in cooking; substitute corn tortillas for flour tortillas to eat with the fajitas.

- Order frijoles a la charra (beans cooked in beer) instead of refried beans.

- Choose a chicken or beef fajita salad or a chicken taco salad and ask that guacamole, cheese, sour cream, and/or salad dressing be served on the side so that you can control the amount used; use salsa as the dressing. Think of the fried tortilla in which the salad is served as a bowl and leave it on the table.

- Ask your waiter or waitress if there are any low-fat specials not on the regular menu, such as broiled or grilled meat, poultry, or fish.

THAI

- Choose fresh (soft) spring rolls instead of fried ones.

- Order stir-fried entrées instead of curry.

- Select plain steamed rice instead of fried rice.

- Choose dishes made without cashews and peanuts, which are high in fat.

VIETNAMESE

- Since Vietnamese restaurants often serve large portions, order fewer entrées than there are people and share.

- Select plain steamed rice instead of fried rice.

- Choose fish soups and entrées instead of sweet-and-sour and curry dishes, which are high in fat.

- Eat foods without the addition of nuts or peanut sauce. Peanut sauce is made with crushed peanuts, peanut oil, and spices; it is served with most appetizers and entrées.

Eating at Parties

Most Americans love to go to parties. Foods high in calories and fat and alcoholic drinks often play a significant role at parties. The following tips will help you choose lower-fat foods when attending a party or other gathering in which you have no control over how the food is prepared.

- If you know that most of the food being served at the party is likely to be high in fat and calories, eat a light meal before you go; it is much easier to control what you eat at a party if you are not very hungry.

- At a party buffet, choose generous servings of low-fat foods such as tossed salad (with a small amount of dressing), fruit, and bread and moderate servings of lean meat, poultry, and fish or shellfish, such as lean roast beef, lean ham, boiled shrimp (high in cholesterol but low in fat), crab fingers, or turkey breast.

- Limit or omit high-fat party foods such as fried appetizers, chips, dips, nachos, high-fat crackers, cheese, croissants, luncheon meats, salads with whipped cream or sour cream, nuts, and pastries.

- If you want to eat dessert, wait until you have eaten the other food before making your choice; choose a moderate portion of one dessert or half portions of two desserts, rather than a full portion of several desserts. Remember, fruit pie and cobbler are fairly low in fat if the crust is not eaten.

- Alcohol contains calories, increases your appetite, and can possibly weaken your decision to control food intake. The Living Heart Diet recommends that if you drink alcoholic beverages, you limit your intake to no more than two drinks per day (see page 60 for definition of one drink).

- If you eat more than you intended to at a party, do not get discouraged: just resume your selection of low-fat foods at your next meal and continue your program of physical activity.

Chapter 9

The Living Heart Guide to Vitamins and Minerals

It is common knowledge that the human body needs vitamins and minerals. Most health experts agree that people can usually obtain sufficient vitamins and minerals from eating a balanced diet instead of depending on supplements. Although there is no recommendation that everyone take a multiple vitamin mineral supplement, if you take one, it should provide no more than 100% of the Reference Daily Intake for any nutrient. People take vitamin and mineral supplements for various reasons, including (1) to supplement a basically healthy diet that they fear may be deficient in some vital nutrient, (2) as a type of insurance that they erroneously believe will compensate for eating a diet that is not balanced, (3) in an attempt to achieve "super-health," and (4) to treat or prevent an illness. Some patients are prescribed specific supplements by their physicians—for example, iron prescribed to women who are pregnant.

Three terms describing daily intakes of vitamins and minerals are mentioned in this section: Recommended Dietary Allowance (RDA), Reference Daily Intake (RDI), and Daily Value (DV). The RDA is the most familiar standard against which the intake of many vitamins and minerals is measured. The RDA for each nutrient is that level that has been judged as adequate to meet the needs of almost all healthy people. The RDAs for most nutrients have been determined by first estimating the average requirement for the nutrient and then adjusting the value to compensate for incomplete utilization in the body and individual differences among people and food sources. The RDAs provide a safety factor that exceeds the actual requirements of most individuals, but they are not designed to meet the needs of people with special nutritional requirements.

The Food and Drug Administration (FDA) requires that the labeling of vitamin and mineral supplements show both the amount of each vitamin and mineral present in a single dose and the percent of the RDI that the dose represents. The RDI is the same as the RDA for many vitamins and minerals, but the FDA has established RDIs for some nutrients that are different from the RDAs. The list below includes the RDIs that are currently in use, as well as those that have been proposed.

REFERENCE DAILY INTAKES

Vitamins	RDI	Minerals	RDI
Approved			
Folate	400 mcg	Biotin	300 mcg
Niacin	20 mg	Calcium	1,000 mg
Pantothenic acid	10 mg	Copper	2 mg
Riboflavin	1.7 mg	Iodine	150 mcg
Thiamine	1.5 mg	Iron	18 mg
Vitamin A	5,000 IU	Magnesium	400 mg
Vitamin B_6	2 mg	Phosphorus	1,000 mg
Vitamin B_{12}	6 mcg	Potassium	3,500 mg
Vitamin C	60 mg	Sodium	2,400 mg
Vitamin D	400 IU	Zinc	15 mg
Vitamin E	30 IU		
Proposed			
Vitamin K	80 mcg	Chloride	3,400 mg
		Chromium	130 mcg
		Fluoride	3 mg
		Manganese	3.5 mg
		Molybdenum	160 mcg
		Selenium	70 mcg

IU = international units; mcg = micrograms; mg = milligrams.

The percent RDI appears on the supplement label as the percent of the Daily Value (DV) for each nutrient; the DV, which was developed by the FDA to be used in food labeling, is a combination of RDIs and similar standards set for other nutrients, such as fat and saturated fat, that appear on food labels.

There are certain special situations in which vitamin and mineral supplementation is recommended. The American Dietetic Association has established the following guidelines for supplement use:

- Infants and children more than 6 months of age may need iron.

- Infants may need vitamin D.

- Women of childbearing age may need folate.

- Adolescent girls and young women may need calcium.

- Women with excessive menstrual blood loss may need iron supplementation.

- Pregnant or lactating women may need iron, folic acid, and calcium supplements.

- Some vegetarians may need supplements of calcium, iron, zinc, and vitamin B_{12}.

- People on very low calorie diets may not be meeting their needs for all nutrients.

- Newborns are often given one dose of vitamin K to prevent abnormal bleeding.

- Some people have different requirements for certain nutrients because they have a disorder or disease or take a medication that interferes with intake, digestion, absorption, metabolism, or excretion of the nutrients.

Some people believe that since vitamins and minerals are necessary for good health, vitamin and mineral supplements must be safe at any level; however, this is not true. Habitually taking large amounts of some vitamins and minerals can be harmful. The following section describes the recommended intake of selected vitamins and minerals, the symptoms indicating that dangerously high amounts of them have been taken, and the best food sources. The vitamins and minerals in this section are those of the greatest current interest in the arena of disease prevention and treatment.

Antioxidants

Many health experts believe that free radicals contribute to the development of atherosclerosis, cancer, immune diseases, cataracts, and other disorders. A free radical is an atom or molecule that is highly reactive because it has an unpaired electron that is seeking another electron with which to pair. Because every molecule has electrons, every molecule is a potential target for a free radical. When a free radical encounters an electron that is easily displaced, it will steal that electron's place (as in a game of musical chairs), creating a new molecule and a new free radical from the displaced electron.

The formation of free radicals is a part of normal plant and animal metabolism; that is, they are formed all the time. For example, free radicals are formed when food is burned for energy or when the body fights infection. Free radicals most often originate in molecules containing oxygen. ("Oxidation" involves the loss of an electron and is the process that occurs when iron rusts or butter turns rancid.) However, the uncontrolled continuation of a free radical chain reaction can be damaging to a biological system, for example, injuring cell membranes or proteins or causing changes in genes, the basic units of inheritance. The body has built-in defenses against the harmful effects of free radicals, including certain enzymes and antioxidants. Antioxidants act to scavenge or "mop up" the loose free radicals and stop their chain reactions. When these antioxidant defenses fail, disease or aging occurs.

Oxidation is an important concept in coronary heart disease (CHD) because it is thought that LDL particles and other lipoproteins that have been oxidized or otherwise chemically modified contribute more to the atherosclerotic process than undamaged lipoproteins. Free radicals may also damage the blood vessels directly. However, to what extent consuming foods with antioxidants such as vitamin A, C, or E or beta-carotene may protect against damage by oxidized lipoproteins or by free radicals is not known. Examination of this question in clinical studies is still in the early stages, and results thus far have been mixed.

Because the role of antioxidants in heart disease is not fully understood, health experts are not recommending at this time that the public begin to take supplements of antioxidant nutrients. Large doses of some of these nutrients can have undesirable side effects in some people, as described in the following sections. However, it is recommended that people consume generous amounts of the fruits and vegetables in which these antioxidant nutrients are naturally found, in order to achieve potential benefits without the possible negative side effects.

VITAMIN A

Vitamin A has several important functions in the body, including acting as an antioxidant. The RDAs for vitamin A are given in micrograms of retinol equivalent, or mcg RE; the labels on many supplements still give the level of vitamin A in international units (IU).

RDA FOR VITAMIN A	
Males, age 11 years & older	1,000 mcg RE (3,330 IU)
Females, age 11 years & older	800 mcg RE (2,664 IU)

IU = international units; mcg RE = micrograms of retinol equivalent.

Vitamin A is often not included in discussions of antioxidants commonly found in food because consuming large amounts of it can present some serious health problems. Vitamin A toxicity can result from a long-term daily intake exceeding about 15,000 mcg RE (50,000 IU) in adults and about 6,000 mcg RE (20,000 IU) in infants and young children; there have been some cases of liver damage in adults at levels of 25,000 IU per day taken over several years. The recommended daily doses of most popular multiple vitamins or vitamin–mineral supplements typically do not exceed 10,000 IU of vitamin A—about three to four times the RDA for adults. Consuming vitamin A in food or getting it in a multiple-vitamin mixture taken in the recommended dosage does not normally result in vitamin A toxicity. However, taking large doses of vitamin A in a single-nutrient supplement for an extended time can potentially lead to nausea, vomiting, fatigue, weakness, headache, lack of appetite, bone abnormalities, or liver damage.

Vitamin A activity in meat and dairy products comes primarily from retinol, for which 1 mcg RE is equal to 3.33 IU; vitamin A activity in fruits and vegetables is primarily in the form of beta-carotene, for which 1 mcg RE is equal to 10 IU. The table below lists good sources of vitamin A from high to low.

VITAMIN A CONTENT OF SELECTED FOODS

Food	Vitamin A	
(½ cup except where noted)	mcg RE	IU
Beef liver, braised (3 oz)	9,012	30,327
Carrot juice, canned	3,167	31,673
Sweet potato, baked	2,182	21,822
Carrots, raw, shredded	1,547	15,471
Spinach, canned, drained	939	9,390
Squash, butternut, baked	714	7,141
Apricots, dried, sulfured, uncooked (about 19 halves)	471	4,706
Cantaloupe, cubed	258	2,579
Milk, 1% low-fat (1 cup)	145	500
Broccoli, cooked, chopped	110	1,099

Adapted from USDA, Composition of Foods, *Agriculture Handbook series no. 8 (Washington, D.C.: USDA, 1976–1992).*
IU = international units; mcg RE = micrograms of retinol equivalent.

BETA-CAROTENE

Beta-carotene is a precursor of vitamin A; it is found in yellow-orange and dark-green leafy vegetables and in yellow-orange fruits. There has been a great deal of interest in beta-carotene because it has been promoted as having the antioxidant benefits of vitamin A without risk at high doses. It has generally been believed that the development of a harmless orange color in the skin, which fades once the intake of beta-carotene is decreased, is the only side effect of consuming large doses of beta-carotene. However, a recent study conducted in Finland found that male smokers who were taking a daily supplement of 20 milligrams (mg), or 33,340 IU, of beta-carotene per day for 5 to 8 years had a higher rate of lung cancer than male smokers who were not taking a beta-carotene supplement. The possible harmful outcome of beta-carotene supplementation in men who smoke supports the caution of the medical community in not recommending general supplementation with beta-carotene. Another recent study showed that a combination of beta-carotene, vitamin C, and vitamin E was no more effective in inhibiting oxidation of LDL than a high dose of vitamin E alone.

However, some of the many research studies examining beta-carotene and its effects on health are reporting more positive results. One large population study suggested that dietary beta-carotene, raw fruits and vegetables, and vitamin E each reduce risk for lung cancer in nonsmoking men and women. Preliminary data from 333 of the 20,000 enrollees in a subset of the Physicians' Health Study, conducted in male physicians, show that those physicians taking 50 mg (83,350 IU) of beta-carotene every other day had a 44% reduction in all major coronary events, such as heart attack, and a 49% reduction in all major vascular events, including heart attack and stroke. The Nurses' Health Study, which involved about 87,000 women, calculated beta-carotene intake from both food and supplements by using diet questionnaires. This study found higher beta-carotene intake to be associated with lower rates of CHD.

A study of more than 1,200 elderly people showed higher beta-carotene intake to be associated with a lower rate of death from cardiovascular disease. The Women's Health Initiative is currently testing the effect of taking 50 mg (83,350 IU) of beta-carotene and 600 mg (894 IU) of vitamin E every other day in more than 44,000 women.

Beta-carotene has no RDA since it is not itself a vitamin but is a source of vitamin A. The average daily intake of beta-carotene in the United States is estimated to be 1.5 to 1.9 mg (2,500 to 3,167 IU). The food sources of beta-carotene in the table below are listed in order of decreasing beta-carotene content.

BETA-CAROTENE CONTENT OF SELECTED FOODS

Food, ½ cup	Beta-Carotene	
	mg	IU
Carrot juice, canned	18.9	31,538
Yams, boiled, mashed	16.7	27,772
Pumpkin, canned	16.2	26,970
Carrots, fresh, cooked	11.5	19,117
Spinach, canned, cooked	5.6	9,374

(continued)

Food, ½ cup	Beta-Carotene	
	mg	IU
Carrots, fresh, grated	5.1	8,495
Apricots, dried, uncooked	2.8	4,708
Squash, acorn, cooked, mashed	2.6	4,349
Beet greens, cooked	2.4	3,951
Mango, fresh, sliced	1.9	3,212
Cantaloupe, fresh, cubed	1.3	2,197
Kale, fresh, cooked	1.1	1,769
Collards, fresh, cooked	1.0	1,740
Broccoli, fresh, cooked	1.0	1,740

Adapted from USDA, Composition of Foods, *Agriculture Handbook series no. 8 (Washington, D.C.: USDA, 1976–1992).*
IU = international units; mg = milligram

VITAMIN E

Vitamin E (alpha-tocopherol) also acts as an antioxidant, neutralizing free radicals. It helps prevent the oxidation of polyunsaturated fatty acids to a form that can damage the tissues of the body and reduces the formation of potentially harmful oxidized LDL. One study reported in 1992 showed that LDL samples taken from people receiving 800 mg (1,192 IU) of vitamin E daily were less susceptible to oxidation. At 10-year follow-up in the Nurses' Health Study, which examined dietary intake in women free from heart disease and cancer at the beginning of the study, the CHD rate was found to be 41% lower in women who reported taking vitamin E supplements for two or more years. Those nurses with the highest daily vitamin E intake (24 mg, or 35.8 IU) as calculated from food and supplementation records were 34% less likely to suffer a heart attack than women with the lowest intake (3.9 mg, or 5.8 IU). These findings were independent of recognized risk factors such as smoking, high blood pressure, and high blood cholesterol levels. The Health Professionals Follow-up Study of more than 51,000 male health professionals provided evidence of an association between a high intake of vitamin E and lower risk for CHD. The maximum result was found in men consuming 67 to 167 mg (100 to 249 IU) per day; no further decrease occurred at higher doses.

In 1991 it was estimated that more than 7 million American adults take a single-nutrient supplement of vitamin E and that an additional 34.5 million get vitamin E in multiple-vitamin supplements. Vitamin E appears to be fairly nontoxic to most adults, even when taken at doses of 100 to 800 mg (149 to 1,192 IU). The health experts who last revised the RDAs (in 1989) did not recommend that the general public take vitamin E supplements.

The RDAs for vitamin E are given as milligrams of alpha-tocopherol equivalents (written as mg α-TE); some supplement labels still list vitamin E in international units (IU).

RDA FOR VITAMIN E

Males, age 11 years & older	10 mg α-TE (15 IU)
Females, age 11 years & older	8 mg α-TE (12 IU)

IU = international units; mg α-TE = milligrams of alpha-tocopherol equivalent.

Sources of vitamin E are shown in the following table, from high to low.

VITAMIN E CONTENT OF SELECTED FOODS

Food	Vitamin E	
(1 tbsp except where noted)	mg α-TE	IU
Wheat-germ oil	24.4	36.4
Sunflower oil	7.3	10.9
Mayonnaise	3.5	5.2
Corn oil	2.3	3.4
Corn oil margarine, soft	1.8	2.7
Soybean oil	1.3	1.9
Avocado (½ medium)	1.1	1.6

Adapted from USDA, Composition of Foods, *Agriculture Handbook series no. 8 (Washington, D.C.: USDA, 1976–1992), and from Nutrition Data System, University of Minnesota, Minneapolis.*
IU = international units; mg α-TE = milligrams of alpha-tocopherol equivalent.

VITAMIN C

Studies of vitamin C suggest that this essential nutrient has two important functions as an antioxidant in relation to heart disease: to prevent the formation of oxidized LDL in the blood and to "spare" vitamin E, thereby making more of this antioxidant available to protect LDL. Some research has suggested that a daily intake of 180 mg of vitamin C (three times the RDA of 60 mg) does not affect the total amount of cholesterol in the blood but that it can increase levels of HDL-cholesterol, or "good" cholesterol, while decreasing LDL-cholesterol, or "bad" cholesterol. Other studies have suggested an association between an intake of vitamin C lower than the RDA and high blood pressure, a major risk factor for heart disease and stroke.

Vitamin C has a long history of being hailed as a cure-all for a number of diseases and conditions. When these claims were subjected to controlled studies, most of them were proved to be either exaggerated or false. While taking extra vitamin C during a cold may decrease the severity of the symptoms, large doses of vitamin C do not prevent the common cold.

RDA FOR VITAMIN C

Both sexes, age 15 years & older	60 mg

There is a widely held, but false, belief that it is not possible to get too much of the water-soluble vitamins: vitamin C and the B-complex vitamins. While research has shown toxic side effects with regularly taking large doses of vitamins A and D, it was thought that any extra water-soluble vitamins consumed would be flushed harmlessly out of the body in urine. There is now evidence suggesting that large doses of vitamin C contribute to the formation of new calcium oxalate urinary stones in some people with a history of these stones and can cause a false-positive test for sugar in the urine. In addition, some individuals taking a daily dose of 500 mg experience stomach upset, diarrhea, dry nose, or nosebleed; this amount of vitamin C is the dosage most often used by people taking a vitamin C supplement and is commonly supplied in one pill. There appears to be a wide range of individual tolerance to vitamin C, and many people are able to take 1,000 mg or more without any obvious problems. However, health experts do not recommend that people take large doses of vitamin C on a regular basis. The following table lists the most common dietary sources of vitamin C, from high to low.

VITAMIN C CONTENT OF SELECTED FOODS

Food (¼ cup)	Vitamin C mg
Peppers, hot chili, raw, chopped	181.9
Peppers, sweet, raw, chopped	64.0
Broccoli, cooked	49.0
Orange juice, frozen, reconstituted	48.5
Brussels sprouts, cooked	48.4
Orange, raw, sections	47.9
Strawberries, fresh	42.3
Grapefruit, raw, sections w/ juice	38.3
Cantaloupe, cubed	33.8
Honeydew melon, cubed	21.1
Tomatoes, ripe, raw, chopped	15.8
Collards, cooked	9.3
Potato, baked	7.8

Adapted from USDA, Composition of Foods, *Agriculture Handbook series no. 8 (Washington, D.C.: USDA, 1976–1992).*

Iron and Heart Disease

In the past the main concern of health experts with regard to iron was to avoid iron deficiency. However, a research study published in 1992 suggested a link between high levels of iron stored in the body and increased risk for heart disease. The Finnish research scientists who conducted the study suggested that one possible explanation for the increased risk is the role of iron as a catalyst in the chemical reactions producing free radicals, which in turn can lead to production of oxidized LDL. It is difficult to determine the possible importance of this finding, because several other research studies failed to show any association between high iron stores and increased risk for heart attack. Most health experts continue to support recommendations that emphasize an adequate iron intake.

There is little risk of consuming too much iron from food; however, iron supplements can easily provide high levels of iron. In the United States about 2,000 young children die of poisoning each year from consuming adult iron supplements. It is estimated that a 2-year-old child can die from ingesting about 3,000 mg of ferrous sulfate (a form of iron); a fatal dose for an adult is about 200 to 250 mg per kilogram (2.2 pounds) of body weight, or approximately 16,000 to 20,000 mg for a 180-pound man.

RDA FOR IRON

Males, age 19 years & older	10 mg
Females, age 11 through 50 years	15 mg
Females, age 51 years & older	10 mg

The RDA for women drops from 15 mg to 10 mg past age 50, which is the approximate age of menopause in women. For both sexes and all age groups, iron supplements are not recommended except when prescribed by a physician. A substantial portion of the iron in the American diet comes from foods such as bread and ready-to-eat cereals that have been fortified as a result of concern about iron deficiency. The following good sources of iron are listed from high to low.

IRON CONTENT OF SELECTED FOODS

Food	Iron mg
Clams, canned (3 oz)	23.8
Fortified oat flakes (1 cup)	13.7
100% bran (1 cup)	8.1
Oatmeal, instant, fortified (1 packet)	6.3

(continued)

Food	Iron mg
Cereals, ready-to-eat & cooked	*
Breads & rolls	*
Beef liver, braised (3 oz)	5.8
Venison, roasted (3 oz)	3.8
Molasses, blackstrap (1 tbsp)	3.5
Beef, bottom round, trimmed, braised (3 oz)	2.9
Baked potato with skin (1 medium)	2.8
Wheat germ, toasted (¼ cup)	2.6
Corn grits, regular and quick, cooked (1 cup)	1.6
Apricots, dried, uncooked (¼ cup)	1.5
Rice, white, medium-grain, cooked (½ cup)	1.4

Adapted from USDA, Composition of Foods, *Agriculture Handbook series no. 8 (Washington, D.C.: USDA, 1976–1992).*
*Iron level will vary with fortification or enrichment.
tbsp = tablespoon

Vitamin B₆ and Premenstrual Syndrome

Premenstrual syndrome, or PMS, is a group of symptoms that some women experience during the days preceding their menstrual period. While some studies have suggested that vitamin B₆ (pyridoxine) helps decrease certain physical and psychological symptoms associated with PMS, others have found it to be of no value.

The attitude of many people toward vitamin B₆ and PMS has been the same as that toward the water-soluble vitamins in general: "Even if it doesn't help, at least it can't hurt." However, this is not always true. There is evidence that consuming daily doses of vitamin B₆ averaging 117 mg per day over several months can result in disorders of the nervous system. Individual tolerance to vitamin B₆ makes it impossible to establish the level of intake above which a person will develop side effects. Side effects associated with high doses include numbing of the hands and feet, tingling and burning sensations of the skin, lack of muscle coordination, and an unsteady gait. Most of these symptoms disappear after supplementation with vitamin B₆ is discontinued; however, there have been cases of lasting damage.

RDA FOR VITAMIN B₆

Males, age 15 years & older	2.0 mg
Females, age 19 years & older	1.6 mg

The following table contains food sources of vitamin B_6, listed from high to low.

VITAMIN B_6 CONTENT OF SELECTED FOODS

Food	Vitamin B_6 mg
Beef liver, braised (3 oz)	0.77
Banana (1 medium)	0.66
Chicken breast, roasted (3 oz)	0.51
Potato, baked, skin not eaten (1 medium)	0.47
Pork loin chop, broiled (3 oz)	0.46
Halibut, cooked, dry heat (3 oz)	0.34
Chicken leg, roasted (3 oz)	0.31
Avocado (½ medium)	0.24
Rice, brown, cooked (⅔ cup)	0.19
Corn, canned (½ cup)	0.05

Adapted from USDA, Composition of Foods, *Agriculture Handbook series no. 8 (Washington, D.C.: USDA, 1976–1992).*

Folate and Health

One of the public health issues of the early 1990s has to do with women's intake of folate, one of the B-complex vitamins, and birth defects. (Folate usually refers to the form of this vitamin in food; the term folic acid is often used for the synthetic form of folate. In this discussion the term folate will be used to mean both forms unless referring specifically to the use of folic acid in fortification.) It is now widely accepted that women who have low levels of folate early in pregnancy have an increased chance of giving birth to a child with neural tube defects, such as spina bifida and anencephaly, which affect the spinal cord and brain. It is estimated that each year approximately 2,500 children are born with neural tube defects.

In October 1993 the FDA proposed that all bread and cereal products be fortified with folic acid at a level of 140 micrograms (mcg) per 100 grams (about 3½ ounces) of bread, flour, rolls, buns, corn grits, cornmeal, rice, farina, or noodles. This proposed measure is designed to help ensure that women consume at least 400 mcg of folate per day during the childbearing years from puberty to menopause; surveys show that at present most women age 19 to 50 get only 200 mcg per day. The FDA approved a health claim on food labels in regard to folic acid intake in women and prevention of neural tube defects. The health claim applies to foods naturally high in folic acid and to supplements.

Folate intake has also been studied in connection with the prevention of cervical cancer. Some studies suggest that women with low levels of folate are more likely to have abnormal cells that, if left untreated, may develop into cancer of the cervix.

Establishing a policy of folic acid supplementation presents some potential problems. Public health experts must weigh the advantages of consuming sufficient folate against certain health concerns. Some studies suggest that high folate levels may decrease the absorption of zinc and may mask the symptoms of pernicious anemia, a disease that, if left untreated, can result in permanent nerve damage. However, there is increasing evidence that a deficiency in folic acid may promote the development of atherosclerotic plaque, which can lead to heart attack or stroke. The FDA subcommittee that updated the RDAs in 1989 did not recommend that people take folate supplements except under the guidance of a physician.

RDA FOR FOLATE

Males, age 15 years & older	200 mcg
Females, age 11 years & older	180 mcg

mcg = micrograms

The RDA, which was established in 1989, is lower than the RDI, which is 400 mcg of folate per day. The following table contains dietary sources of folate, listed from high to low.

FOLATE CONTENT OF SELECTED FOODS

Food (½ cup except where noted)	Folate mcg
Oatmeal, instant, fortified (1 packet)*	150.0
Spinach, frozen	102.1
Wheat germ, toasted (¼ cup)	99.5
Orange juice from frozen concentrate	54.6
Broccoli, fresh, cooked	53.3
Turnip greens, canned	48.2
Orange sections, fresh	27.3
Tangerine juice from frozen concentrate	23.1
Wild rice, cooked	22.0
Cantaloupe, cubed	13.7
Strawberries, fresh	13.2

Adapted from USDA, Composition of Foods, *Agriculture Handbook series no. 8 (Washington, D.C.: USDA, 1976–1992).*
mcg = micrograms
*Regular oatmeal contains 7 mcg folate per ¾ cup prepared.

Calcium and Health

Calcium is the mineral present in the largest amounts in the human body. The best-known function of calcium has to do with the formation and maintenance of bone; all but 1% of the calcium in the body is found in bones and teeth. One of the primary areas of calcium research has to do with osteoporosis, a chronic disease in which bones become brittle and break easily because they have lost too much calcium. Osteoporosis, which affects as many as 20 million Americans, is a major cause of disability in older people, primarily postmenopausal women. There is general agreement among health experts that it is important for people, especially women, to get the RDA for calcium at any age. However, most of the experts do not believe that postmenopausal women can reduce their chances of developing osteoporosis simply by taking calcium supplements; calcium supplements need to be taken in conjunction with vitamin D and/or estrogen in this age group. The human body obtains vitamin D from food and through exposure to sunlight.

Another area of interest is the evidence linking a low intake of calcium to high blood pressure. At present, calcium supplementation for treatment of high blood pressure is not being recommended, although some studies suggest that increasing calcium in the diet may lower blood pressure in some people.

The RDA for calcium is shown in the table below. For purposes of food labeling, a single value of 1,000 mg is used.

RDA For Calcium	
Both sexes, age 11 through 24 years	1,200 mg
Both sexes, age 25 years & older	800 mg

A panel of scientists who met at the National Institutes of Health recommended the following calcium intakes to protect against osteoporosis; these levels are higher than the RDA for calcium.

Males	
Age 25 to 65	1,000 mg
Older than age 65	1,500 mg
Females	
Age 25 to 50	1,000 mg
Age 51 to 65, on estrogen	1,000 mg
Age 51 to 65, not on estrogen	1,500 mg
Older than age 65	1,500 mg

Females age 50 to 65 who are on estrogen have a recommendation of 1,000 mg.

The following table contains good food sources of calcium, listed from high to low.

CALCIUM CONTENT OF SELECTED FOODS

Food	Calcium mg
Yogurt, fat-free, plain (8 oz)	452
Yogurt, low-fat, w/ fruit (8 oz)	383
Milk, skim (1 cup)	302
Tofu, raw, firm (½ cup)	258
Salmon, canned, w/ bones (3 oz)	203
Cheese, fat-free (1 oz)	200
Mozzarella cheese, part-skim (1 oz)	183
Rhubarb, cooked, sweetened (½ cup)	174
Molasses, blackstrap (2 tbsp)	172
Frozen yogurt, fat-free, chocolate (½ cup)	154
Ice milk, hardened (½ cup)	92
Broccoli, fresh, cooked (½ cup)	89
Cottage cheese, 1% fat (½ cup)	69

Adapted from USDA, Composition of Foods, Agriculture Handbook series no. 8 (Washington, D.C.: USDA, 1976–1992), and from Nutrition Data Systems, University of Minnesota, Minneapolis.
tbsp — tablespoon

Zinc and Health

Nutrition surveys of food intake have shown that many Americans, especially women and young children, may be at risk for mild or moderate zinc deficiency; severe zinc deficiency is rare in the United States. Although zinc is a trace mineral—that is, a mineral needed only in tiny amounts—it is essential to many vital metabolic pathways, and any deficiency may have serious consequences to health. It appears to be safe to take most vitamins at levels several times their RDAs, but the margin of safety for many minerals is much smaller. For example, at a daily intake of just above the RDA (18.5 to 25 mg), zinc has been shown to lead to a copper deficiency. A daily zinc intake of 5 times the RDA decreases levels of HDL-cholesterol in the blood; at levels from 10 to 30 times the RDA, abnormally small red blood cells appear and there is a decrease in white blood cells, impairing the body's immune responses.

RDA FOR ZINC

Males, age 11 years & older	15 mg
Females, age 11 years & older	12 mg

The following table lists foods containing zinc, from high to low.

ZINC CONTENT OF SELECTED FOODS

Food (3 oz except where noted)	Zinc mg
Oysters, eastern, cooked, moist heat	62.6
Oysters, Pacific, cooked, moist heat	28.3
Liver, beef, braised	5.2
Wheat germ, toasted (¼ cup)	4.7
Beef, ground, extra-lean, broiled	4.6
Turkey, dark meat	3.8
Crab, blue, canned	3.4
Pecans, dry-roasted (2 oz, or about 30 halves)	3.2
Lobster, cooked, moist heat	2.5
Cheese, ricotta, part-skim (½ cup)	1.7

Adapted from USDA, Composition of Foods, *Agriculture Handbook series no. 8 (Washington, D.C.: USDA, 1976–1992).*

Phytochemicals

Numerous studies have reported that eating more fruits and vegetables is associated with a decrease in cancer risk. The exact source of the protective effect of fruits and vegetables is the subject of much research. Recently, there has been a growing interest in a number of nutritive components called phytochemicals (plant chemicals), which are found in many plant foods. Some studies suggest that these phytochemicals may have important functions in the body, especially in reducing risk for certain cancers. Only a relative few of the thousands of phytochemicals in food have been studied as yet. Among phytochemicals being studied at the time of this printing are those listed below.

PHYTOCHEMICALS

Phytochemical	Food Sources
Allyl sulfides	Garlic & onions
Capsaicin	Chili peppers (hot)
Chlorogenic acid	Tomatoes, green peppers, pineapple, strawberries, & carrots
Ellagic acid	Strawberries, raspberries, & grapes
Flavonoids	Most fruits & vegetables
Genistein	Soybeans
Indole-3-carbinol	Broccoli, cauliflower, & cabbage
p-Coumaric acid	Tomatoes, green peppers, pineapple, strawberries, & carrots
Phenethyl isothiocyanate (PEITC)	Cabbage & turnips
Phytic acid	Grains
Sulforaphane	Broccoli, cauliflower, brussels sprouts, kale, & turnips

The Living Heart
Diet Menus

The menus on the following pages provide maximum flexibility for planning meals. You can choose from 24 breakfast menus, 24 lunch menus, and 24 dinner menus. They can be combined according to your food preferences. The menus provide an easy way to plan a daily intake that is low to moderate in calories, very low to moderate in fat, low in cholesterol, and low to moderate in sodium.

Menus are provided at two different calorie levels for breakfast, lunch, and dinner. The *average* number of calories appears at the top of each set of breakfast, lunch, and dinner menus. The breakfast menus provide about 360 calories each (pages 188–90) or about 500 calories each (pages 194–96). The lunch and dinner menus provide about 570 calories each (pages 190–194) or about 750 calories each (pages 196–200). The lunch and dinner menus are interchangeable—that is, you can substitute a lunch menu for a dinner menu. You can use various combinations of breakfast, lunch, and dinner menus to achieve several calorie levels; examples of combinations are:

	CALORIES	CALORIES	CALORIES	CALORIES
Breakfast	360	360	500	500
Lunch	570	570	570	750
Dinner	570	750	750	750
Total calories	1,500	1,680	1,820	2,000

Many of the recipes in this book have been incorporated into the menus and are indicated by bold print. The nutrient information with each menu is provided for individuals who are counting calories (see pages 73–74), grams of fat and saturated fat (see pages 42–50), or milligrams of sodium (see pages 93–104). For each of the menus, calories can be decreased by reducing the serving sizes or increased by consuming larger servings or by eating additional low-fat foods.

LOW-FAT DIET

Any combination of three menus (breakfast, lunch, and dinner) provides less than 30% of calories from fat, less than 10% of calories from saturated fat, and less than 300 milligrams of cholesterol— that is, conform to the Step I Diet.

VERY LOW FAT DIET

If you are following a very low fat diet, you will need to choose menus providing very low levels of fat. For example, if you consume 1,800 calories per day and your goal is to keep your fat intake at 20% of calories, your maximum grams of fat should be 40. You can use the menus on pages 188–200 to select meals that total 40 grams of fat or less.

LOW-SODIUM DIET

Because a variety of foods and recipes are used in the menus, some of the menus provide more sodium than others. If you select a menu for lunch that is moderately high in sodium, you can compensate by choosing a dinner menu that is lower in sodium. To make choosing lower-sodium meals easier, the menus are arranged from lowest to highest in sodium on each page.

VEGETARIAN DIET

Most of the breakfast menus and several of the lunch and dinner menus do not include meat, poultry, or fish. Recipes for the meatless entrées in the menus are found in this book on pages 244–58.

SNACKS

For simplicity, the following menus are for breakfast, lunch, and dinner only. However, you may wish to save food from meals to eat as a snack. Additional snacks will increase your calorie level.

QUICK AND EASY MENUS

Most of the menus are quick and easy to prepare. The menus that require the least amount of time to prepare are labeled "Quick and Easy." Some of the quick and easy breakfast and lunch menus incorporate the use of frozen single foods (waffles) and meals (pasta dinner). To select a brand of frozen food that is low in fat, saturated fat, and cholesterol, use the guidelines on pages 140–51.

HOLIDAY MENUS

Holiday menus that are lower than traditional holiday meals in calories, fat, saturated fat, cholesterol, and sodium are shown on pages 200 and 201. Recipes printed in bold are from this book.

Breakfast Menus with About 360 Calories Each

Quick and Easy
Oat bran flakes, 1 cup
Brown sugar, 1 tbsp
Skim milk, 1 cup

Cal	Fat g	Sat Fat g	Chol mg	Sod mg
336	3	1	4	136

Quick and Easy
Banana, 1
English muffin, 1
Peanut butter, 1 tbsp

Cal	Fat g	Sat Fat g	Chol mg	Sod mg
355	12	3	2	137

Quick and Easy
Orange juice, ½ cup
Fat-free waffles, 2 (commercially frozen type)
Lite syrup, 3 tbsp

Cal	Fat g	Sat Fat g	Chol mg	Sod mg
378	0	0	0	314

Quick and Easy
Banana, 1
Pancake, 1 (commercially frozen type)
Maple syrup, 2 tbsp
Skim milk, 1 cup

Cal	Fat g	Sat Fat g	Chol mg	Sod mg
378	2	1	5	322

(continued)

tbsp = tablespoon

Breakfast Menus with About 360 Calories Each (cont.)

Quick and Easy
Grapefruit, ⅙
Oatmeal,* 1 cup
Skim milk, 1 cup
Whole-wheat toast, 1 slice
Margarine, 1 tsp

Cal	Fat g	Sat Fat g	Chol mg	Sod mg
361	8	1	4	326

Quick and Easy
Blueberries, ½ cup
Shredded wheat, ¾ cup
Whole-wheat toast, 1 slice
Margarine, 1 tsp
Skim milk, 1 cup

Cal	Fat g	Sat Fat g	Chol mg	Sod mg
346	6	1	4	334

Quick and Easy
Orange juice, 1 cup
English muffin, 1
Margarine, 2 tsp
Jelly, 1 tbsp

Cal	Fat g	Sat Fat g	Chol mg	Sod mg
359	9	2	0	377

Strawberry slices, 1½ cups
Date Bran Muffin, 1
Margarine, 2 tsp
Skim milk, 1 cup

Cal	Fat g	Sat Fat g	Chol mg	Sod mg
350	11	2	5	468

Quick and Easy
Cinnamon-raisin bagel, 1
Low-fat cream cheese, 2 tbsp
Skim milk, 1 cup

Cal	Fat g	Sat Fat g	Chol mg	Sod mg
333	7	4	22	595

Pineapple, 2 slices
Egg and Sausage Burritos, 1 serving
Skim milk, 1½ cups

Cal	Fat g	Sat Fat g	Chol mg	Sod mg
375	4	1	17	783

(continued)

Boldprint = recipe in this book.   *tbsp = tablespoon*   *No salt added in preparation.*
tsp = teaspoon

Breakfast Menus with About 360 Calories Each (cont.)

Cantaloupe, ¼ of 5″ diameter
Breakfast Casserole, 1 serving
Skim milk, 1 cup

Cal	Fat g	Sat Fat g	Chol mg	Sod mg
376	8	3	54	815

Omelet, 1 serving
Whole-wheat toast, 1 slice
Margarine, 1 tsp
Skim milk, 1 cup

Cal	Fat g	Sat Fat g	Chol mg	Sod mg
388	12	4	32	1,336

Lunch Menus with About 570 Calories Each

Low-Sodium Black Bean Soup, 1 serving
Southwest Chicken Salad, 1 serving
Apple, 1

Cal	Fat g	Sat Fat g	Chol mg	Sod mg
584	13	2	67	528

Cottage Cheese–Spinach Casserole,
  3 servings
Onion Bread Squares, 1 serving
Apple, 1

Cal	Fat g	Sat Fat g	Chol mg	Sod mg
554	16	6	39	680

Quick and Easy
Quick and Easy Clam Mushroom Bisque,
  1 serving
Tossed salad with tomato, 1 cup
Avocado, ¼
Caribbean Dressing, 2 tbsp
French roll, 1
Fig bar, 1

Cal	Fat g	Sat Fat g	Chol mg	Sod mg
567	19	3	69	575

Quick and Easy
Frozen pasta with vegetables dinner,
  1 package
Breadsticks, 5
Grapes, 1 cup
Skim milk, 1 cup

Cal	Fat g	Sat Fat g	Chol mg	Sod mg
563	6	2	34	804

(continued)

Boldprint = recipe in this book.   *tbsp = tablespoon*
                                        tsp = teaspoon

Lunch Menus with About 570 Calories Each (cont.)

Meat Loaf, 1 serving
Steamed broccoli,* 1 cup
Mashed potatoes,† ½ cup
Lime sorbet, ½ cup

Cal	Fat g	Sat Fat g	Chol mg	Sod mg
587	15	4	66	828

Quick and Easy
Pop-top can tuna packed in water, 3 oz
Mayonnaise, 1 tbsp
Saltine crackers, 6
Carrot sticks, 4
Celery sticks, 4
Low-fat yogurt with fruit, 8 oz

Cal	Fat g	Sat Fat g	Chol mg	Sodium mg
561	18	4	53	861

Capellini in Red Clam Sauce with
   Parmesan, 1 serving
Steamed zucchini and yellow squash,* ½ cup
French roll, 1
Margarine, 1 tsp
Pear, 1 large

Cal	Fat g	Sat Fat g	Chol mg	Sod mg
579	12	3	25	927

Pasta Salmon Salad with Dill, 1 serving
Melba toast, 6
Dilled Cucumbers, 1 serving
Fruit cocktail, canned in juice, 1 cup

Cal	Fat g	Sat Fat g	Chol mg	Sod mg
569	11	2	39	1,021

Fat-Free Fried Chicken, 1 serving
Living Heart Fettuccine Alfredo, 1 serving
Tossed salad with tomato, 1 cup
Italian Dressing, 2 tbsp
Dinner roll, 1

Cal	Fat g	Sat Fat g	Chol mg	Sod mg
585	16	5	123	1,032

Chicken Fajitas, 1 serving
Fat-free sour cream, 2 tbsp
Southwestern Beans, 1 serving
Shredded lettuce, ½ cup
Chopped tomato, ¼ cup
Guacamole, ¼ cup
Tangerine, 1 large

Cal	Fat g	Sat Fat g	Chol mg	Sod mg
562	13	1	58	1,077

(continued)

Boldprint = recipe in this book.   tbsp = tablespoon   *No salt added in preparation.*
                                      tsp = teaspoon   †*Prepared with skim milk, margarine, and salt.*

Lunch Menus with About 570 Calories Each (cont.)

Quick and Easy

Turkey sandwich
  Wheat bread, 2 slices
  Turkey breast, processed, 2 oz
  Mayonnaise, 1 tbsp
  Tomato, 3 thin slices
  Lettuce, 2 leaves
Angel food cake, 1/12 of 10″ diameter
Frozen fat-free yogurt, ½ cup
Strawberry slices, 1 cup

Cal	Fat g	Sat Fat g	Chol mg	Sod mg
546	17	3	34	1,213

Spinach Quiche, 3 servings
Tossed salad with tomato, 1 cup
Italian Dressing, 2 tbsp
French roll, 1
Margarine, 1 tsp
Peach, canned, packed in juice, 1 cup

Cal	Fat g	Sat Fat g	Chol mg	Sod mg
578	11	5	9	1,231

Dinner Menus with About 570 Calories Each

Lemon Chicken Breast with Mushrooms,
  1 serving
Herbed rice,* ½ cup
Ginger Carrots, 1 serving
Pineapple Freeze, 1 serving

Cal	Fat g	Sat Fat g	Chol mg	Sod mg
533	11	3	77	283

Quick and Easy

Baked potato, 1 large
  Salsa, ¼ cup
  Low-fat cheese, 1 slice
Fat-free whole-wheat crackers, 4
Fruit salad, 1 cup
Skim milk, 1 cup

Cal	Fat g	Sat Fat g	Chol mg	Sod mg
564	7	3	19	625

Veal Scaloppine, 1 serving
Linguine, plain,* 1 cup
Asparagus pieces,* 1 cup
Margarine, 1 tsp for vegetables
Sorbet, ½ cup

Cal	Fat g	Sat Fat g	Chol mg	Sod mg
557	13	3	74	395

Marinated Pork Tenderloin, 1 serving
Cornbread Dressing with pecans, 1 serving
Steamed Brussels sprouts,* 1½ cups
Heavenly Hash, 1 serving

Cal	Fat g	Sat Fat g	Chol mg	Sod mg
554	11	4	115	725

(continued)

Boldprint = recipe in this book.   *tbsp = tablespoon*   **No salt added in preparation.*
                                       tsp = teaspoon

Dinner Menus with About 570 Calories Each (cont.)

Crispy Corny Baked Chicken, 1 serving
Fresh Green Beans and Tomatoes,
   2 servings
Whole-kernel corn,* 1 cup
Blueberries, 1 cup

Cal	Fat g	Sat Fat g	Chol mg	Sod mg
555	9	2	74	810

Mexican Lasagna, 1 serving
Steamed broccoli with lemon juice,* 2 spears
Dinner roll, 1
Cheesecake, 1 serving

Cal	Fat g	Sat Fat g	Chol mg	Sod mg
575	14	6	28	821

Low-Sodium Fish Ragout, 1 serving
Low-Sodium Cornbread, 1 serving
Baked Apple, 1 serving
Skim milk, 1½ cups

Cal	Fat g	Sat Fat g	Chol mg	Sod mg
585	11	3	55	836

Italian Lasagna, 2 servings
Tossed salad with tomato, 2 cups
Italian Dressing, 2 tbsp
French roll, 1
Banana Oatmeal Cookie, 1

Cal	Fat g	Sat Fat g	Chol mg	Sod mg
582	20	9	60	847

Quick and Easy
Quick and Easy Mexican Soup, 2 servings
Melba toast, 4
Tossed salad with tomato, 2 cups
Apple-Cider Vinaigrette Dressing, 1½ tbsp
Frozen fat-free yogurt, ½ cup

Cal	Fat g	Sat Fat g	Chol mg	Sod mg
560	12	2	58	949

Quick and Easy
Quick and Easy Spinach Lasagna, 1 serving
Tomato and cucumber salad, 1½ cups
C'est la Vie Dressing, 2 tbsp
Skim milk, 1½ cups
Cherries, 20

Cal	Fat g	Sat Fat g	Chol mg	Sod mg
569	9	3	25	985

(continued)

Boldprint = recipe in this book.   *tbsp = tablespoon*   **No salt added in preparation.*

Dinner Menus with About 570 Calories Each (cont.)

Living Heart Pepper Steak with rice,
  1 serving
Tossed salad with tomato, 2 cups
Oriental Dressing, 2 tbsp
Unsweetened applesauce, ½ cup

Cal	Fat g	Sat Fat g	Chol mg	Sod mg
572	10	2	75	1,106

Quick and Easy
Quick and Easy Salad Pizza, 2 slices
Mango, ½

Cal	Fat g	Sat Fat g	Chol mg	Sod mg
594	17	7	33	1,382

Breakfast Menus with About 500 Calories Each

Quick and Easy
Grapefruit juice, 1½ cups
Oat bran flakes, 1 cup
Brown sugar, 1 tbsp
Skim milk, 1 cup

Cal	Fat g	Sat Fat g	Chol mg	Sod mg
480	3	1	4	139

Quick and Easy
Banana, 1
Fat-free waffles, 2 (commercially
  frozen type)
Lite syrup, 3 tbsp
Low-fat yogurt with fruit, 8 oz

Cal	Fat g	Sat Fat g	Chol mg	Sod mg
509	1	0	3	412

Quick and Easy
Banana, 1
English muffin, 1
Peanut butter, 1 tbsp
Low-fat yogurt with fruit, 8 oz

Cal	Fat g	Sat Fat g	Chol mg	Sod mg
505	13	3	7	232

Quick and Easy
Orange juice, 1 cup
English muffin, 1
Margarine, 2 tsp
Jelly, 1 tbsp
Low-fat yogurt with fruit, 8 oz

Cal	Fat g	Sat Fat g	Chol mg	Sod mg
509	9	2	5	472

(continued)

Boldprint = recipe in this book.   *tbsp = tablespoon*
                                        tsp = teaspoon

Breakfast Menus with About 500 Calories Each (cont.)

Quick and Easy
Grapefruit, ½
English muffin, 1
Margarine, 2 tsp
Jelly, 1 tbsp
Oatmeal,* 1 cup
Skim milk, 1 cup

Cal	Fat g	Sat Fat g	Chol mg	Sod mg
503	12	2	4	500

Quick and Easy
Banana, 1
Pancakes, 2 (commercially frozen type)
Maple syrup, 3 tbsp
Skim milk, 1 cup

Cal	Fat g	Sat Fat g	Chol mg	Sod mg
511	4	1	6	513

Quick and Easy
Blueberries, ½ cup
Shredded wheat, ¾ cup
Whole-wheat toast, 2 slices
Margarine, 2 tsp
Jelly, 1 tbsp
Skim milk, 1 cup

Cal	Fat g	Sat Fat g	Chol mg	Sod mg
493	11	2	4	542

Quick and Easy
Pineapple juice, 1 cup
Cinnamon raisin bagel, 1
Low-fat cream cheese, 2 tbsp
Skim milk, 1 cup

Cal	Fat g	Sat Fat g	Chol mg	Sod mg
473	7	4	22	597

Strawberry slices, 1½ cups
Date Bran Muffins, 2
Margarine, 2 tsp
Skim milk, 1 cup

Cal	Fat g	Sat Fat g	Chol mg	Sod mg
480	15	2	4	706

Pineapple, 2 slices
Egg and Sausage Burritos, 1 serving
Southwestern Beans, 1 serving
Skim milk, 1½ cups

Cal	Fat g	Sat Fat g	Chol mg	Sod mg
496	6	1	17	1,174

(continued)

Boldprint = recipe in this book.　　tbsp = tablespoon　　*No salt added in preparation.
tsp = teaspoon

Breakfast Menus with About 500 Calories Each (cont.)

Grapes, 1 cup
Omelet, 1 serving
Whole-wheat toast, 1 slice
Margarine, 1 tsp
Skim milk, 1 cup

Cal	Fat g	Sat Fat g	Chol mg	Sod mg
502	13	4	32	1,339

Cantaloupe, ¼ of 5″ diameter
Breakfast Casserole, 2 servings

Cal	Fat g	Sat Fat g	Chol mg	Sod mg
533	16	6	100	1,366

Lunch Menus with About 750 Calories Each

Quick and Easy

Frozen pasta with vegetables dinner,
   1 package
Breadsticks, 5
Low-fat yogurt with fruit, 8 oz
Grapes, 2 cups

Cal	Fat g	Sat Fat g	Chol mg	Sod mg
760	8	4	40	801

Quick and Easy

Quick and Easy Clam Mushroom Bisque,
   1 serving
Tossed salad with tomato, 1 cup
Avocado, ¼
Caribbean Dressing, 2 tbsp
French roll, 1
Fig bars, 2
Skim milk, 1½ cups

Cal	Fat g	Sat Fat g	Chol mg	Sod mg
752	21	4	75	820

Low-Sodium Black Bean Soup, 1 serving
Southwest Chicken Salad, 1 serving
Saltine crackers, 6
Apple, 1
Skim milk, 1 cup

Cal	Fat g	Sat Fat g	Chol mg	Sod mg
748	15	2	71	888

Quick and Easy

Pop-top can tuna packed in water, 3 oz
Mayonnaise, 1 tbsp
Whole-wheat bread, 2 slices
Carrot sticks, 4
Celery sticks, 4
Low-fat yogurt with fruit, 8 oz
Cantaloupe, ½ of 5″ diameter

Cal	Fat g	Sat Fat g	Chol mg	Sod mg
717	19	5	53	948

(continued)

Boldprint = recipe in this book.   *tbsp = tablespoon*
tsp = teaspoon

Lunch Menus with About 750 Calories Each (cont.)

Cottage Cheese–Spinach Casserole,
  3 servings
Onion Bread Squares, 2 servings
Apple, 1
Skim milk, 1½ cups

Cal	Fat g	Sat Fat g	Chol mg	Sod mg
778	19	6	15	1,011

Fat-Free Fried Chicken, 1 serving
Living Heart Fettuccine Alfredo, 1 serving
Tossed salad with tomato, 1 cup
Italian Dressing, 2 tbsp
Dinner roll, 1
Margarine, 1 tsp
Sorbet, ½ cup

Cal	Fat g	Sat Fat g	Chol mg	Sod mg
732	20	6	123	1,079

Pasta Salmon Salad with Dill, 1 serving
Melba toast, 6
Dilled Cucumbers, 1 serving
Apple, sliced, 1
Creamy Cinnamon Dip, 2 tbsp
Skim milk, 1½ cups

Cal	Fat g	Sat Fat g	Chol mg	Sod mg
751	15	4	52	1,339

Capellini with Red Clam Sauce
  with Parmesan, 2 servings
Steamed zucchini and yellow squash,* ½ cup
Pear, 1 large

Cal	Fat g	Sat Fat g	Chol mg	Sod mg
804	10	2	50	1,468

Spinach Quiche, 3 servings
Tossed salad with tomato, 3 cups
Italian Dressing, 4 tbsp
French rolls, 2
Margarine, 2 tsp
Peach, canned, packed in juice, 1 cup

Cal	Fat g	Sat Fat g	Chol mg	Sod mg
747	19	7	10	1,509

Meat Loaf, 1 serving
Steamed broccoli,* 1 cup
Mashed potatoes,† ¾ cup
Key Lime Pie, 1 serving

Cal	Fat g	Sat Fat g	Chol mg	Sod mg
807	22	5	135	1,534

(continued)

Boldprint = recipe in this book.   *tbsp = tablespoon*   *No salt added in preparation.*
                                                    tsp = teaspoon

Lunch Menus with About 750 Calories Each (cont.)

Quick and Easy
Turkey sandwich
 Wheat bread, 2 slices
 Turkey breast, processed, 3 oz
 Mayonnaise, 1 tbsp
 Tomato, 3 thin slices
 Lettuce, 2 leaves
Angel food cake, $\frac{1}{12}$ of 10″ diameter
Frozen fat-free yogurt, $1\frac{1}{2}$ cups
Strawberry slices, 1 cup

Cal	Fat g	Sat Fat g	Chol mg	Sod mg
775	18	3	49	1,590

Chicken Fajitas, 1 serving
Fat-free sour cream, 2 tbsp
Southwestern Beans, 2 servings
Shredded lettuce, $\frac{1}{2}$ cup
Chopped tomato, $\frac{1}{4}$ cup
Guacamole, 2 servings
Rice Pudding, 1 serving

Cal	Fat g	Sat Fat g	Chol mg	Sod mg
791	13	1	59	1,651

Dinner Menus with About 750 Calories Each

Lemon Chicken Breast with Mushrooms,
 1 serving
Herbed rice,* 1 cup
Ginger Carrots, 1 serving
Dinner roll, 1
Margarine, 1 tsp
Pineapple Freeze, 2 servings

Cal	Fat g	Sat Fat g	Chol mg	Sod mg
720	17	5	77	476

Veal Scaloppine, 2 servings
Linguine, plain,* 1 cup
Asparagus pieces,* 1 cup
Margarine, 1 tsp for vegetables
Sorbet, $\frac{1}{2}$ cup

Cal	Fat g	Sat Fat g	Chol mg	Sod mg
734	20	5	148	728

Quick and Easy
Baked potato, 1 large stuffed with:
 Salsa, $\frac{1}{4}$ cup
 Low-fat cheese, 1 slice
Fat-free whole-wheat crackers, 5
Fruit salad, $1\frac{1}{2}$ cups
Skim milk, 1 cup
Souper Raisin Cake with nuts, 1 serving

Cal	Fat g	Sat Fat g	Chol mg	Sod mg
745	10	3	19	839

Italian Lasagna, 2 servings
Tossed salad with tomato, 2 cups
Italian Dressing, 2 tbsp
French roll, 1
Margarine, 1 tsp
Banana Oatmeal Cookies, 3

Cal	Fat g	Sat Fat g	Chol mg	Sod mg
738	28	10	60	1,021

Boldprint = recipe in this book.   *tbsp = tablespoon*   **No salt added in preparation.*   **(continued)**
                                      tsp = teaspoon   *†Prepared with skim milk, margarine, and salt.*

Dinner Menus with About 750 Calories Each (cont.)

Crispy Corny Baked Chicken, 1 serving
Fresh Green Beans and Tomatoes, 2 servings
Whole-kernel corn,* 1 cup
Swirled Blueberry Pie, 1 serving

Cal	Fat g	Sat Fat g	Chol mg	Sod mg
786	15	5	82	1,021

Marinated Pork Tenderloin, 3 servings
Cornbread Dressing with pecans, 1 serving
Steamed Brussels sprouts,* 1½ cups
Heavenly Hash, 1 serving

Cal	Fat g	Sat Fat g	Chol mg	Sod mg
753	16	6	218	1,047

Quick and Easy
Quick and Easy Mexican Soup, 2 servings
Melba toast, 4
Tossed salad with tomato, 2 cups
Apple-Cider Vinaigrette Dressing, 1½ tbsp
Frozen fat-free yogurt, 1½ cups

Cal	Fat g	Sat Fat g	Chol mg	Sod mg
759	12	2	61	1,049

Mexican Lasagna, 2 servings
Steamed broccoli with lemon juice,* 2 spears
Dinner roll, 1
Cheesecake, 1 serving

Cal	Fat g	Sat Fat g	Chol mg	Sod mg
786	21	9	43	1,186

Living Heart Pepper Steak with Rice, 1 serving
Tossed salad with tomato, 2 cups
Oriental Dressing, 2 tbsp
Apple Orange Crumb, 2 servings

Cal	Fat g	Sat Fat g	Chol mg	Sod mg
757	18	4	75	1,194

Low-Sodium Fish Ragout, 2 servings
Cornbread, 1 serving
Baked Apple, 1 serving
Skim milk, 1½ cups

Cal	Fat g	Sat Fat g	Chol mg	Sod mg
729	15	4	103	1,237

(continued)

Boldprint = recipe in this book.   tbsp = tablespoon   *No salt added in preparation.*

Dinner Menus with About 750 Calories Each (cont.)

Quick and Easy

Quick and Easy Spinach Lasagna,
   2 servings
Tomato and cucumber salad,* 1½ cups
C'est la Vie Dressing, 2 tbsp
Cherries, 30

Cal	Fat g	Sat Fat g	Chol mg	Sod mg
763	14	6	38	1,259

Quick and Easy

Quick and Easy Salad Pizza, 2 slices
Skim milk, 1½ cups
Mango, ½

Cal	Fat g	Sat Fat g	Chol mg	Sod mg
723	17	8	40	1,571

Boldprint = recipe in this book.   *tbsp = tablespoon*   **No salt added in preparation.*

HOLIDAY MENU

Living Heart Wassail
Stuffed Mushroom Caps
Roasted Turkey
Cornbread Dressing
Corn Pudding
Fresh Green Beans and Tomatoes
Heavenly Hash
Creamy Cranberry Salad
Dinner Roll
Margarine
Swirled Pumpkin Pie
Coffee
Tea

Cal	Fat g	Sat Fat g	Chol mg	Sod mg
1,176	28	10	97	1,570

Boldprint = recipe in this book. Nutrient analysis includes one serving of each recipe, 3 ounces of fresh-cooked turkey, and 1 teaspoon margarine.

HOLIDAY MENU

Quick and Easy Clam Mushroom Bisque
Baked Ham
Spicy Sweet Potatoes
Broccoli Soufflé
Dinner roll
Margarine
Cranberry Bundt Cake
Frozen Pumpkin Pie
Coffee
Tea

Cal	Fat g	Sat Fat g	Chol mg	Sod mg
1,047	28	10	121	2,265

Boldprint = recipe in this book. Nutrient analysis includes one serving of each recipe, 3 ounces of ham, and 1 teaspoon of margarine.

The Living Heart Diet Recipes

All the recipes in this book are moderately low in calories, fat, saturated fat, cholesterol, and sodium. With the exception of the entrées, most of the recipes provide no more than 3 grams of fat per serving; most of the entrées provide no more than 9 grams of fat per serving.

Except for the entrées, almost all the recipes contain less than 360 mg of sodium; most of the entrées contain less than 480 mg of sodium. Low-sodium variations are included for most of the recipes that exceed these guidelines. The following footnote is included for most of the recipes that exceed the guidelines and do not have a low-sodium variation: *This recipe is high in sodium; select other foods throughout the day that are very low in sodium.*

Ingredients used in the recipes were selected using the guidelines that begin on page 140. For example, when a recipe calls for oil, you can use any oil that meets the guideline of no more than 2 grams of saturated fat per tablespoon; these oils include canola, olive, safflower, sunflower, corn, and soybean.

Information on exchanges is provided for each recipe that is appropriate for a diabetic to use. Recipes that contain more sugar than is recommended for a diabetic diet have the following note instead of exchange information: *Not applicable for this recipe.* Many of the recipes in this book have been included in the Living Heart Diet menus, which begin on page 186.

Preparation of Dried Legumes

1. Sort through the dried legumes carefully, removing any rocks and moldy or discolored beans.
2. Place the dried legumes in a colander and rinse thoroughly with cold water. Use one of the following methods for cooking legumes:

Overnight Soaking Method	*Boiling and Cooking Method*	*Pressure Cooking Method*
3. In a large container, soak the washed legumes overnight (preferably in the refrigerator) in water 3 to 4 times their volume.	3. In a large saucepan, place the washed legumes in water 3 to 4 times their volume and bring to a full boil. Continue boiling for 2 minutes.	3. Place the washed legumes in a pressure cooker with water 3 to 4 times their volume.
4. Transfer the soaked legumes and the water used for soaking to a large saucepan.	4. Remove from heat. Cover tightly and let stand for 1 hour or more.	4. Cover and bring the pressure cooker to 15 pounds of pressure.
5. Heat the legumes and liquid to boiling. Lower the heat and simmer, partially covered (adding water if necessary), until the legumes are tender and well done. See package for cooking times.	5. Same as for the overnight soaking method.	5. Length of cooking time varies by legume (see package). Cook as directed and cool immediately.

6. Drain the cooked legumes. They are now ready for use in any recipe.

Helpful Hints: It is important that legumes be covered with liquid at all times—both during soaking and during cooking. Oil the inside and top edge of the pan to prevent liquid from boiling over. Keep the saucepan partially uncovered during cooking—the legumes will boil over if the saucepan is tightly covered. Do not add salt to the legumes until they have cooked to the desired tenderness; adding salt during cooking may make them tough. Save the drained liquid to use as a base for soups or gravies.

Tofu

Tofu, also known as soybean curd, is made from curdled soy milk, extracted from ground cooked soybeans. Tofu is an excellent source of protein and contains no cholesterol; it is a good substitute for meat. Fresh tofu packed in water may be purchased in the produce section of most supermarkets.

We recommend that you try fresh tofu before trying the canned, dried, or frozen varieties. Fresh tofu has a very mild, subtle flavor and a soft, light texture, slightly denser than gelatin and less dense than soft cheese. The texture varies slightly from brand to brand. Very soft tofu crumbles easily and is not as satisfactory for cutting into small cubes as a denser, drier tofu. As soon as you bring tofu home, rinse it in cold water and repack it in your own container (plastic, glass, or stainless steel, not aluminum), covering it completely with cold water. Tofu should have very little odor; if it has a strong or sour smell, return it to the store because it is probably spoiled. Keep tofu refrigerated at all times; it should remain fresh for at least a week. Rinse the tofu every 2 days and cover it with cold water to preserve its fresh, delicate flavor. As tofu ages, it develops a stronger taste and aroma. Older tofu may be used in more strongly flavored dishes in which the slightly stronger taste will not be noticed. To restore the freshness of tofu, cut the tofu into cubes, place it in enough cold water to cover it, bring it to a boil, and allow it to simmer over low heat for a few minutes.

If tofu is beginning to age and you are not ready to use it, place it in a plastic bag and freeze it for up to 3 months. Tofu that has been frozen is somewhat drier than fresh tofu and rather meat-like, a characteristic many people prefer.

Because tofu has such a mild flavor, it is frequently marinated or combined with other foods. It has an exceptional ability to absorb flavors and will taste almost exactly like the seasoned sauce in which it is cooked or marinated. For example, marinate cubes of tofu for about half an hour in soy sauce plus vinegar, then combine the marinated tofu with stir-fried vegetables. You can broil or sauté tofu in seasoned liquid for a simple side dish, or combine it with almost any vegetable. You can broil an entire cake of tofu whole, or cut it into 1-inch cubes, which will allow it to absorb more of the sauce. Tofu cubes that have been creatively marinated add a nice flavor to fruit or vegetable salads. Plain tofu cubes make an excellent appetizer when served with several dipping sauces.

Before using tofu in any recipe, drain excess water that has accumulated in the tofu cake by placing it on a paper towel for 15 to 30 minutes.

CRUMBLED TOFU

Crumbled tofu is very similar in texture to crumbly cooked hamburger and can be used in place of hamburger in your favorite recipes.

1. Combine tofu and 2 cups of water in a saucepan. Break the tofu into very small pieces with a wooden spoon or spatula while bringing the water to a boil. Cook until tofu is heated through.

2. Place a colander in the sink and line it with a large cloth. Pour the heated tofu onto the cloth. Hold the corners of the cloth to form a sack, then twist closed. Press the sack of tofu firmly against the bottom of the

colander, expelling as much water as possible. Empty the pressed tofu into a large bowl and cool for several minutes.

3. With fingertips or a spoon, crumble the tofu into very small pieces.

PRESSED TOFU

1. Drain tofu and place it on top of a dry towel.

2. Cover the tofu with another dry towel and place a 2- to 3-pound weight on top.

3. Replace the damp towels with dry ones after 30 minutes. Press the tofu for a minimum of 60 minutes.

Appetizers

TRAIL MIX

3 cups air-popped popcorn, prepared with
   no fat

½ cup dried apricot halves, quartered

½ cup diced dried pineapple

½ cup raisins

½ cup dates

¼ cup pecan pieces

1.   Preheat oven to 350°F.

2.   Combine all ingredients and mix well.

3.   Line jelly roll pan or cookie sheet with foil;
spread popcorn and fruit mixture.

4.   Bake 10 minutes.

Yield: 5 cups

¼ cup contains:

Cal	Carb g	Fat g	Sat Fat g	Chol mg	Sod mg	Fib g
107	23	2	0	0	4	2

Exchanges: Not applicable for this recipe

GUACAMOLE

2 cups frozen green peas, thawed

2 avocados, peeled and pitted

2 tomatoes, diced

½ small onion, finely chopped

2 tablespoons lemon juice

1 jalapeño pepper, seeded and chopped

1.   Purée peas in blender or food processor until
smooth.

2.   Mash avocados with fork or potato masher to
desired consistency.

3.   Add peas and mix well.

4.   Stir in tomatoes, onion, lemon juice, and
jalapeño.

5.   Refrigerate 4 hours or overnight to allow flavors to blend. Garnish with lemon slices and
serve with baked tortilla chips.

Yield: 12 servings

¼ cup contains:

Cal	Carb g	Fat g	Sat Fat g	Chol mg	Sod mg	Fib g
70	7	5	1	0	24	3

Exchanges: ¼ cup = 1 vegetable, 1 fat

Abbreviations: Cal = Calories; Carb = Carbohydrates; Sat Fat = Saturated Fat; Chol = Cholesterol; Sod = Sodium; Fib = Fiber; < = less than.

BROCCOLI CHEESE DIP

1 tablespoon tub margarine

2 cloves garlic, minced

2 stalks celery, chopped

1 small onion, chopped

¼ pound fresh mushrooms, chopped

¼ cup all-purpose flour

2 cups skim milk

10 ounces processed yellow cheese (no more than 5 grams fat per ounce)

1 package (10 ounces) frozen chopped broccoli, cooked and drained

2 drops Tabasco

⅛ teaspoon ground red pepper (cayenne pepper)

⅛ teaspoon Worcestershire sauce

⅛ teaspoon black pepper

1.   Heat margarine in skillet. Add garlic, celery, onion, and mushrooms and cook until celery and onion are soft. Set aside.

2.   In large microwave-safe container, whisk together flour and milk until smooth. Heat in microwave at 80% power 4–5 minutes or until thickened, stirring thoroughly at 1-minute intervals while it is cooking. Watch the mixture carefully during last 2 minutes; it boils over quickly once thickened.

3.   Add cheese to white sauce, stirring thoroughly until melted.

4.   Add sauce to vegetable mixture. Stir in remaining ingredients.

5.   Pour into chafing dish to serve hot or refrigerate and serve cold.

6.   Serve with fresh vegetables or baked tortilla chips.

Yield: 18 servings

¼ cup contains:

Cal	Carb g	Fat g	Sat Fat g	Chol mg	Sod mg	Fib g
71	6	3	2	9	260	1

Exchanges: ¼ cup = 1 vegetable, 1 fat

CREAMY CINNAMON DIP

8 ounces low-fat cream cheese

8 ounces fat-free cream cheese

1½ teaspoons ground cinnamon

3 tablespoons white sugar

1 cup firmly packed brown sugar

½ teaspoon vanilla extract

1.   Combine all ingredients in food processor or blender and process just until smooth.

2.   Refrigerate and serve with fresh fruit, bagels, or low-fat muffins.

Yield: 10 servings

¼ cup contains:

Cal	Carb g	Fat g	Sat Fat g	Chol mg	Sod mg	Fib g
168	27	4	3	15	271	0

Exchanges: Not applicable for this recipe

BRAVO BLACK BEAN DIP

8 ounces dried black beans

1 chicken bouillon cube

3 cloves garlic (or to taste)

½ tablespoon fat-free mayonnaise

2 tablespoons minced red onion

¼ cup chopped tomato

⅛ teaspoon Cajun or Creole seasoning

¼ teaspoon fresh lemon juice

⅛ teaspoon Tabasco

1. Clean beans; cover with water and soak overnight.

2. Drain beans, rinse, and add 4 cups fresh water and bouillon cube. Bring beans to a rolling boil; reduce heat, cover, and simmer 1–2 hours or until tender.

3. Drain beans and reserve all liquid.

4. Combine beans and remaining ingredients in blender or food processor; cover and process until smooth, gradually adding reserved liquid while blending. Mixture will thicken after being refrigerated.

5. Serve with low-fat chips.

Yield: 16 servings

¼ cup contains:

Cal	Carb g	Fat g	Sat Fat g	Chol mg	Sod mg	Fib g
51	9	0	0	0	72	2

Exchanges: ¼ cup = 1 starch/bread

QUICK AND EASY CLAM DIP

2 tablespoons finely chopped onion

1 can (7 ounces) minced clams, drained

1 tablespoon catsup

2–3 drops Tabasco or to taste

1 cup low-fat sour cream

1 teaspoon Worcestershire sauce

1. Combine all ingredients and chill overnight.

2. Serve with fresh vegetables or baked tortilla chips.

Yield: 5 servings

¼ cup contains:

Cal	Carb g	Fat g	Sat Fat g	Chol mg	Sod mg	Fib g
99	9	4	2	29	116	0

Exchanges: ¼ cup = 1 meat

SPINACH AND SOUR CREAM DIP

2 cups low-fat sour cream

½ cup reduced-fat mayonnaise

1 package (10 ounces) frozen chopped spinach, thawed and well drained

½ cup finely chopped red bell pepper

¼ cup finely chopped green bell pepper

2 tablespoons instant dried minced onions

2 cloves garlic, minced

½ teaspoon salt

¼ teaspoon ground red pepper (cayenne pepper)

1.   Stir all ingredients together.

2.   Cover and chill overnight.

3.   Serve with low-fat crackers, baked chips, or fresh vegetables. Another attractive way to serve this dip is to remove the center from an uncut round loaf of bread; fill the hole in the bread with dip. Tear the bread that has been removed into bite-size chunks for dipping and arrange the chunks of bread around the loaf.

Yield: 12 servings

¼ cup contains:

Cal	Carb g	Fat g	Sat Fat g	Chol mg	Sod mg	Fib g
92	8	6	2	16	202	<1

Exchanges: ¼ cup = 2 vegetables, 1 fat

TROPICAL CHEESE SPREAD

½ cup low-fat cream cheese

¼ cup crushed pineapple, drained

1 teaspoon lemon juice

2 teaspoons sugar

1.   Combine all ingredients in food processor or blender and process until smooth.

2.   Serve as a sandwich filling or spread on toast or low-fat crackers.

Yield: 12 servings

1 tablespoon contains:

Cal	Carb g	Fat g	Sat Fat g	Chol mg	Sod mg	Fib g
27	2	2	1	6	55	0

Exchanges: 1 tablespoon = Free

HERBED ARTICHOKES

¼ cup finely chopped onion

1 clove garlic, minced

1 cup reduced-sodium chicken broth

1 package (10 ounces) frozen artichoke hearts, thawed

2 tablespoons lemon juice

¼ teaspoon pepper

½ teaspoon dried oregano

¼ teaspoon dried basil

1. Cook onion and garlic in broth until tender.

2. Add remaining ingredients and simmer 5 minutes.

3. Drain and chill.

4. Serve speared with toothpicks.

Yield: 4 servings

1 serving contains:

Cal	Carb g	Fat g	Sat Fat g	Chol mg	Sod mg	Fib g
33	7	0	0	0	78	2

Exchanges: 1 serving = 1 vegetable

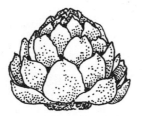

OKAY DEVILED EGGS

1 teaspoon tub margarine

¾ cup egg substitute

2 tablespoons fat-free mayonnaise

2 teaspoons prepared mustard

1 tablespoon chopped sweet pickles

1 tablespoon minced onion

⅛ teaspoon pepper

¼ teaspoon dry mustard

6 eggs, hard-cooked and cooled

paprika

1. Heat margarine in skillet. Add egg substitute; stir frequently until cooked.

2. Mash egg substitute with fork until smooth.

3. In blender, mix egg substitute with mayonnaise, prepared mustard, pickles, onion, pepper, and dry mustard. Cover and refrigerate until chilled.

4. Halve eggs lengthwise and discard yolks.

5. Fill each egg-white half with chilled egg substitute mixture and sprinkle with paprika.

6. Refrigerate until ready to serve.

Yield: 6 servings

2 egg halves contain:

Cal	Carb g	Fat g	Sat Fat g	Chol mg	Sod mg	Fib g
44	3	1	0	0	222	0

Exchanges: 2 egg halves = 1 meat

TORTILLA BITES

4 ounces fat-free cream cheese

½ of 4-ounce can chopped green chilies

1 can (15 ounces) pinto beans with jalapeños, drained

1 teaspoon chili powder

12 corn tortillas

1. In small bowl, mix cream cheese and chilies until smooth. Set aside.

2. In small saucepan, mash beans with fork; add chili powder and heat. Remove from heat and set aside.

3. Wrap corn tortillas in paper towels and microwave for 1 minute, or wrap in foil and heat in oven at 350°F for about 10 minutes.

4. Spread tortilla with a thin layer of beans and then a thin layer of cheese mixture. Roll up into a cigar shape and cut into 4 equal pieces. Repeat with remaining tortillas. Serve immediately.

Yield: 48 pieces

4 pieces contain:

Cal	Carb g	Fat g	Sat Fat g	Chol mg	Sod mg	Fib g
87	15	1	0	1	203	3

Exchanges: 4 pieces = 1 starch/bread

STUFFED MUSHROOM CAPS

½ pound fresh mushrooms

2 tablespoons tub margarine

1 clove garlic, minced

¼ teaspoon salt

⅛ teaspoon pepper

2 tablespoons chopped fresh parsley

2 tablespoons minced onion

¼ cup fine dry bread crumbs

1. Preheat oven to 350°F.

2. Clean mushrooms, removing stems.

3. Chop stems finely and cook in margarine with garlic until mushroom pieces are soft.

4. Add salt, pepper, parsley, and onion. Remove from heat and add bread crumbs.

5. Fill each mushroom cap with stuffing and place in a shallow baking dish.

6. Bake 10–15 minutes in conventional oven or 2 minutes in microwave.

Yield: 20 mushroom caps

2 mushroom caps contain:

Cal	Carb g	Fat g	Sat Fat g	Chol mg	Sod mg	Fib g
37	3	2	1	0	100	<1

Exchanges: 2 mushroom caps = 1 vegetable

Beverages

BURNIECE'S HOLIDAY WASSAIL

1 tablespoon whole cloves

1 can (48 ounces) orange juice

1 can (48 ounces) apple juice

1 can (48 ounces) pineapple juice

½ cup sugar

2 sticks cinnamon

½ teaspoon ground cinnamon

1 teaspoon ground allspice

½ cup (about 6 ounces) red hot candies

1. Place cloves in tea ball. In large pan, combine all ingredients.

2. Cover and heat about 30 minutes, stirring frequently to prevent candy from sticking before it dissolves. Remove tea ball before serving.

Yield: 24 servings

6 ounces contains:

Cal	Carb g	Fat g	Sat Fat g	Chol mg	Sod mg	Fib g
125	31	0	0	0	5	<1

Exchanges: Not applicable for this recipe

CHOCOLATE STRAWBERRY COOLER

½ cup sliced strawberries

2 tablespoons sugar

4 teaspoons chocolate extract or cocoa powder

1 cup skim milk, divided in half

½ cup chilled, clear carbonated beverage

2 fresh strawberries (optional)

1. In blender, place strawberries, sugar, cocoa, and half of milk (½ cup) and process until smooth.

2. Add remaining milk and carbonated beverage. Whip until well mixed. Garnish with a strawberry if desired and serve.

Yield: 2 servings

1 serving contains:

Cal	Carb g	Fat g	Sat Fat g	Chol mg	Sod mg	Fib g
142	31	1	<1	2	67	2

Exchanges: Not applicable for this recipe

Abbreviations: Cal = Calories; Carb = Carbohydrates; Sat Fat = Saturated Fat; Chol = Cholesterol; Sod = Sodium; Fib = Fiber; < = less than.

LIVING HEART WASSAIL

2 quarts apple cider

2 cups orange juice

1 cup lemon juice

5 cups pineapple juice

⅓ cup sugar or honey to taste

1½ teaspoons whole cloves

1 stick cinnamon

1 orange, unpeeled and diced (optional)

1 lemon, unpeeled and diced (optional)

1 red apple, unpeeled, cored, and diced (optional)

1. Combine juices and sugar or honey in large pan. Place cloves in tea ball. Add cloves and cinnamon stick to juice.

2. Cover and simmer 1 hour.

3. Serve in punch bowl with diced orange, diced lemon, and diced apple floating for garnish if desired.

Yield: 21 servings

6 ounces without garnish contains:

Cal	Carb g	Fat g	Sat Fat g	Chol mg	Sod mg	Fib g
103	26	0	0	0	7	0

Exchanges: Not applicable for this recipe

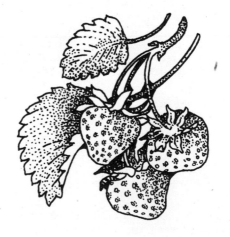

Salads and Salad Dressings

SUGAR-FREE CRANBERRY SALAD

1 cup hot water

1 package (0.3 ounce) sugar-free strawberry gelatin

½ cup cold water

1 cup raw cranberries, finely chopped

1.   Add hot water to gelatin and stir until dissolved. Add cold water and stir.

2.   Add cranberries to gelatin.

3.   Pour into mold and chill until set.

Yield: 4 servings

⅔ cup contains:

Cal	Carb g	Fat g	Sat Fat g	Chol mg	Sod mg	Fib g
20	3	0	0	0	56	1

Exchanges: ⅔ cup = Free

HEAVENLY HASH

1 can (20 ounces) pineapple tidbits packed in juice, drained

1 can (16 ounces) mandarin orange sections, drained

¾ cup miniature marshmallows

1 jar (6 ounces) maraschino cherries, drained, cut in halves

½ cup low-fat sour cream

1 banana, sliced

1.   Mix all ingredients together.

2.   Cover and refrigerate overnight.

Yield: 7 servings

1 serving contains:

Cal	Carb g	Fat g	Sat Fat g	Chol mg	Sod mg	Fib g
120	27	1	1	6	23	2

Exchanges: Not applicable for this recipe

Abbreviations: Cal = Calories; Carb = Carbohydrates; Sat Fat = Saturated Fat; Chol = Cholesterol; Sod = Sodium; Fib – Fiber; < = less than.

MOM'S FROZEN FRUIT SALAD

1 packet (¼ ounce) unflavored gelatin

6 tablespoons cold water

3 tablespoons powdered (confectioners') sugar

¼ cup lemon juice

2 tablespoons maraschino cherry juice

1 cup canned evaporated skim milk, chilled

⅔ cup fat-free sour cream

1 banana, cubed

1 can (20 ounces) crushed pineapple packed in juice, drained

1 jar (10 ounces) maraschino cherries, quartered

lettuce leaves (optional)

1.   In small saucepan, sprinkle gelatin over cold water. Stir over low heat until gelatin dissolves.

2.   Add powdered sugar, lemon juice, and maraschino cherry juice.

3.   In mixing bowl, whip chilled evaporated milk until soft peaks form.

4.   Fold sour cream into whipped milk. (Do this step immediately or whipped milk will get runny.)

5.   Fold in gelatin mixture. Fold in fruits.

6.   Pour into refrigerator trays, loaf pan, or large mold and place in freezer, stirring once before mixture gets firm.

7.   Freeze 4–5 hours or overnight.

8.   Slice and serve on lettuce leaves if desired.

Yield: 24 servings

1 serving contains:

Cal	Carb g	Fat g	Sat Fat g	Chol mg	Sod mg	Fib g
42	9	0	0	<1	19	<1

Exchanges: Not applicable for this recipe.

CREAMY CRANBERRY SALAD

1½ cups water

1 package (3 ounces) cherry gelatin

1 can (16 ounces) whole-berry cranberry sauce

8 ounces low-fat sour cream

2 tablespoons chopped pecans (optional)

1.   In medium pan, heat water to boiling.

2.   Remove from heat and add gelatin; stir until dissolved.

3.   Stir in cranberry sauce.

4.   Stir in sour cream and pecans.

5.   Pour into glass serving bowl. Cover with plastic wrap and refrigerate until firm.

Yield: 8 servings

½ cup without pecans contains:

Cal	Carb g	Fat g	Sat Fat g	Chol mg	Sod mg	Fib g
167	35	2	1	9	71	1

Exchanges: Not applicable for this recipe

½ cup with pecans contains:

Cal	Carb g	Fat g	Sat Fat g	Chol mg	Sod mg	Fib g
179	35	3	1	9	71	1

ARTICHOKE PASTA SALAD

1 package (12 ounces) tricolor pasta, uncooked

1 can (14 ounces) artichoke hearts, drained
and quartered

1 can (14 ounces) hearts of palm, drained
and sliced into 1-inch slices

2 tomatoes, cut into wedges (may substitute
cherry tomatoes, halved)

20 large ripe olives, pitted, sliced

2 slices ($\frac{1}{4}$ inch thick) purple onion, quartered and separated into rings

2 tablespoons olive oil

1 tablespoon garlic wine vinegar

$\frac{1}{2}$ teaspoon sugar

$\frac{1}{4}$ teaspoon salt

8 lettuce leaves

1. Cook pasta according to package directions,
omitting salt and fat. Drain and rinse with cold
water. Set aside in large mixing bowl.

2. Add artichokes, hearts of palm, tomatoes,
olives, and onion. Toss lightly.

3. In small bowl, combine oil, vinegar, sugar,
and salt; mix well. Add to pasta mixture; mix
well.

4. Refrigerate until thoroughly chilled, preferably overnight.

5. Serve on lettuce leaves.

Yield: 8 servings

1 cup contains:

Cal	Carb g	Fat g	Sat Fat g	Chol mg	Sod mg	Fib g
248	43	6	1	0	332	4

Exchanges: 1 cup = 2 starch/breads, 2 vegetables, 1 fat

VARIATION:

Low-Sodium Artichoke Pasta Salad: Omit salt and
olives.

1 cup contains:

Cal	Carb g	Fat g	Sat Fat g	Chol mg	Sod mg	Fib g
235	42	4	1	0	170	4

CALICO LENTIL SALAD

$\frac{1}{2}$ cup dried lentils

3 cups water

2 tablespoons fresh lemon juice

1 tablespoon minced fresh dill or 1 teaspoon
dried dill weed

$\frac{1}{4}$ teaspoon salt

$\frac{1}{2}$ teaspoon pepper

4 green onions, finely chopped

1 red bell pepper, finely chopped

1 medium carrot, grated

$\frac{1}{3}$ cup shredded part-skim mozzarella cheese

1. Combine lentils and water in saucepan;
bring to a boil. Reduce heat to low and cook 30
minutes or until lentils are tender. Drain; let cool.

2. In bowl, combine lentils, lemon juice, dill,
salt, and pepper; mix together.

3. Add green onions, bell pepper, and carrot;
toss well. Gently toss cheese with other ingredients and chill.

4. Serve cold.

Yield: 6 servings

$\frac{1}{2}$ cup contains:

Cal	Carb g	Fat g	Sat Fat g	Chol mg	Sod mg	Fib g
85	13	1	1	3	131	3

Exchanges: $\frac{1}{2}$ cup = 1 starch/bread

CHICKEN AND RICE SALAD

2 cups cooked rice, prepared without salt or fat, cooled

2 cups chopped cooked chicken (3 deboned chicken breast halves, skin and fat removed)

1 package (10 ounces) frozen peas

5 stalks celery, chopped

½ green bell pepper, chopped

2 tablespoons finely chopped onion

¾ cup low-fat mayonnaise

½ teaspoon salt

¼ teaspoon pepper

2 tablespoons lemon juice

2 tablespoons chopped fresh parsley

1. Combine rice, chicken, peas, celery, bell pepper, and onion. Set aside.

2. Combine remaining ingredients.

3. Toss chicken mixture with mayonnaise mixture.

4. Chill well before serving. Serve with fruit salad and bread.

Yield: 8 servings

1 serving contains:

Cal	Carb g	Fat g	Sat Fat g	Chol mg	Sod mg	Fib g
214	20	8	1	34	342	3

Exchanges: 1 serving = 1 starch/bread, 1 meat, 1 fat

CHICKEN CAESAR SALAD

CHICKEN AND CROUTONS

2 teaspoons olive oil

2 cloves garlic, minced

1 tablespoon chopped fresh parsley

¼ teaspoon coarsely ground pepper

4 deboned chicken breast halves, skin and fat removed

4 slices French bread, cut into ½-inch cubes

DRESSING

1 ounce lean ham, minced

2 cloves garlic, minced

1½ tablespoons fresh lemon juice

1 tablespoon red wine vinegar

½ cup egg substitute

1 tablespoon olive oil

1 small head romaine lettuce, torn into pieces

2 tablespoons grated Parmesan cheese

coarsely ground pepper

CHICKEN AND CROUTONS

1. In shallow dish, combine oil, garlic, parsley, and pepper. Add chicken and turn to coat with oil.

2. Preheat skillet. Cook chicken 4 minutes on each side or until well done. Remove chicken from pan and cool to room temperature.

3. Preheat oven to 350°F. Toast bread for 10–15 minutes to make croutons. Set aside.

DRESSING

1. In small bowl, mix ham, garlic, lemon juice, vinegar, and egg substitute. Gradually whisk in oil. Set aside.

2. Cut chicken into thin strips and dip in dressing. Set aside.

3. In large bowl, toss together lettuce, croutons, Parmesan cheese, and remaining dressing.

4. Divide salad among 4 plates and top with chicken strips and pepper.

Yield: 4 servings

1 serving contains:

Cal	Carb g	Fat g	Sat Fat g	Chol mg	Sod mg	Fib g
339	18	11	3	83	417	2

Exchanges: 1 serving = 1 starch/bread, 4 meats

CHICKEN SALAD

4 deboned chicken breast halves, skin and fat removed

3 tablespoons sliced almonds

1 stalk celery, finely chopped

2 tablespoons low-fat mayonnaise

2 tablespoons low-fat sour cream

1 cup grapes, sliced lengthwise, or ½ cup pineapple tidbits packed in juice, drained

6 leaves lettuce or 3 medium tomatoes

1. Cook chicken. Tear or cut into small chunks.

2. Preheat oven to 350°F. Spread almonds evenly in cake pan. Bake about 10 minutes or until lightly browned. Cool.

3. In large bowl, mix chicken, almonds, and celery.

4. In small bowl, combine mayonnaise and sour cream; stir into chicken mixture.

5. Add grapes or pineapple; stir gently.

6. Serve on bed of lettuce or in tomato half.

Yield: 6 servings

½ cup with tomato half contains:

Cal	Carb g	Fat g	Sat Fat g	Chol mg	Sod mg	Fib g
182	10	6	1	55	94	1

Exchanges: ½ cup with tomato half = 3 meats

VARIATION

Chicken Salad with Water Chestnuts: Substitute 3 tablespoons chopped water chestnuts for almonds.

½ cup with tomato half and water chestnuts contains:

Cal	Carb g	Fat g	Sat Fat g	Chol mg	Sod mg	Fib g
167	10	5	1	55	94	1

Exchanges: ½ cup with tomato half and water chestnuts = 3 meats

COBB SALAD

1 head Boston lettuce

1 head romaine lettuce

3 hard-cooked eggs, yolks discarded

4 green onions, chopped

4 ounces Cheddar cheese (no more than 5 grams fat per ounce), diced

1 large tomato, chopped

¼ cup imitation bacon chips

1 avocado, peeled, pitted, and diced

2 deboned chicken breast halves, skin and fat removed, cooked and cubed (optional)

1 recipe Apple Cider Vinaigrette Dressing (page 230)

1. Arrange lettuce on large platter.

2. Decoratively arrange other ingredients on top in spokes or rings as desired.

3. Serve with Apple Cider Vinaigrette.

Yield: 6 servings

1 serving without chicken contains:

Cal	Carb g	Fat g	Sat Fat g	Chol mg	Sod mg	Fib g
186	12	11	3	10	351	3

Exchanges: 1 serving without chicken = 1 meat, 2 vegetables, 1 fat

1 serving with chicken contains:

Cal	Carb g	Fat g	Sat Fat g	Chol mg	Sod mg	Fib g
241	12	12	4	36	375	3

Exchanges: 1 serving with chicken = 2 meats, 2 vegetables, 1 fat

COUSCOUS SALAD

1 cup couscous, uncooked

¾ teaspoon salt

1 cup snow peas

1 tablespoon balsamic vinegar

1 tablespoon olive oil

1 teaspoon dried basil or 1 tablespoon minced fresh basil

1 clove garlic, minced

3 green onions, sliced

12 cherry tomatoes, halved

1. Prepare couscous according to package directions, using ¾ teaspoon salt. Cool.

2. Cook snow peas in boiling water for 1 minute or in microwave in covered dish without water for 1 minute. Drain and set aside.

3. Combine vinegar, oil, basil, and garlic.

4. Add couscous, green onions, tomatoes, and snow peas. Toss lightly.

5. Chill before serving.

Yield: 6 servings

¾ cup contains:

Cal	Carb g	Fat g	Sat Fat g	Chol mg	Sod mg	Fib g
156	28	3	0	0	275	2

Exchanges: ¾ cup = 2 starch/breads

GARDEN RICE SALAD

2 cloves garlic, minced

1 onion, chopped

2 carrots, chopped

1 stalk celery, chopped

⅓ cup chopped fresh parsley

2 teaspoons dried basil

1 teaspoon dried oregano

¼ cup water

2 tomatoes, chopped

1 can (16 ounces) vegetarian baked beans

5 cups cooked rice, prepared without salt or fat

¼ cup seasoned rice vinegar

1 teaspoon salt

¾ teaspoon pepper

2 teaspoons sugar

2 teaspoons olive oil

1.   Cook garlic, onion, carrots, celery, parsley, basil, and oregano in ¼ cup boiling water until vegetables are tender. Add tomatoes, beans, and rice.

2.   Combine vinegar, salt, pepper, sugar, and oil. Toss with vegetables.

3.   Chill overnight before serving.

Yield: 18 servings

½ cup contains:

Cal	Carb g	Fat g	Sat Fat g	Chol mg	Sod mg	Fib g
109	22	1	0	2	273	2

Exchanges: ½ cup = 1 starch/bread

IMITATION CRAB PASTA SALAD

1 package (12 ounces) vermicelli, uncooked

1 onion, grated or minced

1 stalk celery, finely chopped

1 package (10 ounces) frozen peas

⅓ cup low-fat mayonnaise

1 tablespoon apple cider vinegar

1 pound imitation crabmeat, sliced

lettuce leaves

avocado, peeled, pitted, and sliced (optional)

cherry tomatoes, halved (optional)

fresh basil, chopped (optional)

1.   Cook vermicelli according to package directions, omitting salt and fat. Drain and rinse under cold water. Place in large mixing bowl.

2.   Mix next 6 ingredients in small mixing bowl; add to vermicelli and stir to mix. Cover and chill well, preferably overnight.

3.   Serve on bed of lettuce with avocado, cherry tomatoes, and fresh basil if desired.

Yield: 13 servings

1 cup without optional ingredients contains:

Cal	Carb g	Fat g	Sat Fat g	Chol mg	Sod mg	Fib g
175	28	3	0	12	357	2

Exchanges: 1 cup = 2 starch/breads, 1 meat

LENTIL AND JICAMA SALAD

1 cup dried lentils

2 cups water

2 tablespoons olive oil

½ cup chopped onion

4 large serrano peppers, seeded and minced

1 medium ear corn, kernels cut off

½ cup diced jicama

¼ large bell pepper, any color

1 tablespoon chopped fresh cilantro

½ teaspoon dried basil

¼ teaspoon ground ginger

⅛ teaspoon pepper

⅛ teaspoon salt

1. Cook lentils in water for 15 minutes or until tender. Drain.

2. Heat oil in saucepan over medium heat. Add onion and serrano peppers. Cook until onion is soft.

3. Add remaining ingredients and cook 5 more minutes.

4. Serve warm or cold.

Yield: 4 servings

1 serving contains:

Cal	Carb g	Fat g	Sat Fat g	Chol mg	Sod mg	Fib g
277	41	8	1	0	81	10

Exchanges: 1 serving = 2 starch/breads, 1 meat, 1 vegetable, 1 fat

PASTA SALAD AT ITS BEST

DRESSING

¾ cup water

¾ cup tarragon vinegar

1½ tablespoons corn oil

¾ teaspoon garlic powder

¾ teaspoon dried oregano

¾ teaspoon dried basil

¼ teaspoon salt

1½ teaspoons sugar

1½ teaspoons pepper

¾ teaspoon minced onion

SALAD

2 cups fresh snow peas

1½ cups broccoli florets

2½ cups cherry tomato halves

2 cups sliced fresh mushrooms

2 cans (3 ounces each) sliced black olives

12 ounces fusilli pasta, uncooked

1 tablespoon grated Parmesan cheese

1. In jar with tight-fitting lid, combine all ingredients for dressing; shake vigorously and refrigerate.

2. In saucepan, bring water to a boil and drop in snow peas. Boil 1 minute and remove with a slotted spoon.

3. Place broccoli in boiling water; boil 1 minute and drain.

4. Combine peas, broccoli, tomatoes, mushrooms, and olives.

5.   Cook pasta according to package directions, omitting fat and salt; drain and cool slightly.

6.   In large bowl, combine vegetables, pasta, Parmesan cheese, and dressing; toss well. Chill several hours before serving.

Yield: 12 servings

1 cup contains:

Cal	Carb g	Fat g	Sat Fat g	Chol mg	Sod mg	Fib g
168	29	4	1	0	153	2

Exchanges: 1 cup = 2 starch/breads, 1 fat

LINGUINE BLACK BEAN SALAD

¼ cup pine nuts

½ of 12-ounce package linguine, uncooked

¼ tablespoon olive oil

½ cup chopped green onions

½ teaspoon dried oregano

⅛ teaspoon salt

pinch ground red pepper

pinch coarsely ground black pepper

1 clove garlic, minced

1 can (14½ ounces) tomatoes, chopped, undrained

1 can (15 ounces) black beans, drained

½ of 14-ounce can artichoke hearts, packed in water, drained, cut into bite-size pieces

5 tablespoons grated Parmesan cheese

2 tablespoons rehydrated sun-dried tomatoes (packaged dry, not in oil)

1.   Preheat oven to 375°F. Place pine nuts on baking sheet and toast in oven for 10 minutes.

2.   Cook linguine according to package directions, omitting salt and fat; do not overcook. Drain and rinse in cold water.

3.   In large nonstick skillet, heat oil over medium heat and add green onions, oregano, salt, red and black pepper, garlic, and tomatoes. Reduce heat, cover, and simmer for 10 minutes.

4.   Add beans and simmer, covered, for 5 minutes.

5.   Combine pasta and bean mixture; add artichokes and toss well to prevent beans from sinking to bottom of bowl.

6.   Before serving, add Parmesan, pine nuts, and sun-dried tomatoes to each plate.

Yield: 5 servings

1 cup contains:

Cal	Carb g	Fat g	Sat Fat g	Chol mg	Sod mg	Fib g
313	50	8	2	4	513	8

Exchanges: 1 cup = 3 starch/breads, 1 vegetable, 1 fat

VARIATION

Low-Sodium Linguine Black Bean Salad: Omit salt and Parmesan cheese.

1 cup contains:

Cal	Carb g	Fat g	Sat Fat g	Chol mg	Sod mg	Fib g
291	50	6	1	0	364	8

Exchanges: 1 cup = 3 starch/breads, 1 vegetable, 1 fat

SALMON SALAD

1 can (14 ounces) red salmon, drained

5 Roma or plum tomatoes, chopped (may
    substitute cherry tomatoes cut into halves)

4 green onions, chopped

½ cucumber, unpeeled, chopped

2 tablespoons apple cider vinegar

coarsely ground pepper

1.   Combine all ingredients and toss lightly.

2.   Serve on chilled plates.

Yield: 6 servings

⅔ cup contains:

Cal	Carb g	Fat g	Sat Fat g	Chol mg	Sod mg	Fib g
108	5	4	1	34	350	1

Exchanges: ⅔ cup = 2 meats

SEAFOOD SALAD

seafood seasoning or crab boil

½ pound uncooked large shrimp, unpeeled

1 tablespoon sliced almonds

¼ pound crabmeat

3 cups chopped lettuce

1 cup chopped spinach

15 small mushrooms, sliced

1 small onion, sliced

2 cups bean sprouts

2 medium carrots, grated

8 radishes, sliced

4 stalks celery, sliced diagonally

¼ small head red cabbage, shredded

1 medium green bell pepper, diced

¼ cup shredded Cheddar cheese (no more
    than 5 grams fat per ounce)

¼ cup shredded part-skim mozzarella cheese

1.   Add seafood seasoning to water according to package directions and bring to a boil. Add shrimp and stir. When water returns to a boil, remove from heat and pour through strainer. Cover shrimp with ice and refrigerate until ready to serve.

2.   Spread almonds on cookie sheet and toast in 350°F oven for 3 minutes or until golden brown. Set aside.

3.   Peel shrimp and mix with crabmeat.

4.   In large salad bowl or trifle bowl, layer remaining ingredients in order listed, with shrimp and crabmeat as last layer.

5.   Sprinkle with almonds.

6.   Serve with favorite dressing.

Yield: 6 servings

3 cups without dressing contains:

Cal	Carb g	Fat g	Sat Fat g	Chol mg	Sod mg	Fib g
119	10	3	1	60	250	4

Exchanges: 3 cups = 1 meat, 2 vegetables

PASTA SALMON SALAD WITH DILL

8 ounces (3 cups) spiral pasta, uncooked

2 tablespoons tarragon vinegar

1 can (16 ounces) salmon, drained, skin removed

2 tablespoons chopped onion

1½ cups fresh pea pods, cut into thirds, or 1 package (16 ounces) frozen pea pods, thawed and drained

½ cup low-fat mayonnaise

¼ cup plain low-fat yogurt

2 teaspoons chopped fresh dill or 1 teaspoon dried dill weed

¼ teaspoon salt

¼ teaspoon pepper

1 teaspoon lemon juice

6 leaves lettuce (optional)

fresh dill (optional)

1. Cook pasta according to package directions, omitting salt and fat. Drain and rinse under cold water.

2. In large bowl, toss pasta with vinegar to coat

3. Add salmon, onion, and pea pods to pasta.

4. In small bowl, blend mayonnaise, yogurt, dill, salt, pepper, and lemon juice.

5. Spoon dressing over salmon and pasta mixture; toss gently.

6. Refrigerate until thoroughly chilled.

7. Serve on lettuce leaves and garnish with fresh dill if desired. Serve immediately. Leftovers do not keep well.

Yield: 6 servings

1 cup contains:

Cal	Carb g	Fat g	Sat Fat g	Chol mg	Sod mg	Fib g
317	36	10	2	39	559	2

Exchanges: 1 cup = 2 starch/breads, 2 meats, 1 fat

VARIATION

Low-Sodium Pasta Salmon Salad with Dill: Omit salt.

1 cup has same analysis as above, except 470 mg sodium.

CREAMY SPINACH SALAD

¼ cup low-fat sour cream

2 tablespoons low-fat mayonnaise

1 bunch fresh spinach leaves, torn in pieces (about 5 ounces)

1 red apple, unpeeled, cored and diced

½ cup chopped green onions

1. Mix sour cream and mayonnaise.

2. In separate bowl, mix spinach, apple, and green onions.

3. Lightly toss all ingredients together.

Yield: 6 servings

1 serving contains:

Cal	Carb g	Fat g	Sat Fat g	Chol mg	Sod mg	Fib g
49	7	2	1	5	59	1

Exchanges: 1 serving = 1 fruit

TACO SALAD

1 pound lean ground beef

1 medium onion, chopped

1 medium green bell pepper, chopped

¼ cup water

2 teaspoons chili powder

2 teaspoons ground cumin

½ teaspoon salt

½ teaspoon pepper

1 teaspoon garlic powder

¼ cup chopped fresh cilantro

5 cups shredded lettuce

2 large tomatoes, chopped

1. In large saucepan, bring about 1 quart water to a boil. Crumble ground beef into water and stir constantly. When water starts to boil again, pour water and meat into colander or large strainer sitting in sink.

2. Place ground beef in skillet; add onion, bell pepper, and water. Simmer 10 minutes or until onion is soft.

3. Add chili powder, cumin, salt, pepper, and garlic powder; cook about 5 minutes.

4. Add cilantro. Remove from heat.

5. Arrange lettuce in bowl; add meat mixture and top with tomato.

Yield: 6 servings

½ cup meat with lettuce and tomato contains:

Cal	Carb g	Fat g	Sat Fat g	Chol mg	Sod mg	Fib g
153	7	6	2	43	238	2

Exchanges: ½ cup meat with lettuce and tomato = 2 meats, 1 vegetable

VARIATION

Low-Sodium Taco Salad: Omit salt.

½ cup meat with lettuce and tomato has same analysis as above, except 60 mg sodium.

SOUTHWEST CHICKEN SALAD

1 pound deboned chicken breast halves, skin and fat removed

¼ cup plus 1 tablespoon low-fat mayonnaise

¼ cup plain fat-free yogurt

2 teaspoons curry powder

3 stalks celery, chopped

3 tablespoons imitation bacon chips

½ cup raisins

½ cup unpeeled apple, cored and cut into 1-inch chunks

½ cup chopped fresh cilantro

1. Cook chicken thoroughly and tear or cut into small chunks.

2. In small bowl, mix mayonnaise, yogurt, and curry powder.

3. In large bowl, lightly toss remaining ingredients except cilantro.

4. Add mayonnaise mixture to chicken mixture and mix lightly.

5. Chill thoroughly and garnish with cilantro.

Yield: 4 servings

1 serving contains:

Cal	Carb g	Fat g	Sat Fat g	Chol mg	Sod mg	Fib g
296	24	10	2	67	313	2

Exchanges: 1 serving = 4 meats, 1 fruit

DILLED CUCUMBERS

2 medium cucumbers

½ teaspoon salt

1 teaspoon sugar

½ cup vinegar (any type)

¼ cup chopped fresh dill or 2 tablespoons dried dill weed

1.   Peel cucumbers and slice thinly. Put in small bowl and sprinkle with salt. Let stand at least 30 minutes, stirring occasionally to distribute salt on all slices.

2.   Discard water from bowl. Press cucumbers lightly with paper towel to remove excess moisture.

3.   In separate bowl, combine sugar, vinegar, and dill; pour over cucumbers. Cover and refrigerate 1–3 hours to blend flavors.

Yield: 4 servings

1 serving contains:

Cal	Carb g	Fat g	Sat Fat g	Chol mg	Sod mg	Fib g
26	7	0	0	0	208	1

Exchanges: 1 serving = Free

TURKEY SALAD WITH YOGURT DRESSING

DIJON YOGURT DRESSING

½ cup plain fat-free yogurt

1 tablespoon finely chopped fresh parsley

¼ teaspoon salt

¼ teaspoon celery seed

3 tablespoons skim milk

2 teaspoons Dijon mustard

1 teaspoon lemon juice

SALAD

2 cups torn iceberg lettuce

2 cups torn romaine lettuce

2 cups cooked turkey breast, cubed (not processed turkey)

2 cups broccoli florets

¼ red onion, thinly sliced and separated into rings

1 tomato, sliced

½ cup green grapes, halved

1.   In small bowl, combine dressing ingredients. Refrigerate at least 1 hour to blend flavors.

2.   In large bowl, combine salad ingredients, or arrange ingredients on 4 salad plates.

3.   Pour dressing over salad.

Yield: 4 servings

2½ cups with dressing contains:

Cal	Carb g	Fat g	Sat Fat g	Chol mg	Sod* mg	Fib g
182	12	3	1	55	264	2

*Analysis is for fresh turkey breast (not processed).

Exchanges: 2½ cups with dressing = 3 meats, 2 vegetables

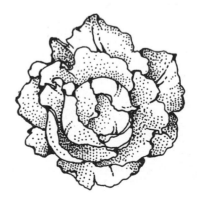

WILD RICE SALAD

SALAD

2 deboned chicken breast halves, skin and fat removed, or 1 pound shrimp without heads

1 cup wild rice, uncooked

3 green onions, sliced

1 red bell pepper, diced

½ cup sliced almonds

1 can (11 ounces) mandarin orange sections, chilled and drained

1 avocado, peeled, pitted, and cut into chunks

24 leaves romaine lettuce

MUSTARD VINAIGRETTE DRESSING

2 large cloves garlic, minced

1½ tablespoons Dijon or regular prepared mustard

½ teaspoon salt

¼ teaspoon sugar

¼ teaspoon pepper

¼ cup seasoned rice vinegar

2 tablespoons olive oil

1. Simmer chicken in small amount of water until meat is done. Cut into bite-size pieces; set aside to cool. If using shrimp, boil, peel, devein, and cut into bite-size pieces.

2. Cook rice according to package directions, omitting salt. Grains of rice will open when done; taste to be sure rice is desired tenderness before removing from heat.

3. While rice is cooking, combine all dressing ingredients in food processor or blender and process until smooth. Set aside.

4. Drain any excess liquid from rice. In large serving bowl, combine rice, chicken, green onions, and bell pepper. Add dressing and toss. Cover and refrigerate at least 2 hours. Chill plates on which salad will be served.

5. Preheat oven to 350°F. Spread almonds in cake pan. Bake, uncovered, about 10 minutes or until almonds are toasted. Set aside to cool.

6. Just before serving, add orange sections, avocado, and almonds to rice salad; toss lightly.

7. Arrange 3 lettuce leaves on each plate and top with scoop of salad. Serve immediately.

Yield: 8 servings

1 cup contains:

Cal	Carb g	Fat g	Sat Fat g	Chol mg	Sod mg	Fib g
254	27	11	2	19	329	3

Exchanges: 1 cup = 1 starch/bread, 1 meat, 1 vegetable, 2 fats

GEORGIA'S POTATO SALAD

3½ pounds red potatoes, cooked in skins, cut into ½-inch pieces

1 medium onion, chopped

2 cups chopped bread-and-butter pickles

½ cup imitation bacon chips

1 cup low-fat mayonnaise

¼ cup Dijon mustard

¼ cup skim milk

½ tablespoon coarsely ground pepper

1 tablespoon mustard seed

paprika

1. In large bowl, combine potatoes, onion, pickles, and imitation bacon chips.

2. In small bowl, combine mayonnaise, mustard, milk, pepper, and mustard seed.

3. Carefully mix dressing into potato mixture to avoid mashing the potatoes.

4. Sprinkle with paprika when ready to serve. Can be made ahead of time to allow flavors to blend.

Yield: 18 servings

⅔ cup contains:

Cal	Carb g	Fat g	Sat Fat g	Chol mg	Sod mg	Fib g
160	27	5	1	3	353	2

Exchanges: ⅔ cup = 1 starch/bread, 1 vegetable, 1 fat

VARIATION

Low-Sodium Georgia's Potato Salad: Substitute no-salt-added cucumber pickles for bread-and-butter pickles. Reduce imitation bacon chips to 2 tablespoons.

⅔ cup contains:

Cal	Carb g	Fat g	Sat Fat g	Chol mg	Sod mg	Fib g
132	21	4	1	3	146	2

Exchanges: ⅔ cup = 1 starch/bread, 1 fat

TABBOULEH

2 cups boiling water

1 cup bulgur, uncooked

4 small or 2 large green onions with tops, finely chopped

½ small red onion, sliced very thin, separated into rings

1 cup chopped fresh parsley (about 1 bunch)

¼ cup chopped fresh mint or 1 tablespoon mint flakes

1 cup coarsely chopped cucumber (about 1 small or ⅔ medium)

1½ tablespoons olive oil

¼ cup lemon juice

¼ teaspoon ground cumin

¼ teaspoon pepper

1 teaspoon salt

½ tablespoon lemon zest or grated lemon rind (optional)

1. In large bowl, pour boiling water over bulgur; stir and let stand until water is absorbed (about 1 hour).

2. In medium bowl, combine green onions, red onion, parsley, mint, and cucumber; add to bulgur.

3. In small bowl, combine olive oil, lemon juice, cumin, pepper, salt, and lemon zest; stir into bulgur and vegetable mixture and mix well.

4. Refrigerate 4 hours or overnight to allow flavors to blend.

Yield: 12 servings

½ cup contains:

Cal	Carb g	Fat g	Sat Fat g	Chol mg	Sod mg	Fib g
84	15	2	0	0	186	4

Exchanges: ½ cup = 1 starch/bread

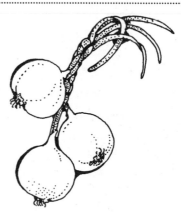

APPLE CIDER VINAIGRETTE

½ cup apple cider

3 tablespoons tarragon wine vinegar

2 tablespoons lemon juice

1 tablespoon Dijon mustard

¼ teaspoon salt

1 tablespoon corn oil

1. In small jar with tight-fitting lid, place all ingredients; shake until combined.

Yield: 11 servings

1½ tablespoons contain:

Cal	Carb g	Fat g	Sat Fat g	Chol mg	Sod mg	Fib g
19	2	1	0	0	66	0

Exchanges: 1½ tablespoons = Free

FIESTA SLAW

½ small head green cabbage, shredded

¼ small head red cabbage, shredded

4 medium carrots, grated

½ medium onion, chopped

2 medium apples, unpeeled, diced

½ cup low-fat mayonnaise

½ cup fat-free mayonnaise

½ cup apple juice

¼ cup skim milk

⅓ cup cider vinegar

1 tablespoon sugar

½ tablespoon celery seed

2 tablespoons dried tarragon

½ cup raisins (optional)

1. In large bowl, combine cabbage, carrots, onion, and apples.

2. In small bowl, combine mayonnaise, apple juice, milk, vinegar, sugar, celery seed, and tarragon. For a more tart coleslaw, increase vinegar to ½ cup.

3. Toss vegetables with dressing and add raisins if desired. Chill until ready to serve.

Yield: 12 servings

⅔ cup without raisins contains:

Cal	Carb g	Fat g	Sat Fat g	Chol mg	Sod mg	Fib g
87	15	3	<1	2	206	2

Exchanges: ⅔ cup = 2 vegetables, 1 fat

⅔ cup with raisins contains:

Cal	Carb g	Fat g	Sat Fat g	Chol mg	Sod mg	Fib g
106	20	3	<1	2	208	3

Exchanges: ⅔ cup = 1 fruit, 1 vegetable, 1 fat

CARIBBEAN DRESSING

½ cup plain fat-free yogurt

1½ tablespoons chili sauce

1 tablespoon chopped dill pickle

1–2 tablespoons finely chopped celery

1 tablespoon finely chopped fresh parsley

⅛ teaspoon ground red pepper (cayenne pepper)

⅛ teaspoon dry mustard

1. Combine all ingredients.

2. Chill before serving on tossed greens.

Yield: 6 servings

2 tablespoons contain:

Cal	Carb g	Fat g	Sat Fat g	Chol mg	Sod mg	Fib g
16	3	0	0	0	81	0

Exchanges: 2 tablespoons = Free

CILANTRO AND JALAPEÑO DRESSING

1 cup fat-free sour cream
½ teaspoon garlic powder
1 tablespoon finely chopped fresh cilantro
1 jalapeño pepper, seeded and finely chopped
¼ teaspoon pepper
¼ teaspoon salt
2 tablespoons skim milk
¼ cup lime juice

1. Combine all ingredients in covered container.

2. Shake well and refrigerate several hours.

Yield: 12 servings

2 tablespoons contain:

Cal	Carb g	Fat g	Sat Fat g	Chol mg	Sod mg	Fib g
15	3	0	0	0	63	0

Exchanges: 2 tablespoons = Free

ORIENTAL DRESSING

1 teaspoon sesame seeds
½ cup red wine vinegar
½ cup pineapple juice
2 tablespoons reduced-sodium soy sauce
1 tablespoon sesame oil
½ teaspoon ground ginger
¼ teaspoon pepper
¼ teaspoon garlic powder

1. Preheat oven to 350°F. Spread sesame seeds in cake pan and toast in oven about 5 minutes or until golden brown.

2. Combine all ingredients in covered container.

3. Shake vigorously several seconds; refrigerate several hours.

4. Serve on salads containing meat.

Yield: 10 servings

2 tablespoons contain:

Cal	Carb g	Fat g	Sat Fat g	Chol mg	Sod mg	Fib g
25	3	2	0	0	120	0

Exchanges: 2 tablespoons = Free

C'EST LA VIE DRESSING

¼ cup plain fat-free yogurt

¼ cup catsup

1 tablespoon seasoned rice wine vinegar

¼ teaspoon salt

¼ teaspoon pepper

⅛ teaspoon Tabasco

⅛ teaspoon garlic powder

⅛ teaspoon Worcestershire sauce

1. Combine all ingredients.

2. Chill before serving on tossed greens.

Yield: 5 servings

2 tablespoons contains:

Cal	Carb g	Fat g	Sat Fat g	Chol mg	Sod mg	Fib g
23	5	0	0	0	316	0

Exchanges: 2 tablespoons = Free

GINGERED PINEAPPLE DRESSING

1 teaspoon firmly packed brown sugar

½ cup fat-free sour cream

½ cup pineapple juice

¼ teaspoon ground ginger

1. Combine all ingredients in covered container.

2. Shake well and refrigerate several hours.

Yield: 8 servings

2 tablespoons contains:

Cal	Carb g	Fat g	Sat Fat g	Chol mg	Sod mg	Fib g
20	4	0	0	0	12	0

Exchanges: 2 tablespoons = Free

ITALIAN DRESSING

½ cup water

½ cup tarragon vinegar

1 tablespoon corn oil

½ teaspoon garlic powder

½ teaspoon dried oregano

½ teaspoon dried basil

¼ teaspoon salt

1 teaspoon sugar

1 teaspoon pepper

½ teaspoon minced onion

1. Combine all ingredients in covered container.

2. Shake vigorously; refrigerate several hours.

Yield: 8 servings

2 tablespoons contain:

Cal	Carb g	Fat g	Sat Fat g	Chol mg	Sod mg	Fib g
21	2	2	0	0	67	0

Exchanges: 2 tablespoons = Free

HERBED FRENCH DRESSING

¾ cup seasoned rice vinegar

1 can (10¾ ounces) condensed tomato soup

1 clove garlic, minced

2 tablespoons finely chopped dill pickle

2 tablespoons finely chopped celery

2 tablespoons finely chopped fresh parsley

1 tablespoon Worcestershire sauce

1 teaspoon paprika

½ teaspoon dry mustard

1. Combine all ingredients in large jar. Cover tightly and shake well.

2. Store in refrigerator. Shake well before serving.

Yield: 20 servings

2 tablespoons contain:

Cal	Carb g	Fat g	Sat Fat g	Chol mg	Sod mg	Fib g
23	5	0	0	0	287	0

Exchanges: 2 tablespoons = Free

ORANGE POPPY-SEED DRESSING

¼ cup seasoned rice wine vinegar

1 cup orange juice

1 teaspoon dry mustard

1 tablespoon corn oil

1 teaspoon poppy seeds

1 tablespoon firmly packed brown sugar

1. Combine all ingredients in covered container.

2. Shake vigorously several seconds; refrigerate several hours.

Yield: 12 servings

2 tablespoons contain:

Cal	Carb g	Fat g	Sat Fat g	Chol mg	Sod mg	Fib g
32	5	1	0	0	90	0

Exchanges: Not applicable for this recipe

TOMATO DRESSING

1 can (10¾ ounces) condensed tomato soup

¼ cup water

1 tablespoon lime juice

1 tablespoon lemon juice

2 teaspoons grated onion

½ teaspoon prepared mustard

¼ teaspoon pepper

1. Combine all ingredients in container with tightly fitting cover. Shake until blended.

2. Chill well before serving over crisp salad greens.

Yield: 16 servings

2 tablespoons contain:

Cal	Carb g	Fat g	Sat Fat g	Chol mg	Sod mg	Fib g
14	3	0	0	0	135	0

Exchanges: 2 tablespoons = Free

Soups

AUTUMN VEGETABLE BEEF SOUP*

½ pound very lean ground beef

1 small onion, chopped

3 stalks celery, chopped

2 small potatoes, unpeeled, diced

1 teaspoon salt

¼ teaspoon pepper

½ bay leaf, crumbled

¼ teaspoon dried basil

¼ teaspoon minced fresh chives

⅛ teaspoon garlic powder

¼ teaspoon dried thyme

½ jalapeño pepper, seeded and chopped (optional)

1 can (14½ ounces) tomatoes, chopped, undrained

2 medium carrots, thinly sliced

2 cups hot water

1.   In large saucepan, bring about 1 quart water to a boil. Crumble ground beef into water and stir constantly. When water starts to boil again, pour water and meat into large strainer in sink.

2.   Return meat to pan; add remaining ingredients.

3.   Bring to a boil and simmer, covered, about 30 minutes or until vegetables are tender.

Yield: 6 servings

1 cup contains:

Cal	Carb g	Fat g	Sat Fat g	Chol mg	Sod mg	Fib g
119	14	3	1	22	520	2

Exchanges: 1 cup = 1 starch/bread, 1 meat

*This recipe is moderately high in sodium; select other foods throughout the day that are very low in sodium.

BLACK-EYED PEA AND CHICKEN SOUP

4 deboned chicken breast halves, skin and fat removed

1 teaspoon olive oil

1 large onion, chopped

3 cloves garlic, chopped

1 teaspoon chili powder

1 can (14½ ounces) tomatoes, chopped, undrained

1 can (14½ ounces) chicken broth

Abbreviations: Cal = Calories; Carb = Carbohydrates; Sat Fat = Saturated Fat; Chol = Cholesterol; Sod = Sodium; Fib = Fiber; < = less than.

1 can (3 ounces) diced mild green chilies

1 teaspoon dried oregano

1 teaspoon ground coriander

1 teaspoon ground cumin

2 cans (15 ounces each) black-eyed peas
(without bacon or fat), undrained

½ teaspoon salt

½ teaspoon pepper

juice of 1 lime

½ cup chopped fresh cilantro

1.   Poach chicken in water until tender. Pull chicken apart with fork into bite-size pieces.

2.   Heat oil in large saucepan. Add onion and garlic and cook until soft.

3.   Add remaining ingredients except lime juice and cilantro. Bring to a boil; reduce heat and simmer about 20 minutes.

4.   Add lime juice and stir.

5.   Cilantro can be stirred into whole recipe just before serving or added to individual soup bowls.

Note: Recipe can be doubled very successfully.

Yield: 9 servings

1 cup contains:

Cal	Carb	Fat	Sat Fat	Chol	Sod	Fib
	g	g	g	mg	mg	g
176	18	3	1	34	713	7

Exchanges: 1 cup = 1 starch/bread, 2 meats

VARIATION

Low-Sodium Black-Eyed Pea and Chicken Soup:
Substitute 1 can (14½ ounces) no-salt-added tomatoes for regular canned tomatoes. Substitute 1 can (14½ ounces) reduced-sodium chicken broth for regular canned chicken broth. Substitute 1 fresh jalapeño pepper (seeded and chopped) for canned chilies. Omit salt.

1 cup has same analysis as above, except 310 mg sodium.

BLACK BEAN SOUP

1 tablespoon oil

2 cloves garlic, minced

1 medium onion, chopped

1 medium carrot, thinly sliced

3 cans (15 ounces each) black beans, undrained

1 can (14½ ounces) tomatoes, chopped, undrained

1 can (14½ ounces) reduced-sodium chicken broth

1 teaspoon ground cumin

¼ teaspoon pepper

8 ounces plain fat-free yogurt

1.   Heat oil in large saucepan. Add garlic, onion, and carrot; cook until onion is soft.

2.   Add beans, tomatoes, broth, cumin, and pepper.

3.   Bring to a boil, reduce heat, and simmer, uncovered, 1 hour.

4.   Pour part of soup in food processor or blender and process to desired consistency. Repeat with remaining soup.

5.   Return to pan and heat. Add water to thin if necessary.

6.   Top each serving with dollop of yogurt.

Yield: 6 servings

1 cup contains:

Cal	Carb	Fat	Sat Fat	Chol	Sod	Fib
	g	g	g	mg	mg	g
261	43	4	1	1	864	11

Exchanges: 1 cup = 3 starch/breads, 1 meat

LOW-SODIUM BLACK BEAN SOUP

1 pound dried black beans

1 tablespoon oil

4 cloves garlic, minced

1 large onion, chopped

2 medium carrots, thinly sliced

1 can (14½ ounces) tomatoes, chopped, undrained

1 can (14½ ounces) reduced-sodium chicken broth

1½ teaspoons ground cumin

½ teaspoon pepper

8 ounces plain fat-free yogurt

1. Soak dried beans in water overnight (see "Preparation of Dried Legumes," page 204).

2. Drain beans and cook in 8 cups water, covered, for about 1½ hours.

3. In separate pan, heat oil; add garlic, onion, and carrots and cook until onion is soft.

4. Transfer garlic, onion, and carrots to beans and add tomatoes, chicken broth, cumin, and pepper. Simmer, uncovered, 1½ hours or until beans are tender, adding more water if necessary.

5. Pour part of soup in food processor or blender and process to desired consistency. Repeat with remaining soup.

6. Return to pan and heat.

7. Top each serving with dollop of yogurt.

Yield: 10 servings

1 cup contains:

Cal	Carb g	Fat g	Sat Fat g	Chol mg	Sod mg	Fib g
207	35	2	0	0	214	9

Exchanges: 1 cup = 2 starch/breads, 1 meat

BLACK BEAN AND VEGETABLE CHILI

nonstick cooking spray

1 teaspoon olive oil

1 large onion, chopped

2 cloves garlic, minced

3 medium parsnips, peeled and chopped

2 medium yellow squash, cut in half lengthwise and sliced

2 medium zucchini, chopped

½ pound fresh mushrooms, sliced

1 large green bell pepper, chopped

2 cans (14½ ounces each) tomatoes, chopped, undrained

2 large stalks celery, chopped

1 fresh jalapeño pepper, seeded and chopped very fine

1 can (14½ ounces) vegetable broth

1 tablespoon chili powder

1 teaspoon ground cumin

1 teaspoon dried oregano, crumbled

⅛ teaspoon ground red pepper (cayenne pepper)

3 cans (16 ounces each) black beans, undrained

1 cup plain fat-free yogurt

3 ounces shredded Cheddar cheese (no more than 5 grams fat per ounce)

1. Coat large saucepan with nonstick spray. Add oil and place over medium heat. Add onion and garlic; cook until onion is soft.

2. Add remaining ingredients except beans, yogurt, and cheese. Bring to a boil; reduce heat, cover, and simmer 20 minutes.

3. Stir in beans; cover and simmer an additional 15 minutes.

4. Spoon into individual bowls and top with yogurt and cheese.

Note: A variety of other vegetables can be used, such as carrots, broccoli, green beans, or corn. Other beans, such as pinto beans or kidney beans, can be substituted for black beans.

Yield: 15 servings

1 cup contains:

Cal	Carb g	Fat g	Sat Fat g	Chol mg	Sod mg	Fib g
159	27	2	1	3	438	7

Exchanges: 1 cup = 2 starch/breads

VARIATION

Low-Sodium Black Bean and Vegetable Chili: Use 2 cans (14½ ounces each) no-salt-added canned tomatoes, 3 cans (15 ounces each) very-low-sodium black beans, and omit cheese.

1 cup contains:

Cal	Carb g	Fat g	Sat Fat g	Chol mg	Sod mg	Fib g
144	27	1	0	0	124	7

Exchanges: 1 cup = 2 starch/breads

CABBAGE AND MUSHROOM SOUP

1 tablespoon tub margarine

½ medium onion, diced

1 stalk celery, diced

2 cloves garlic, chopped

½ small head green cabbage, chopped

2 tablespoons all-purpose flour

2 cans (14½ ounces each) reduced-sodium chicken broth

1 deboned chicken breast half, skin and fat removed

4 large fresh mushrooms, sliced

2 tablespoons chopped fresh parsley

¼ teaspoon pepper

1. Heat margarine in soup pan and add onion, celery, and garlic. Cook until vegetables are nearly tender.

2. Add cabbage and simmer 5 minutes, stirring occasionally.

3. Add flour and blend well. Cook 2 minutes.

4. Add broth gradually and mix until smooth.

5. Cut chicken into bite-size pieces; add to soup and simmer 15 minutes.

6. Add mushrooms, parsley, and pepper. Simmer 5 minutes.

Yield: 5 servings

1 cup contains:

Cal	Carb g	Fat g	Sat Fat g	Chol mg	Sod mg	Fib g
106	9	4	1	16	97	2

Exchanges: 1 cup = 1 meat, 2 vegetables

COLD CUCUMBER YOGURT SOUP

2 small cucumbers, peeled (remove seeds if large)

3 cups plain fat-free yogurt

2 cloves garlic, minced

2 tablespoons tarragon vinegar

1 teaspoon lemon zest or grated peel

2 teaspoons finely chopped fresh dill or ½ teaspoon dried dill weed

ground red pepper (cayenne pepper) to taste

1 tablespoon sugar

¼ cup chopped fresh parsley

1. Grate cucumber into bowl and set aside.

2. In blender, combine remaining ingredients except parsley. Blend until smooth.

3. Pour into bowl containing cucumber.

4. Add chopped parsley and stir.

5. Refrigerate 4 hours or more before serving.

Yield: 5 servings

1 cup contains:

Cal	Carb g	Fat g	Sat Fat g	Chol mg	Sod mg	Fib g
102	16	0	0	3	116	<1

Exchanges: 1 cup = 1 milk

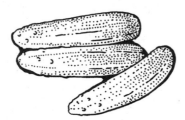

GAZPACHO

3 tomatoes

1 green bell pepper

1 small onion

1 cucumber, peeled

1¼ cups tomato juice

2 cloves garlic

1 teaspoon salt

½ teaspoon pepper

½ teaspoon dried oregano

½ teaspoon dried basil

1 tablespoon olive oil

12 drops Tabasco (more for a spicier taste)

1. Cut vegetables in large chunks.

2. Place half of tomato juice, half of vegetables, and garlic in blender and process at low speed to desired consistency. Repeat process with remaining tomato juice and vegetables.

3. Combine blended mixture, salt, pepper, oregano, basil, olive oil, and Tabasco.

4. Cover and chill.

Yield: 6 servings

1 cup contains:

Cal	Carb g	Fat g	Sat Fat g	Chol mg	Sod mg	Fib g
57	8	3	0	0	551	2

Exchanges: 1 cup = 2 vegetables

VARIATION

Low-Sodium Gazpacho: Omit salt and increase oregano and basil to ¾ teaspoon each.

1 cup has same analysis as above, except 195 mg sodium.

IRANIAN YOGURT SOUP

½ cup raisins

2 cups water

2 cups fat-free yogurt

1 cup canned evaporated skim milk

1 cup peeled, seeded, and chopped cucumber

½ cup chopped walnuts

1 hard-boiled egg, chopped

½ cup thinly sliced scallions

½ teaspoon salt

½ teaspoon pepper

chopped fresh parsley

chopped fresh dill

1. Soak raisins in water for 10 minutes.

2. Combine remaining ingredients except parsley and dill, add to raisins and water

3. Chill at least 3 hours. Garnish with parsley and dill just prior to serving.

Yield: 7 servings

1 cup contains:

Cal	Carb g	Fat g	Sat Fat g	Chol mg	Sod mg	Fib g
171	21	6	1	33	263	1

Exchanges: 1 cup = 1 fruit, 1 milk, 1 fat

LENTIL AND VEGETABLE SOUP

1 cup dried lentils

6 cups water

1 can (24 ounces) tomatoes, chopped, undrained

1 package (10 ounces) frozen whole-kernel corn

3 medium carrots, sliced

2 cloves garlic, minced

1 medium onion, chopped

2 stalks celery, chopped

2 medium yellow squash, chopped

2 medium zucchini, chopped

1 medium green bell pepper, chopped

1 can (4 ounces) sliced mushrooms, drained

¼ teaspoon ground cumin

½ teaspoon dried oregano, crumbled

1 teaspoon beef bouillon granules

1 bay leaf

1. Rinse lentils and place in large saucepan with remaining ingredients.

2. Bring to a boil, reduce heat, and simmer, covered, for 45 minutes, stirring occasionally. Remove bay leaf. Serve hot.

Yield: 12 servings

1 cup contains:

Cal	Carb g	Fat g	Sat Fat g	Chol mg	Sod mg	Fib g
117	24	1	0	0	260	6

Exchanges: 1 cup = 1 starch/bread, 1 vegetable

HARVEST CHICKEN SOUP

1 tablespoon corn oil

¼ cup chopped onion

½ cup chopped lean ham

3 cloves garlic, minced

2 cups fresh green beans, cut diagonally
  in 2-inch pieces

3 carrots, sliced

6 green onions, white part only, sliced

1 stalk celery, chopped

3 cans (14½ ounces each) reduced-sodium
  chicken broth

1 tablespoon chopped fresh parsley

¼ teaspoon dried thyme

¼ teaspoon dried basil

¼ teaspoon white pepper

½ teaspoon black peppercorns, cracked

2 deboned chicken breast halves, skin and fat
  removed

1 tablespoon prepared mustard

1. Heat oil in soup pan; add onion, ham, and garlic. Cook 2–3 minutes.

2. Add green beans, carrots, green onions, celery, and broth. Bring to a boil.

3. Add parsley, thyme, basil, pepper, and peppercorns. Reduce heat, cover, and simmer 20 minutes or until vegetables are desired tenderness.

4. Cut chicken into bite-size pieces.

5. Add chicken and mustard to soup; simmer about 10 minutes or until chicken is tender.

Yield: 8 servings

1 cup contains:

Cal	Carb g	Fat g	Sat Fat g	Chol mg	Sod mg	Fib g
115	7	4	1	25	232	2

Exchanges: 1 cup = 1 meat, 1 vegetable

VARIATION

Low-Sodium Harvest Chicken Soup: Omit ham and use only 1 can (14½ ounces) reduced-sodium chicken broth plus 2 cans water.

1 cup contains:

Cal	Carb g	Fat g	Sat Fat g	Chol mg	Sod mg	Fib g
90	7	3	1	19	78	2

Exchanges: 1 cup = 1 meat, 1 vegetable

QUICK AND EASY CLAM MUSHROOM BISQUE

1 pound fresh mushrooms, chopped

2 tablespoons tub margarine

¼ cup all-purpose flour

4 cans (6½ ounces each) minced clams in
  clam juice, undrained

1 cup canned evaporated skim milk

¼ teaspoon pepper

1. Cook mushrooms in margarine until soft.

2. Stir in flour. Add clams. Simmer 5 minutes.

3. Add milk and pepper; heat through. Serve hot.

Yield: 4 servings

1 cup contains:

Cal	Carb g	Fat g	Sat Fat g	Chol mg	Sod mg	Fib g
304	24	8	1	69	266	2

Exchanges: 1 cup = 1 starch/bread, 3 meats, 1 vegetable, 1 fat

SPICY TOMATO VEGETABLE SOUP BASE

1 tablespoon olive oil

1 medium onion, chopped

3 cloves garlic, minced

2 green bell peppers, chopped

4 stalks celery, thinly sliced

5 medium carrots (if soup base will be used for soup, slice carrots; if soup base will be used for gumbo, finely chop carrots in food processor)

2 cans (14½ ounces each) tomatoes, chopped, undrained

1 package (9 ounces) frozen cut okra or 1½ teaspoons gumbo filé

1 teaspoon Worcestershire sauce

2 teaspoons Creole seasoning

¼ teaspoon pepper

2 bay leaves

2 cups water

1 jalapeño pepper, seeded and finely chopped (optional)

1. Heat oil in large soup pan that will hold 1½ gallons. Cook onion and garlic until soft.

2. Add bell peppers, celery, and carrots; stir until hot.

3. Add tomatoes with juice, okra, Worcestershire sauce, Creole seasoning, pepper, bay leaves, water, and jalapeño to vegetable mixture.

4. Bring to a boil; reduce heat, cover and simmer 1 hour.

Notes: Can be stored in container with tight-fitting lid 1 week. Raw seafood (see Seafood Soup or Gumbo on page 243) or chicken (see variation below) can be added.

Yield: 12 servings

1 serving contains:

Cal	Carb g	Fat g	Sat Fat g	Chol mg	Sod mg	Fib g
56	10	1	0	0	367	3

Exchanges: 1 serving = 2 vegetables

VARIATION

Spicy Tomato Vegetable Soup with Chicken. Substitute 1 potato, peeled and diced, for okra or gumbo filé. Cut 4 deboned chicken breast halves, skin and fat removed, into small pieces; add to Spicy Tomato Vegetable Soup Base and cook about 30 minutes or until chicken is tender.

Yield: 16 servings with chicken

1 serving with chicken contains:

Cal	Carb g	Fat g	Sat Fat g	Chol mg	Sod mg	Fib g
85	8	2	0	19	298	2

Exchanges: 1 serving with chicken = 1 meat, 1 vegetable

QUICK AND EASY MEXICAN SOUP

1 pound ground turkey

2 medium onions, chopped

5 cloves garlic, minced

1 package taco seasoning mix (dry)

1 can (14½ ounces) tomatoes, chopped, undrained

1 can (15½ ounces) yellow hominy, drained

1 can (15 ounces) kidney beans, drained

1 package (10 ounces) frozen whole-kernel corn

¼ teaspoon pepper

4 cups water

fresh cilantro, chopped (optional)

1. In soup pan, cook turkey, onions, and garlic until turkey is cooked.

2. Add remaining ingredients except cilantro. Stir well. Bring to a boil, reduce heat, and cook over low heat 1 hour, stirring occasionally.

3. If desired, put cilantro in bottom of soup bowls before adding soup.

Yield: 11 servings

1 cup contains:

Cal	Carb g	Fat g	Sat Fat g	Chol mg	Sod mg	Fib g
168	20	5	1	28	325	4

Exchanges: 1 cup = 1 starch/bread, 1 meat, 1 vegetable

OLD-FASHIONED MUSHROOM SOUP

2 tablespoons tub margarine

1 pound fresh mushrooms, sliced

4 large carrots, sliced

3 stalks celery, chopped

2 medium onions, chopped

2 cloves garlic, minced

2 cans (14½ ounces each) beef broth

4 cups water

3 tablespoons tomato paste

¼ teaspoon salt

⅛ teaspoon pepper

¼ teaspoon Worcestershire sauce

2 tablespoons chopped fresh parsley

2 tablespoons chopped celery leaves

2 bay leaves

¼ cup dry sherry

1. In soup pan, heat margarine; add mushrooms and cook until soft. Remove half of mushrooms and set aside.

2. Add carrots, celery, onions, and garlic and cook until onions are tender.

3. Stir in remaining ingredients except sherry and reserved mushrooms.

4. Bring to a boil. Reduce heat, cover, and simmer for 45 minutes.

5. Remove bay leaves and purée in blender or food processor to desired consistency. Return to pan.

6. Add sherry and reserved mushrooms to soup. Briefly reheat; do not boil.

Yield: 12 servings

1 cup contains:

Cal	Carb g	Fat g	Sat Fat g	Chol mg	Sod mg	Fib g
67	10	2	<1	0	306	2

Exchanges: 1 cup = 2 vegetables

SEAFOOD SOUP OR GUMBO

1 recipe Spicy Tomato Vegetable Soup Base (page 241)

1 pound fish fillets, skinned and cut into small pieces

1 pound uncooked shrimp without heads, peeled and deveined

1 pound cooked crabmeat

1. Bring Spicy Tomato Vegetable Soup Base to a boil. Add fish and shrimp, stirring frequently. Just before soup returns to a boil, add crab. Continue heating until soup boils and all shrimp turn pink.

2. Store leftovers in container with tight-fitting lid in refrigerator for up to 2 days. Reheat only the amount that will be eaten, so as not to overcook the seafood.

Yield: 16 servings

1 cup contains:

Cal	Carb g	Fat g	Sat Fat g	Chol mg	Sod mg	Fib g
110	8	2	0	70	414	2

Exchanges: 1 cup = 2 meats, 1 vegetable

SPLIT PEA SOUP

3 cups dried split green peas

1 pound lean ham, finely chopped

13 cups water

1 large onion, minced

2 stalks celery with tops, chopped

1 medium carrot, chopped

1 teaspoon dried basil

2 bay leaves

¼ teaspoon dried marjoram

2 cloves garlic, minced, or ½ teaspoon garlic powder

1 teaspoon salt

¼ teaspoon pepper

1. Wash peas in cold water and drain.

2. Place peas in soup pan; add remaining ingredients and bring to a boil, uncovered. Reduce heat, cover, and simmer 1 hour.

Yield: 19 servings

1 cup contains:

Cal	Carb g	Fat g	Sat Fat g	Chol mg	Sod mg	Fib g
146	21	2	<1	13	408	3

Exchanges: 1 cup = 1 starch/bread, 1 meat

Meatless Entrées

BEAN-FILLED PITAS

2 cans (16 ounces each) white kidney, Great
    Northern, or navy beans, drained

2 tablespoons lemon juice

½ cup plain fat-free yogurt

1 teaspoon dried oregano

¼ teaspoon salt

½ teaspoon ground cumin

¼ teaspoon pepper

¼ cup low-fat cottage cheese, drained

2 tomatoes, coarsely chopped

1 cucumber, peeled and chopped

4 pita breads

1.   In large bowl, toss beans, lemon juice, yogurt, oregano, salt, cumin, and pepper. Gently stir
in cottage cheese, tomatoes, and cucumber.

2.   Cover and chill about 2 hours.

3.   Fill pita breads.

Yield: 4 servings

1 serving contains:

Cal	Carb g	Fat g	Sat Fat g	Chol mg	Sod mg	Fib g
358	65	2	<1	2	746	9

Exchanges: 1 serving = 4 starch/breads, 1 meat

VARIATION

Low-Sodium Bean-Filled Pitas: Substitute no-salt-
added canned beans for regular canned beans. Omit
salt.

1 serving has same analysis as above, except 312
mg sodium.

CHILI-STUFFED PEPPERS

nonstick cooking spray

6 green bell peppers

1 medium onion, chopped

1 teaspoon oil

1 cup cooked rice, prepared without salt
    or fat

1 can (15 ounces) kidney beans, drained

1 tablespoon chili powder

1 can (8 ounces) whole-kernel corn, drained, with liquid reserved

1 can (16 ounces) tomatoes, chopped, drained

1 tablespoon cornstarch

1. Preheat oven to 350°F. Spray 9 × 13-inch baking dish with nonstick spray.

2. Cut tops off peppers. Remove seeds and membranes. Cook peppers in boiling water 5–10 minutes or until tender. Drain.

3. Cook onion in oil until soft.

4. Mix onion, rice, beans, chili powder, corn, and tomatoes.

5. Mix cornstarch with 1 tablespoon reserved corn liquid; add to vegetable mixture.

6. Fill peppers and stand upright in dish. Bake 30 minutes.

Yield: 6 servings

1 stuffed pepper contains:

Cal	Carb g	Fat g	Sat Fat g	Chol mg	Sod mg	Fib g
161	32	2	0	0	268	7

Exchanges: 1 stuffed pepper = 2 starch/breads

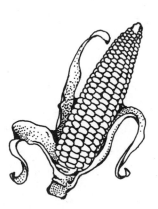

COTTAGE CHEESE–SPINACH CASSEROLE

nonstick cooking spray

2 cups fat-free cottage cheese

¾ cup egg substitute

3 tablespoons all-purpose flour

4 ounces part-skim mozzarella cheese, shredded

½ of 10-ounce package frozen chopped spinach, partially thawed and drained

1. Preheat oven to 350°F. Spray 8 × 8-inch casserole dish with nonstick spray.

2. Combine cottage cheese, egg substitute, and flour.

3. Add mozzarella cheese and spinach.

4. Place in casserole dish and bake, uncovered, about 1 hour or until lightly browned.

Yield: 6 servings

1 serving contains:

Cal	Carb g	Fat g	Sat Fat g	Chol mg	Sod mg	Fib g
126	6	4	2	13	179	1

Exchanges: 1 serving = 2 meats, 1 vegetable

EGGPLANT PARMIGIANA*

nonstick cooking spray

1 medium eggplant

¾ cup egg substitute

⅛ teaspoon garlic powder

2 teaspoons olive oil, divided

1 jar (26 ounces) fat-free, reduced-sodium
    spaghetti sauce

8 ounces part-skim mozzarella cheese, shredded

1.   Preheat oven to 350°F. Spray 10-inch casserole dish with nonstick spray.

2.   Cut eggplant into ¼-inch slices, then cut
slices into quarters.

3.   Combine egg substitute and garlic powder;
dip eggplant in mixture.

4.   Heat 1 teaspoon oil in skillet; brown half of
eggplant. Repeat with remaining oil and eggplant.

5.   Cover bottom of dish with ½ cup spaghetti
sauce. Add layer of eggplant, spaghetti sauce, and
cheese. Continue layering until all ingredients
are used, ending with cheese.

6.   Bake 30 minutes. Serve hot.

Yield: 6 servings

1 serving contains:

Cal	Carb g	Fat g	Sat Fat g	Chol mg	Sod mg	Fib g
201	18	8	4	20	641	4

Exchanges: 1 serving = 2 meats, 3 vegetables

*This recipe is moderately high in sodium; select other foods
throughout the day that are very low in sodium.*

GRILLED VEGETABLES BY CHEF BAKER

VEGETABLES

7 small new potatoes, unpeeled

4 small zucchini, cut lengthwise in quarters

2 medium eggplant, cut in ¼-inch slices

2 red bell peppers, cut into 8 pieces

2 yellow bell peppers, cut into 8 pieces

3 green bell peppers, cut into 8 pieces

1 pound mushrooms, whole

28 cherry tomatoes, whole

7 small carrots, cut in half

MARINADE

2 teaspoons salt

1 teaspoon paprika

1 teaspoon onion powder

1 teaspoon garlic powder

1 teaspoon pepper

3 cloves garlic

½ bunch fresh parsley, chopped (about 1 cup)

½ bunch fresh basil, chopped (about 1 cup),
    or 1 tablespoon dried basil

½ teaspoon coriander seeds or ¼ teaspoon
    ground coriander

½ cup olive oil

½–1 cup water

1. Cook potatoes in boiling water until soft. Slice in ¼-inch rounds.

2. In food processor or blender, combine all marinade ingredients except water and process until very finely chopped. Add water to make marinade thin enough to coat all vegetables.

3. Pour marinade over vegetables and shake gently to coat. Allow vegetables to marinate 1 hour.

4. Spread vegetables on grill and cook to desired doneness.

Yield: 14 servings

1 serving contains:

Cal	Carb g	Fat g	Sat Fat g	Chol mg	Sod mg	Fib g
184	26	8	1	0	331	5

Exchanges: 1 serving = 1 starch/bread, 1 vegetable, 2 fats

LIVING HEART FETTUCCINE ALFREDO

2 tablespoons tub margarine

1 tablespoon all-purpose flour

3 large cloves garlic, minced

1 can (12 ounces) evaporated skim milk

½ pound fresh mushrooms, sliced

¾ cup grated reduced-fat Parmesan cheese

¼ cup white wine

1 teaspoon chopped fresh basil or ½ teaspoon dried basil

1 teaspoon chopped fresh parsley

1 package (9 ounces) fettuccine, cooked according to package directions, omitting salt and fat

1. In nonstick skillet, melt margarine and simmer 1–2 minutes to evaporate moisture. Add flour and cook over low heat, stirring constantly, until it stops bubbling and becomes a golden paste.

2. Add garlic and continue stirring until garlic softens.

3. Add evaporated milk and simmer over medium heat, stirring constantly, until milk thickens.

4. Add mushrooms and continue cooking over low heat until mushrooms soften.

5. Add Parmesan cheese and stir well. Simmer, stirring often, until cheese melts and is blended thoroughly. Remove skillet from heat.

6. Stir in wine, basil, and parsley. Toss with hot fettuccine and serve immediately.

Yield: 6 cups

1 cup contains:

Cal	Carb g	Fat g	Sat Fat g	Chol mg	Sod mg	Fib g
282	39	8	3	46	385	3

Exchanges: 1 cup = 2 starch/breads, 1 milk, 2 fats

PASTA WITH FRESH TOMATO BASIL SAUCE

nonstick cooking spray

¼ small onion, chopped

1 clove garlic, minced

¼ small green bell pepper, chopped

3 cups chopped ripe tomatoes

½ cup chopped fresh basil

1 cup part-skim ricotta cheese

2 tablespoons olive oil

¼ teaspoon pepper

1 pound shaped pasta, uncooked

1.   Spray large skillet with nonstick spray; cook onion, garlic, and bell pepper until onion is soft.

2.   Combine with tomatoes and basil. Stir in ricotta cheese, oil, and pepper.

3.   Cook pasta according to package directions, omitting salt and fat.

4.   Toss hot pasta with sauce and serve at once.

Yield: 12 servings

1 cup contains:

| Cal | Carb | Fat | Sat Fat | Chol | Sod | Fib |
	g	g	g	mg	mg	g
206	33	5	1	6	32	2

Exchanges: 1 cup = 2 starch/breads, 1 vegetable, 1 fat

LINGUINE WITH BASIL SAUCE

½ cup chopped fresh parsley, loosely packed

½ cup chopped fresh basil, loosely packed

1 tablespoon olive oil

1 tablespoon malt vinegar

1 teaspoon sugar

2 tablespoons reduced-sodium chicken broth (more if thinner sauce is desired)

1 clove garlic

3 tablespoons chopped walnuts

¼ teaspoon pepper

12 ounces linguine, uncooked

1.   Combine all ingredients except linguine in food processor or blender. Process to desired consistency.

2.   Cook linguine according to package directions, omitting salt and fat. Drain and return to pan.

3.   Add sauce to linguine and stir gently. Serve hot.

Yield: 4 servings

1 serving contains:

| Cal | Carb | Fat | Sat Fat | Chol | Sod | Fib |
	g	g	g	mg	mg	g
417	72	9	1	0	33	3

Exchanges: 1 serving = 5 starch/breads, 2 fats

NEW ENGLAND BAKED SOYBEANS

2 cups dried soybeans

nonstick cooking spray

2 whole cloves

1 onion

½ teaspoon salt

½ teaspoon dry mustard

¼ cup molasses

2–3 drops Worcestershire sauce

1. Cover beans with cold water and soak overnight (see "Preparation of Dried Legumes," page 204). Simmer until tender, about 2 hours.

2. Preheat oven to 275°F. Spray casserole dish with nonstick spray. Stick cloves in onion and place in dish.

3. Add beans with their cooking liquid and remaining ingredients. (Reserve some of the liquid if beans are soupy.)

4. Cover dish and bake 8 hours. Add reserved bean liquid or hot water if needed.

5. Uncover and bake 30–40 minutes longer to brown.

Yield: 13 servings

1 serving contains:

Cal	Carb g	Fat g	Sat Fat g	Chol mg	Sod mg	Fib g
171	14	8	1	0	85	2

Exchanges: 1 serving = 1 starch/bread, 1 meat, 1 fat

MEXICAN LASAGNA

nonstick cooking spray

1 teaspoon olive oil

1 medium onion, chopped (about 1 cup)

3 cloves garlic, minced

1 medium green bell pepper, chopped

4 medium carrots, grated (about 2 cups)

1 medium tomato, chopped

1 can (16 ounces) tomato sauce

1 can (16 ounces) pinto, red, or kidney beans, undrained

2 tablespoons (½ of 4½-ounce can) chopped green chilies

1 teaspoon chili powder

½ teaspoon ground cumin

¼ teaspoon pepper

6 corn tortillas

2 cups shredded part-skim mozzarella cheese

1. Preheat oven to 350°F. Spray 8 × 11-inch casserole dish with nonstick spray.

2. In large skillet, heat oil; add onion, garlic, and bell pepper and cook until soft, stirring frequently.

3. Add carrots; cover and cook 5 minutes. Stir in tomato, tomato sauce, beans, chilies, chili powder, cumin, and pepper. Bring to a boil. Reduce heat and simmer until mixture thickens slightly, about 5 minutes.

4. Place 2 corn tortillas on bottom of casserole dish. Add ⅓ of vegetable mixture and ⅓ of cheese. Repeat layers, except set aside last ⅓ of cheese.

5. Bake until hot throughout (about 30 minutes).

continued

6.   Add remaining cheese to top and return to oven until cheese melts (about 5 minutes).

Note: Can be made ahead through Step 4 and refrigerated. Bake about 45 minutes, add cheese to top, and return to oven until cheese melts (about 5 minutes).

Yield: 8 servings

1 serving contains:

Cal	Carb g	Fat g	Sat Fat g	Chol mg	Sod mg	Fib g
211	27	7	3	15	691	6

Exchanges: 1 serving = 1 starch/bread, 1 meat, 2 vegetables, 1 fat

VARIATION

Low-Sodium Mexican Lasagna: Substitute no-salt-added tomato sauce for regular tomato sauce.

1 serving has same analysis as above, except 365 mg sodium.

QUICK AND EASY SALAD PIZZA*

3 cups torn spinach

6 cherry tomatoes, sliced

1 can (2½ ounces) sliced pitted ripe olives, drained

6 fresh mushrooms, sliced

½ cup low-fat cottage cheese

2 teaspoons chopped fresh oregano or 1 teaspoon dried oregano

3 tablespoons skim milk

1 low-fat pizza crust†

1 cup commercial low-fat pizza sauce

8 ounces part-skim mozzarella cheese, shredded

1.   Set top rack of oven about 5 inches from broiler.

2.   Preheat oven to 375°F.

3.   In large mixing bowl, combine spinach, tomatoes, olives, and mushrooms.

4.   In small mixing bowl, stir together cottage cheese, oregano, and milk. Drizzle over spinach mixture. Toss to coat well.

5.   Place crust on ungreased pizza pan; generously prick with fork. Bake 5 minutes or until lightly browned.

6.   Remove crust from oven and spread with pizza sauce. Bake 5 minutes more or until hot.

7.   Remove pizza from oven and spread salad mixture over top.

8.   Sprinkle cheese evenly over salad and crust. Broil 1–2 minutes or until cheese starts to melt. Cut pizza into wedges. Serve immediately.

Yield: 8 servings

1 serving contains:

Cal	Carb g	Fat g	Sat Fat g	Chol mg	Sod mg	Fib g
263	32	8	4	17	691	3

Exchanges: 1 serving = 2 starch/breads, 1 meat, 1 fat

*This recipe is moderately high in sodium; select other foods throughout the day that are very low in sodium.
†Other forms of crust, such as Afghanistan bread, can be used. Analyzed with crust containing 1 gram fat per ⅛ of crust (50 grams).

QUICK AND EASY LINGUINE CASSEROLE

nonstick cooking spray

6 ounces linguine, uncooked

1 package (10 ounces) frozen green beans, slightly thawed

1 can (8 ounces) sliced water chestnuts, drained

2 green onions, sliced

1 jar (14 ounces) fat-free reduced-sodium spaghetti sauce

¼ cup shredded part-skim mozzarella cheese

1. Preheat oven to 350°F. Spray 13 × 8-inch casserole dish with nonstick spray.

2. Cook linguine according to package directions, omitting salt and fat.

3. Place linguine on bottom of casserole dish.

4. Add green beans, water chestnuts, and onions in layers.

5. Top with spaghetti sauce and sprinkle with cheese.

6. Bake 40 minutes or until hot throughout, or microwave 12 minutes.

Yield: 8 servings

1 cup contains:

Cal	Carb g	Fat g	Sat Fat g	Chol mg	Sod mg	Fib g
130	26	1	<1	2	180	3

Exchanges: 1 cup = 1 starch/bread, 2 vegetables

QUICK AND EASY SPINACH LASAGNA

nonstick cooking spray

1 package (10 ounces) frozen chopped spinach, thawed and drained

¼ teaspoon ground nutmeg

½ teaspoon pepper

1 carton (15 ounces) fat-free small-curd cottage cheese

1 jar (26 ounces) fat-free reduced-sodium spaghetti sauce

1 cup water

1 small box (8 ounces or 9 pieces) lasagna noodles, uncooked

8 ounces part-skim mozzarella cheese, shredded

3 tablespoons chopped fresh parsley (optional)

1. Preheat oven to 350°F. Spray 12 × 7-inch baking dish with nonstick spray. (If lasagna will be cooked in microwave, use microwave-safe baking dish.)

2. In mixing bowl, combine spinach, nutmeg, pepper, and cottage cheese.

3. In separate bowl, combine spaghetti sauce and water.

4. Pour 1 cup sauce in baking dish; arrange 3 pieces uncooked noodles over sauce. Continue to layer sauce, spinach mixture, and noodles, ending with sauce.

5. Top with cheese and, if desired, parsley.

continued

6. *Conventional oven:* Bake, covered, 45 minutes. Remove cover and bake 15 more minutes. *Microwave oven:* Cover with microwaveable wrap and cook on high 8 minutes. Then microwave on medium 17–20 minutes or until lasagna is tender when pierced with fork.

Yield: 8 servings

1 serving contains:

Cal	Carb g	Fat g	Sat Fat g	Chol mg	Sod mg	Fib g
274	33	6	3	19	463	3

Exchanges: 1 serving = 2 starch/breads, 2 meats

RATATOUILLE PASTA

2 teaspoons olive oil

2 cloves garlic, minced

1 large onion, cut into thin slices

½ of 12-ounce package tricolor spiral pasta

1 can (16 ounces) tomatoes, chopped, undrained

1 tablespoon Italian seasoning

1 teaspoon salt

1 teaspoon sugar

1 medium eggplant, cut into 1-inch cubes

1 large green bell pepper, cut into strips

1 large or 2 small zucchini, cut into strips

1 large or 2 small yellow squash, cut into strips

4 medium Roma tomatoes, cut into quarters

1. In Dutch oven, heat oil and cook garlic and onion until soft (8–10 minutes).

2. While cooking garlic and onion, in separate pan cook pasta according to package directions, omitting salt and fat.

3. Add canned tomatoes with liquid, Italian seasoning, salt, and sugar to garlic and onion and heat 2 minutes.

4. Stir eggplant and bell pepper into mixture and heat 2 minutes.

5. Add squashes to mixture; cover and cook over low to medium heat 8–10 minutes or until crisp-tender.

6. Stir cooked, drained pasta into vegetable mixture.

7. Place Roma tomatoes on top and heat slightly before serving.

Yield: 10 servings

1 cup contains:

Cal	Carb g	Fat g	Sat Fat g	Chol mg	Sod mg	Fib g
134	27	2	0	0	295	4

Exchanges: 1 cup = 1 starch/bread, 2 vegetables

TOFU SANDWICH SPREAD

8 ounces tofu, squeezed dry

¾ cup egg substitute, cooked and diced

2 tablespoons lemon juice

⅛ teaspoon garlic powder

2 teaspoons prepared mustard

¾ tablespoon chopped green onion

⅛ teaspoon pepper

1½ tablespoons chopped fresh parsley

1.   Combine all ingredients except parsley in blender. Blend until smooth.

2.   Stir in parsley and spread mixture over bread.

Yield: Filling for 4 sandwiches

1 serving contains:

Cal	Carb g	Fat g	Sat Fat g	Chol mg	Sod mg	Fib g
69	3	3	0	0	127	1

Exchanges: 1 serving = 1 meat

SOYBEAN STEW*

1 cup dried soybeans (2½ cups cooked)

1 can (8 ounces) tomato sauce

⅓ cup chopped onions

1 cup frozen green peas

1 clove garlic, minced

2 carrots, chopped

1 stalk celery, chopped

½ teaspoon ground cumin

½ teaspoon salt

½ cup finely chopped green bell pepper

¼ cup grated Parmesan cheese

1.   Place dried beans in water and soak overnight (see "Preparation of Dried Legumes," page 204). Simmer 4 hours and drain.

2.   In Dutch oven, combine soybeans with remaining ingredients except green pepper and cheese. Cook 30 minutes over low heat, adding water if needed.

3.   Remove from heat and stir in bell pepper and cheese.

Yield: 6 servings

1 serving contains:

Cal	Carb g	Fat g	Sat Fat g	Chol mg	Sod mg	Fib g
224	19	10	2	3	503	5

Exchanges: 1 serving = 1 starch/bread, 2 meats, 1 fat

*This recipe is moderately high in sodium; select other foods throughout the day that are very low in sodium.

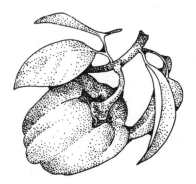

SOUTHWESTERN BEANS

1 pound dried kidney, pinto, or red beans

3½ teaspoons salt, divided

1 tablespoon olive oil

1 large onion, chopped

1 green bell pepper, chopped

2 cloves garlic, minced

1–2 jalapeño peppers, sliced thin

1 tablespoon chili powder

½ teaspoon ground cumin

½ teaspoon sugar

1 large bay leaf

½ teaspoon Tabasco (optional)

1 tomato, chopped (optional)

1–2 shallots, chopped (optional)

fresh cilantro, chopped (optional)

1. Sort and wash beans in cold water (see "Preparation of Dried Legumes," page 204). Put beans in large pot with 2 quarts water and 1½ teaspoons salt; cover and heat to a rolling boil.

2. Turn off heat and keep pan covered; soak 1 hour. (For high altitude, boil beans 1 hour and soak 1 hour.) Drain and rinse.

3. Add 2 quarts water and remaining salt (2 teaspoons) and heat to boiling.

4. Heat oil in skillet; add onion, bell pepper, garlic, and jalapeños. Cook until onion is soft. Add to beans.

5. Add chili powder, cumin, sugar, bay leaf, and Tabasco, if desired. Cover and simmer 1–2 hours or until beans are soft. (Add more water if needed.)

6. Garnish with tomato, shallots, and cilantro if desired.

Yield: 14 servings

¾ cup contains:

Cal	Carb g	Fat g	Sat Fat g	Chol mg	Sod mg	Fib g
121	21	2	0	0	391	7

Exchanges: ¾ cup = 2 starch/breads

VARIATIONS

Southwestern Hoppin' John: Spoon ¾ cup beans with juice over ¼ cup cooked rice. Garnish with tomato, shallots, and cilantro.

Yield: 14 servings

1 cup contains:

Cal	Carb g	Fat g	Sat Fat g	Chol mg	Sod mg	Fib g
174	32	2	0	0	392	7

Exchanges: 1 cup = 2 starch/breads

Chalupas: Preheat oven to 350°F. Drain 1 cup Southwestern Beans; put in food processor or blender and process until smooth. Bake 8 corn tortillas on rack in oven for about 10 minutes or until crisp. Spread 2 tablespoons beans over each tortilla. Garnish each with ⅓ cup shredded lettuce, 2 tablespoons chopped tomato, and 1 teaspoon chopped onion; top each with 1 teaspoon shredded Cheddar cheese (no more than 5 grams fat per ounce).

Yield: 8 servings

1 chalupa contains:

Cal	Carb g	Fat g	Sat Fat g	Chol mg	Sod mg	Fib g
84	15	2	0	1	123	3

Exchanges: 1 chalupa = 1 starch/bread

STUFFED MANICOTTI

nonstick cooking spray

1 package (10 ounces) frozen chopped spinach, thawed

1 tablespoon chopped green onions

¼ teaspoon ground nutmeg

1 cup low-fat cottage cheese, drained

¼ cup skim milk

2 teaspoons chopped fresh parsley

1 egg white

2 cups tomato sauce

¼ cup tomato paste

½ teaspoon garlic powder

¾ teaspoon dried oregano

½ teaspoon dried basil

12 manicotti pasta shells, cooked and drained

2 tablespoons grated Parmesan cheese

1.   Preheat oven to 350°F. Spray baking dish with nonstick spray.

2.   Cook spinach, green onions, and nutmeg in small amount of water and drain.

3.   Mash cottage cheese; stir in milk and parsley. Add to spinach mixture.

4.   Beat egg white with fork until frothy; add to spinach mixture.

5.   In separate pan, combine remaining ingredients except manicotti shells and Parmesan cheese and cook over low heat 3–5 minutes.

6.   Stuff spinach mixture into manicotti shells.

7.   Cover bottom of dish with some tomato sauce. Arrange stuffed shells on top. Pour remaining sauce over manicotti and sprinkle with Parmesan cheese.

8.   Bake 30 minutes.

Yield: 6 servings

2 manicotti contain:

Cal	Carb g	Fat g	Sat Fat g	Chol mg	Sod mg	Fib g
175	29	2	1	5	807	3

Exchanges: 2 manicotti = 2 starch/breads, 1 meat

VARIATION

Low-Sodium Stuffed Manicotti: Substitute no-salt-added tomato sauce for regular tomato sauce. Omit Parmesan cheese.

2 manicotti have same analysis as above, except 306 mg sodium.

STUFFED PEPPERS

nonstick cooking spray

6 green bell peppers

¼ cup chopped onion

1 tablespoon tub margarine

1 cup regular white or brown rice, uncooked

2 cups water

1 teaspoon garlic power

1 teaspoon paprika

2 teaspoons Worcestershire sauce

1 can (16 ounces) tomatoes, chopped, undrained

1 teaspoon dried oregano

1 teaspoon dried basil

1 cup frozen peas, thawed

½ cup shredded part-skim mozzarella cheese

1.   Preheat oven to 350°F. Spray 9 × 13-inch baking dish with nonstick spray.

continued

2. Cut tops off peppers. Remove seeds and membranes. Cook peppers in boiling water 5–10 minutes or until tender. Drain and set aside.

3. In large saucepan, cook onion in margarine until tender.

4. Add rice, water, garlic powder, paprika, Worcestershire sauce, tomatoes, oregano, and basil to saucepan. Cover and cook until rice absorbs the liquid and is tender.

5. Stir peas and cheese into rice mixture.

6. Stuff peppers and stand upright in dish. Bake 30 minutes.

Yield: 6 servings

1 stuffed pepper contains:

Cal	Carb g	Fat g	Sat Fat g	Chol mg	Sod mg	Fib g
225	40	4	2	5	234	4

Exchanges: 1 stuffed pepper = 2 starch/breads, 1 vegetable, 1 fat

VEGETABLE BEAN NOODLE BAKE

1 cup dried soybeans (2 cups cooked)

6 ounces noodles, uncooked (3 cups cooked)

1 onion, chopped

½ stalk celery, chopped

5 tablespoons all-purpose flour

2 cups water

2 carrots, sliced

1 potato, cubed

½ package (10 ounces) frozen corn

4 tomatoes, 1 chopped and 3 sliced

1 teaspoon salt

¼ teaspoon pepper

½ teaspoon dry mustard

½ teaspoon dried sage

2 teaspoons dried basil

nonstick cooking spray

⅓ cup finely chopped fresh parsley

1. Place dried beans in water and soak overnight (see "Preparation of Dried Legumes," page 204). Simmer 4 hours and drain.

2. Preheat oven to 350°F.

3. Cook noodles and drain.

4. In saucepan, simmer onion and celery in small amount of water until tender. Stir in flour and cook several minutes over medium heat, stirring constantly.

5. Slowly add 2 cups water, stirring constantly over low heat.

6. Add carrots, potato, corn, chopped tomato, salt, pepper, mustard, sage, and basil. Bring to a boil to thicken, stirring constantly. Remove from heat.

7. Spray 9 × 13-inch baking dish with nonstick spray. Alternate layers of beans, noodles, and vegetables, pouring some of the juice from vegetables over each layer. Liquid should come almost to top of dish.

8. Arrange sliced tomatoes on top.

9. Sprinkle with parsley. Bake 1 hour.

Yield: 8 servings

1 serving contains:

Cal	Carb g	Fat g	Sat Fat g	Chol mg	Sod mg	Fib g
270	37	8	1	18	289	5

Exchanges: 1 serving = 2 starch/breads, 1 meat, 1 vegetable, 1 fat

SPINACH AND CHEESE CALZONES

DOUGH

1 package (¼ ounce) active dry yeast

1⅓ cups lukewarm water (95°–105°F)

3 tablespoons corn oil

4½ cups all-purpose flour

1 teaspoon salt

SPINACH FILLING

2 cloves garlic, minced

1 small onion, chopped

1 small green bell pepper, chopped

1 teaspoon tub margarine

2 pounds fresh spinach, chopped

16 ounces fat-free cottage cheese

8 ounces fat-free mozzarella cheese, shredded

1 teaspoon pepper

cornmeal

1 jar (14 ounces) commercial low-fat
   pizza sauce

DOUGH

1. In large bowl, dissolve yeast in lukewarm water. Add oil and stir in flour and salt.

2. Turn onto lightly floured surface and knead until smooth.

3. Place dough back in bowl. Cover and let rise until doubled in bulk, 1½–2 hours. Punch dough down. (Can be refrigerated up to 2 days.)

SPINACH FILLING

4. Cook garlic, onion, and bell pepper in margarine 2 minutes. Add spinach and mix well; cover and cook until tender.

5. Drain spinach mixture and allow to cool.

6. Add cottage cheese, mozzarella cheese, and pepper. Mix well and set aside.

ASSEMBLY

7. Preheat oven to 425°F.

8. Punch dough down and knead 2–3 minutes. If dough has been refrigerated, knead 5–6 minutes. Divide dough into 14 portions.

9. On lightly floured surface, use rolling pin to roll out each portion of dough into circle about 5 inches in diameter.

10. Spread ⅓ cup spinach–cheese mixture over half of each circle.

11. Fold over and seal by pressing edges with tines of fork.

12. Sprinkle cornmeal in bottom of baking sheet to keep calzones crisp on bottom.

13. Use spatula to move calzones to baking sheet. Use fork to poke holes in top of each calzone to allow steam to evaporate. Bake 25 minutes. Serve with pizza sauce on top.

Yield: 14 servings

1 calzone contains:

Cal	Carb g	Fat g	Sat Fat g	Chol mg	Sod mg	Fib g
265	39	5	1	3	584	4

Exchanges: 1 calzone = 2 starch/breads, 1 meat, 1 vegetable

VARIATION

Low-Sodium Spinach and Cheese Calzones: Omit pizza sauce.

1 calzone contains:

Cal	Carb g	Fat g	Sat Fat g	Chol mg	Sod mg	Fib g
247	37	4	1	3	463	3

Exchanges: 1 calzone = 2 starch/breads, 1 meat, 1 vegetable

TOFU BURGERS

1 onion, finely chopped

24 ounces tofu, crumbled

2 cups water

½ cup fine dry bread crumbs

2 tablespoons Worcestershire sauce

½ teaspoon salt

⅛ teaspoon pepper

nonstick cooking spray

1. Cook onion in small amount of water until soft. Remove from heat and cool.

2. Mix onion with remaining ingredients except nonstick spray and form into 8 patties.

3. Spray nonstick skillet with nonstick spray and heat.

4. Add 4 patties, cover, and cook over low heat about 5 minutes per side.

5. Repeat for remaining 4 patties.

Yield: 8 servings

1 patty contains:

Cal	Carb g	Fat g	Sat Fat g	Chol mg	Sod mg	Fib g
97	8	4	1	0	223	2

Exchanges: 1 patty = 1 meat

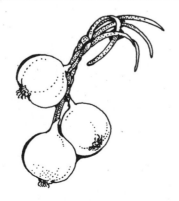

TWO-BEAN CASSEROLE*

¼ cup dried garbanzo beans (½ cup cooked)

nonstick cooking spray

⅓ cup dried soybeans (1 cup cooked)

1 can (8 ounces) whole-kernel corn, drained

1 medium tomato, chopped

¼ teaspoon paprika

¼ teaspoon salt

½ teaspoon sugar

1 teaspoon finely chopped onion

1 teaspoon chili powder

½ teaspoon ground cumin

¼ cup catsup

2 ounces Cheddar cheese (no more than 5 grams fat per ounce), shredded

1. Place dried beans in water and soak overnight (see "Preparation of Dried Legumes," page 204). Simmer 4 hours and drain.

2. Preheat oven to 350°F. Spray casserole dish with nonstick spray.

3. Combine all ingredients except cheese in casserole dish. Top with cheese.

4. Bake 45 minutes.

Yield: 4 servings

1 serving contains:

Cal	Carb g	Fat g	Sat Fat g	Chol mg	Sod mg	Fib g
217	25	8	2	8	503	4

Exchanges: 1 serving = 1 starch/bread, 1 meat, 1 vegetable, 1 fat

This recipe is moderately high in sodium; select other foods throughout the day that are very low in sodium.

Entrées with Meat, Poultry, and Fish

OVEN-DRIED BEEF JERKY

2–2½ pounds flank steak or lean roast,
   fat trimmed off

1 cup water

2 tablespoons liquid smoke

2 teaspoons salt

¼ teaspoon pepper

1 teaspoon garlic powder (optional)

1 teaspoon onion powder (optional)

1. Cut meat into strips 4–6 inches long, ½–1 inch wide, and ⅛–¼ inch thick. (Meat is easier to work with if partially frozen.) For chewy jerky, cut with grain of meat. For more tender jerky, cut across grain.

2. Mix water and seasonings; marinate beef in mixture overnight in refrigerator.

3. Drain beef strips and pat dry with paper towels.

4. Cover bottom rack of oven with aluminum foil or baking sheet.

5. Hang or lay strips on top oven rack so they do not touch or overlap.

6. Dry meat at lowest oven temperature (150°–200°F) until it has turned brown, feels hard, and is dry to the touch, about 4–5 hours.

7. Let cool, then remove from rack.

8. Store in cool, dry place in tightly covered container.

Yield: 24 strips (approximately)

1 strip contains:

Cal	Carb g	Fat g	Sat Fat g	Chol mg	Sod mg	Fib g
73	0	3	1	27	77	0

Exchanges: 1 strip = 1 meat

FRIED RICE

1½ cups rice, uncooked

3 tablespoons peanut oil

4 cloves garlic, minced

1 egg, lightly beaten

½ cup chopped onion

½ cup chopped celery

½ cup water chestnuts, chopped

⅔ cup frozen green peas

1 cup finely chopped cooked lean pork

2 tablespoons dark soy sauce

continued

Abbreviations: Cal = Calories; Carb = Carbohydrates; Sat Fat = Saturated Fat; Chol = Cholesterol; Sod = Sodium; Fib = Fiber; < = less than.

2 5 9

1 tablespoon light soy sauce

2 green onions, cut lengthwise into
  3-inch slivers

1.   Rinse rice in strainer under running water to remove excess starch.

2.   In large saucepan, bring 2 cups water to a boil. Add rice and cook, uncovered, until water cooks down and rice is slightly pitted. Cover rice and let simmer 10–12 minutes longer. Turn off heat; let rice sit for 10–12 minutes longer; set aside to cool. (Rice can be cooked a day ahead and stored in refrigerator.)

3.   Heat oil in wok or skillet over medium heat. Add garlic; cook until soft. Place oil and garlic mixture in small bowl and set aside.

4.   Pour ½ tablespoon oil and garlic mixture back into wok. Add egg, rolling it around like a crêpe until cooked in thin layer. Remove egg from wok and cut into small pieces; set aside.

5.   Increase heat to high. Pour ½ tablespoon oil and garlic mixture into wok. Add onion, celery, and water chestnuts. Cook until onion is soft, stirring constantly. Remove from wok and set aside.

6.   Add frozen peas to wok and cook 1–2 minutes or until peas are thawed. Remove peas from wok and set aside.

7.   Pour ½ teaspoon oil and garlic mixture into wok. Add pork and cook until done. Remove from wok and set aside.

8.   Pour remaining oil and garlic mixture into wok. Add cooked rice; stir until rice is coated with oil. When rice begins to warm, add dark and light soy sauces. Add all ingredients that have been set aside. Toss thoroughly.

9.   Serve from wok or pour into large serving bowl. Garnish with green onion slivers.

Yield: 16 servings

½ cup contains:

Cal	Carb g	Fat g	Sat Fat g	Chol mg	Sod mg	Fib g
131	18	4	1	21	214	1

Exchanges: ½ cup = 1 starch/bread, 1 fat

BURGUNDY FLANK STEAK

¾ cup dry red or rosé wine

1 onion, sliced

1 clove garlic, minced

1 teaspoon salt

1 teaspoon pepper

¼ teaspoon dried rosemary

1 bay leaf

1½ pounds flank steak

1.   Combine first 7 ingredients and pour over flank steak. Marinate 2–3 hours at room temperature, turning steak frequently. Drain, reserving marinade.

2.   Place meat on broiler rack and broil 3 inches from heat 3–4 minutes on each side, basting frequently with marinade.

3.   Slice diagonally into very thin slices before serving.

Yield: 6 servings

1 serving contains:

Cal	Carb g	Fat g	Sat Fat g	Chol mg	Sod mg	Fib g
176	0	8	3	65	186	0

Exchanges: 1 serving = 3 meats

LIVING HEART PEPPER STEAK*

1 pound top sirloin steak, ¾–1 inch thick, fat trimmed off

6 tablespoons reduced-sodium soy sauce

2 tablespoons balsamic vinegar

1 teaspoon dried thyme

1 teaspoon paprika

½ teaspoon ground ginger

½ teaspoon coarsely ground pepper

2 teaspoons olive oil

2 cloves garlic, minced

1 bunch green onions, cut lengthwise
    into strips

1 large green bell pepper, cut into strips

1 large red bell pepper or 1 small red and 1
    small yellow bell pepper, cut into strips

4 ounces fresh or frozen snow peas
    or pea pods

1¼ cups sliced fresh mushrooms

2 teaspoons cornstarch

½ cup water

4 cups cooked rice, prepared without salt
    or fat (optional)

1. Slice beef across grain in thin slices. (Partially freezing meat makes slicing easier.)

2. In medium bowl, combine beef, soy sauce, vinegar, thyme, paprika, ginger, and pepper; marinate 10–15 minutes.

3. Heat oil in large nonstick skillet and cook garlic. Lift meat from marinade (reserve marinade) and add to skillet. Cook meat just until pink disappears, about 2–3 minutes; remove meat from skillet and put aside. Keep meat warm.

4. Add green onions, bell peppers, snow peas, and mushrooms to skillet and cook about 3–4 minutes.

5. In small bowl, blend cornstarch into water, stirring until smooth; add to marinade. Add marinade to vegetable mixture in skillet and heat until sauce thickens slightly.

6. Add meat to vegetable mixture and stir until meat is hot.

7. Serve with rice if desired.

Yield: 4 servings

1½ cups without rice contains:

Cal	Carb g	Fat g	Sat Fat g	Chol mg	Sod mg	Fib g
252	14	7	2	75	961	3

Exchanges: 1½ cups without rice = 3 meats, 3 vegetables

1½ cups meat and vegetables with 1 cup rice contains:

Cal	Carb g	Fat g	Sat Fat g	Chol mg	Sod mg	Fib g
465	60	8	2	75	965	4

Exchanges: 1½ cups meat and vegetables with 1 cup rice = 3 starch/breads, 3 meats, 3 vegetables

This recipe is high in sodium; select other foods throughout the day that are very low in sodium.

APPLESAUCE MEAT LOAF

nonstick cooking spray

1½ pounds very lean ground beef

¾ cup fine dry bread crumbs

½ cup unsweetened applesauce

¾ teaspoon salt

½ teaspoon pepper

½ cup catsup, divided

1. Preheat oven to 350°F. Spray 9 × 5-inch loaf pan with nonstick spray.

2. Combine all ingredients except ¼ cup catsup.

3. Press meat into pan.

4. Bake about 1½ hours or until brown. Remove from oven; drain off any fat or juice that has cooked out. Spread remaining ¼ cup catsup on top and return to oven until catsup is hot and meat is done. Serve hot.

Yield: 6 servings

continued

1 serving contains:

Cal	Carb g	Fat g	Sat Fat g	Chol mg	Sod mg	Fib g
255	17	9	3	65	654	1

Exchanges: 1 serving = 1 starch/bread, 3 meats

VARIATION

Low-Sodium Applesauce Meat Loaf: Omit salt.
1 serving has same analysis as above, except 388 mg sodium.

SKINNY BEEF STROGANOFF

1 pound top sirloin steak, ¾–1 inch thick, fat trimmed off

8 ounces noodles, uncooked

1 tablespoon beef bouillon granules

1 cup boiling water

1 teaspoon Worcestershire sauce

¼ teaspoon ground nutmeg

1 teaspoon dry mustard

¼ teaspoon coarsely ground pepper

2 teaspoons olive oil

3 cups sliced fresh mushrooms (about 12 ounces)

1 medium onion, sliced thin

1 tablespoon cornstarch

½ cup golden sherry or burgundy

16 ounces low-fat sour cream

1. Slice beef across grain in thin slices. (Partially freezing meat makes slicing easier.)

2. Cook noodles according to package directions, omitting salt and fat.

3. In small bowl, dissolve bouillon in boiling water and add Worcestershire sauce, nutmeg, mustard, and pepper.

4. In large nonstick skillet, heat oil; cook meat until pink disappears and it is lightly browned. Remove meat from skillet and keep warm.

5. Add bouillon mixture to skillet and bring to a boil. Add mushrooms and onion; cook until crisp-tender.

6. Add cornstarch to wine and stir until smooth; add to vegetables in skillet and heat, stirring, until slightly thickened.

7. Add meat to mixture in skillet and heat; turn off heat and let mixture cool slightly.

8. Stir sour cream into meat and vegetable mixture until well blended. *Note: If reheating is necessary before serving, do not heat to boiling.*

9. Serve over cooked noodles.

Yield: 6 servings

⅔ cup stroganoff with ⅔ cup noodles contains:

Cal	Carb g	Fat g	Sat Fat g	Chol mg	Sod mg	Fib g
384	40	11	5	107	766	3

Exchanges: ½ cup stroganoff with ⅔ cup noodles = 3 starch/breads, 3 meats

VARIATION

Low-Sodium Skinny Beef Stroganoff: Omit bouillon granules; use 1 cup water as stated in step 3 of recipe for Skinny Beef Stroganoff and use burgundy instead of sherry.

⅔ cup stroganoff with ⅔ cup noodles has same analysis as above, except 129 mg sodium.

CHILI

1 pound very lean ground beef

1 medium onion, chopped

1 clove garlic, minced

4 teaspoons chili powder

½ teaspoon salt

1 can (8 ounces) tomato sauce

1 can (14½ ounces) chopped tomatoes, undrained

½ green bell pepper, chopped

1 cup water

1. In large pan, bring about 1 quart water to a boil. Crumble ground beef into water and stir constantly. When water starts to boil again, pour water and meat into large strainer in sink.

2. Place ground beef in skillet, add onion and garlic, and cook until onion is soft.

3. Add chili powder and stir until hot, being careful not to let it stick.

4. Add remaining ingredients.

5. Cover and simmer 30 minutes, stirring occasionally.

Yield: 4 servings

1 cup contains:

Cal	Carb g	Fat g	Sat Fat g	Chol mg	Sod mg	Fib g
236	13	9	3	65	862	3

Exchanges: 1 cup = 1 starch/bread, 3 meats

VARIATIONS

Chili with Beans: Add 2 cans (16 ounces each) undrained kidney or pinto beans.

Yield: 6 servings

1 cup contains:

Cal	Carb g	Fat g	Sat Fat g	Chol mg	Sod mg	Fib g
266	28	6	2	43	915	9

Exchanges: 1 cup = 2 starch/breads, 2 meats

Low-Sodium Chili (without beans): Omit salt and substitute 1 can (8 ounces) low-sodium tomato sauce for regular tomato sauce.

1 cup without beans has same analysis as original recipe, except 270 mg sodium.

ITALIAN LASAGNA

8 ounces lasagna noodles, uncooked

½ cup egg substitute

1 pound part-skim ricotta cheese

⅛ teaspoon ground nutmeg

¼ cup minced fresh parsley

1 recipe Italian Meat Sauce (see recipe, page 264)

½ pound shredded part-skim mozzarella

⅓ cup grated Parmesan cheese (optional)

1. Cook noodles according to package directions, omitting salt and fat. Drain, rinse, and let noodles stand in cold water.

2. Preheat oven to 375°F.

3. Beat egg substitute into ricotta cheese; add nutmeg and parsley.

4. Cover bottom of 9 x 13-inch nonstick baking dish with 2 cups meat sauce and layer as follows: half of noodles, half of remaining meat sauce (about 1¾ cups), half of ricotta cheese mixture, half of mozzarella cheese. Repeat layers, starting with noodles and ending with mozzarella cheese; top with Parmesan cheese if desired.

5. Bake 35–40 minutes or until cheese melts and is golden brown.

Yield: 18 servings

1 serving without Parmesan cheese contains:

Cal	Carb g	Fat g	Sat Fat g	Chol mg	Sod mg	Fib g
187	16	7	3	29	246	1

Exchanges: 1 serving = 1 starch/bread, 1 meat, 1 fat

1 serving with Parmesan cheese contains:

Cal	Carb g	Fat g	Sat Fat g	Chol mg	Sod mg	Fib g
193	16	7	4	30	274	1

ITALIAN MEAT SAUCE

1 pound very lean ground beef

1 large onion, chopped

2 cloves garlic, minced

1 can (14½ ounces) chopped tomatoes, undrained

11 ounces tomato juice

1 teaspoon fennel seed

½ cup chopped fresh parsley

¼ teaspoon coarsely ground pepper

½ tablespoon dried oregano

½ teaspoon dried basil

½ teaspoon dried thyme

¼ teaspoon dried marjoram

⅓ cup dry red wine, such as chianti

1. In large pan, bring about 1 quart water to a boil. Crumble ground beef into water and stir constantly. When water starts to boil again, pour water and meat into large strainer in sink.

2. Place meat in large saucepan or Dutch oven; add onion and garlic and cook until onion is tender.

3. Add remaining ingredients except wine. Bring to a boil; reduce heat, cover with lid ajar, and simmer 1½ hours, stirring occasionally.

4. Add wine and simmer 30 minutes, stirring occasionally.

5. Meat sauce can be served with pasta or used to make Italian Lasagna (see page 263).

Yield: 8 servings

⅔ cup contains:

Cal	Carb g	Fat g	Sat Fat g	Chol mg	Sod mg	Fib g
119	7	4	2	32	257	2

Exchanges: ⅔ cup = 2 meats, 1 vegetable

VARIATION

Low-Sodium Italian Meat Sauce: Substitute no-salt-added canned tomatoes for regular canned tomatoes and no-salt-added tomato juice for regular tomato juice.

⅔ cup has same analysis as above, except 43 mg sodium.

MEAT LOAF

nonstick cooking spray

1 pound very lean ground beef

¼ cup egg substitute

1 cup skim milk

3 slices bread, toasted and cubed

½ cup chopped onion

1 clove garlic, minced

2 stalks celery, chopped

¼ teaspoon pepper

2 teaspoons chili powder

½ cup catsup

1. Preheat oven to 350°F. Spray 9 × 5-inch loaf pan with nonstick spray.

2. Combine all ingredients except catsup.

3. Press meat into pan. Cover with foil.

4. Bake 50 minutes.

5. Remove foil, drain fat, and top with catsup. Return to oven and bake uncovered 15 minutes. Serve hot.

Yield: 4 servings

1 serving contains:

Cal	Carb g	Fat g	Sat Fat g	Chol mg	Sod mg	Fib g
302	24	9	3	66	601	2

Exchanges: 1 serving = 1 starch/bread, 3 meats, 2 vegetables

VARIATIONS

Turkey Meat Loaf: Substitute ground turkey breast for ground beef.

1 serving contains:

Cal	Carb g	Fat g	Sat Fat g	Chol mg	Sod mg	Fib g
270	24	4	1	69	605	2

Exchanges: 1 serving = 1 starch/bread, 3 meats, 2 vegetables

Low-Sodium Meat Loaf: Substitute low-sodium catsup for regular catsup.

1 serving has same analysis as original recipe, except 251 mg sodium.

SPAGHETTI SAUCE WITH BEEF

1 pound very lean ground beef

1 tablespoon oil

1 green bell pepper, chopped

1 stalk celery, chopped

1 medium onion, chopped

2 cloves garlic, minced

1 teaspoon chili powder

½ teaspoon cumin seed

½ teaspoon dried thyme or 1 teaspoon minced fresh thyme

1 can (6 ounces) tomato paste

1 can (8 ounces) tomato sauce

2 cans (14½ ounces each) chopped tomatoes, undrained

1 can (4 ounces) sliced mushrooms, drained

¼ cup sliced black olives, drained

½ cup dry sherry

½ teaspoon sugar

¼ teaspoon salt

¼ teaspoon pepper

8 drops Tabasco

1 package (12 ounces) thin spaghetti, uncooked

1. In large pan, bring about 1 quart water to a boil. Crumble ground beef into water and stir constantly. When water starts to boil again, pour water and meat into large strainer in sink.

2. Heat oil in skillet. Add bell pepper, celery, onion, and garlic; cook until onion is soft. Add meat and remaining ingredients except spaghetti; mix well. Simmer 1½–2 hours, stirring occasionally.

3. Cook spaghetti according to package directions, omitting salt and fat. Drain and rinse under cold water.

4. Mix sauce with cooked spaghetti or ladle it on top.

Yield: 12 servings

1 cup contains:

Cal	Carb g	Fat g	Sat Fat g	Chol mg	Sod mg	Fib g
233	33	5	1	22	473	3

Exchanges: 1 cup = 2 starch/breads, 1 meat, 1 vegetable

VARIATION

Low-Sodium Spaghetti Sauce with Beef: Substitute no-salt-added canned tomatoes for regular canned tomatoes. Omit salt.

1 cup has same analysis as above, except 326 mg sodium.

SHISH KABOB

MARINADE

¼ cup olive oil

½ cup vinegar

½ cup water

¼ teaspoon Liquid Smoke

¼ cup Worcestershire sauce

½ onion, finely chopped

½ teaspoon pepper

½ teaspoon dried tarragon

1 tablespoon catsup

¼ teaspoon lemon pepper

MEAT AND VEGETABLES

2 pounds lean beef or lamb, cut into
   1-inch cubes

16 small onions, quartered

1 green bell pepper, cut into chunks

16 fresh mushrooms

16 cherry tomatoes

1. In medium bowl, mix all marinade ingredients; beat with a fork. Pour over meat and vegetables. Cover and marinate several hours or overnight in refrigerator.

2. Remove meat and vegetables from marinade and thread on 8 skewers. Brush with marinade.

3. Broil or grill 6–8 minutes or until done, turning once.

Yield: 8 servings

1 kabob contains:

Cal	Carb g	Fat g	Sat Fat g	Chol mg	Sod mg	Fib g
266	18	8	2	73	117	4

Exchanges: 1 kabob = 3 meats, 3 vegetables

CHICKEN AND SPINACH PINWHEELS

nonstick cooking spray

4 ounces fresh spinach

1 cup water

⅛ teaspoon pepper

1 teaspoon chopped fresh oregano or ½ teaspoon dried oregano

¼ cup part-skim ricotta cheese

¼ cup shredded part-skim mozzarella cheese

4 deboned chicken breast halves, skin and fat removed

¼ teaspoon lemon pepper, divided

Mushrooms in White Wine Sauce (see variation, page 308)

1. Preheat oven to 350°F. Spray 8 × 8-inch covered casserole dish with nonstick spray.

2. Wash spinach and remove stems. Boil water and add spinach; cook 1 minute. Drain and chop spinach.

3. Combine pepper, oregano, ricotta, and mozzarella cheese with spinach and mix thoroughly.

4. Flatten chicken breasts. Sprinkle with half of lemon pepper (⅛ teaspoon). Place spinach mixture in center of each and roll up; secure with toothpicks.

5. Place chicken breasts, seam side down, in covered casserole dish and sprinkle with remaining lemon pepper (⅛ teaspoon). Add ½ cup water; cover and bake 25–30 minutes or until chicken is tender. Serve with Mushrooms in White Wine Sauce.

Yield: 4 servings

1 pinwheel with sauce contains:

Cal	Carb g	Fat g	Sat Fat g	Chol mg	Sod mg	Fib g
269	10	8	3	86	197	2

Exchanges: 1 pinwheel with sauce = 4 meats, 2 vegetables

CHICKEN STIR-FRY

nonstick cooking spray

1½ pounds boneless chicken breasts or turkey breasts, skin and fat removed, sliced into strips

1 bunch fresh broccoli, divided into florets

1 large onion, sliced

½ pound fresh mushrooms, sliced

1 tablespoon reduced-sodium soy sauce

1 tablespoon white wine

1 tablespoon Worcestershire sauce

1. Spray wok or stir-fry pan with nonstick spray.

2. Cook chicken or turkey until brown, stirring often.

3. Add broccoli and onion; cook until onion is soft.

4. Add mushrooms, soy sauce, wine, and Worcestershire sauce; stir well to coat vegetables.

5. Cook until vegetables are crisp-tender, stirring frequently.

6. Serve hot.

Yield: 6 servings

1 cup contains:

Cal	Carb g	Fat g	Sat Fat g	Chol mg	Sod mg	Fib g
166	7	3	1	62	210	2

Exchanges: 1 cup = 3 meats, 1 vegetable

CHICKEN FAJITAS*

1 pound deboned chicken breasts, skin and fat removed, cut into strips

1 large onion, cut into thin rings

2 large green bell peppers, cut into strips

juice of 3 limes

⅛ teaspoon salt

½ teaspoon garlic powder

½ teaspoon pepper

¼ cup water

¼ cup chopped fresh cilantro

½ cup taco sauce

8 corn tortillas

1. Combine all ingredients except cilantro, taco sauce, and tortillas; marinate overnight.

2. Preheat large skillet (preferably cast-iron). Add chicken only and cook at medium-high temperature, stirring frequently to prevent sticking.

3. Add marinade, including onion and bell pepper; cook until liquid has evaporated and vegetables are soft.

4. Garnish with cilantro and taco sauce. Serve in warm corn tortillas.

Yield: 4 servings

1 serving contains:

Cal	Carb g	Fat g	Sat Fat g	Chol mg	Sod mg	Fib g
275	33	5	1	58	511	5

Exchanges: 1 serving = 1 starch/bread, 3 meats, 2 vegetables

This recipe is moderately high in sodium; select other foods throughout the day that are very low in sodium.

CHICKEN WITH PINEAPPLE SAUCE

4 deboned chicken breast halves, skin and
    fat removed

½ teaspoon dried basil

½ teaspoon dried thyme

½ teaspoon ground cumin

2 cloves garlic, minced

2 teaspoons chopped fresh parsley

1 teaspoon salt

½ teaspoon pepper

1. Pound chicken breasts slightly on both sides to flatten.

2. Combine remaining ingredients and sprinkle on both sides of chicken.

3. Place in nonstick skillet and cover.

4. Cook 7 minutes over medium heat.

5. Turn chicken and continue cooking 5–7 minutes.

6. Remove lid and allow moisture to evaporate and chicken to brown.

PINEAPPLE SAUCE

1 can (20 ounces) pineapple tidbits packed
    in juice

4 teaspoons chopped shallots or red onions

4 teaspoons chopped fresh parsley

4 teaspoons fresh lemon juice

4 teaspoons cornstarch

4 teaspoons tub margarine

1. Drain pineapple, reserving juice; set pineapple aside. Add water to juice to make 2 cups.

2. In saucepan, combine juice with all ingredients except margarine and pineapple.

3. Simmer about 5 minutes or until about ½ of volume has evaporated.

4. Add margarine and pineapple; simmer 1 minute. Spoon over cooked chicken.

Yield: 4 servings

1 serving contains:

Cal	Carb g	Fat g	Sat Fat g	Chol mg	Sod mg	Fib g
302	26	8	2	77	659	3

Exchanges: 1 serving = 4 meats, 2 fruits

VARIATION

Low-Sodium Chicken with Pineapple Sauce: Omit salt.

1 serving has same analysis as above, except 127 mg sodium.

CHICKEN CRÊPES

1 tablespoon olive oil

1 small onion, chopped

¼ pound fresh mushrooms, sliced

3 tablespoons all-purpose flour

1 teaspoon chicken bouillon granules

1 teaspoon salt

¼ teaspoon pepper

¼ cup chopped fresh parsley

3 cups skim milk

⅓ cup white wine

3½ cups chopped cooked chicken (prepared
    without salt or fat)

1 recipe Basic Crêpes (see page 310)

1. Preheat oven to 350°F.

2. Heat oil in skillet; add onion and mushrooms and cook until soft.

3. Sprinkle with flour; add bouillon granules, salt, pepper, and parsley.

4. Gradually stir in milk and cook, stirring constantly, until mixture thickens.

5. Add wine and cook 5 minutes longer.

6. Add half of sauce mixture to chicken.

7. Place ¼ cup chicken mixture on each crêpe.

8. Roll crêpes up and place seam side down in 9 × 13-inch baking dish.

9. Top with remaining sauce, cover, and bake 20–30 minutes in oven or 4 minutes in microwave on high.

Yield: 9 crêpes

1 crêpe contains:

Cal	Carb g	Fat g	Sat Fat g	Chol mg	Sod mg	Fib g
217	16	6	1	44	522	1

Exchanges: 1 crêpe = 1 starch/bread, 2 meats

VARIATIONS

Low-Sodium Chicken Crêpes: Omit salt.

1 crêpe has same analysis as above, except 285 mg sodium.

Chicken Tetrazzini: Complete main recipe through Step 5. Cook 6 ounces of fettuccine or linguine according to package directions, omitting fat and salt, and combine with sauce and chicken. Bake 20–30 minutes or microwave for 4 minutes on high.

Yield: 6 servings

1 serving contains:

Cal	Carb g	Fat g	Sat Fat g	Chol mg	Sod mg	Fib g
327	30	7	2	90	698	2

Exchanges: 1 serving = 2 starch/breads, 3 meats

Low-Sodium Chicken Tetrazzini: Omit salt.

1 serving has same analysis as above, except 342 mg sodium.

Chicken and Rice Casserole: Complete main recipe through Step 5. Combine sauce and chicken with 2 cups cooked rice and bake 20–30 minutes or microwave 4 minutes on high.

Yield: 6 servings

1 serving contains:

Cal	Carb g	Fat g	Sat Fat g	Chol mg	Sod mg	Fib g
300	27	6	1	66	694	1

Exchanges: 1 serving = 2 starch/breads, 3 meats

Low-Sodium Chicken and Rice Casserole: Omit salt.

1 serving has same analysis as above, except 338 mg sodium.

CHICKEN FETTUCCINE ALFREDO

2 tablespoons tub margarine

1 pound deboned chicken breasts, skin and fat removed, cut into bite-size pieces

1 tablespoon all-purpose flour

3 large cloves garlic, minced

1 can (12 ounces) evaporated skim milk

½ pound fresh mushrooms, sliced

¾ cup grated reduced-fat Parmesan cheese

¼ cup white wine

1 teaspoon chopped fresh basil or ½ teaspoon dried basil

1 teaspoon chopped fresh parsley

1 package (9 ounces) fettuccine, prepared according to package directions, omitting salt and fat

1. In nonstick skillet, melt margarine; add chicken and cook until tender. Remove chicken from skillet and set aside.

2. Add flour and cook over low heat, stirring constantly, until it stops bubbling and becomes a golden paste.

3. Add garlic and continue stirring until garlic softens.

4. Add evaporated milk and simmer over medium heat, stirring constantly, until milk thickens.

5. Add mushrooms and continue cooking over low heat until mushrooms soften.

6. Add Parmesan cheese and stir well. Simmer, stirring often, until cheese melts and is blended thoroughly. Remove from heat.

7. Stir in wine, basil, parsley, and chicken; stir until hot. Toss with hot fettuccine and serve immediately.

Yield: 8 cups

1 cup contains:

Cal	Carb g	Fat g	Sat Fat g	Chol mg	Sod mg	Fib g
278	29	7	3	66	317	2

Exchanges: 1 cup = 2 starch/breads, 2 meats

CHINESE CHICKEN

2 tablespoons soy sauce

2 tablespoons dry sherry

1 piece (2 inches) fresh ginger, peeled and grated

3 cloves garlic, minced

4 deboned chicken breast halves, skin and fat removed, cut into bite-size pieces

1 teaspoon olive oil

½ pound fresh mushrooms, sliced

4 stalks celery, thinly sliced

4 green onions, thinly sliced

1 package (7 ounces) frozen snow peas

1 can (8 ounces) sliced water chestnuts, drained

1 tablespoon cornstarch

1 cup water

1. Blend soy sauce, sherry, ginger, and garlic. Divide in half.

2. Marinate chicken in half of mixture 30 minutes in refrigerator. Drain.

3. Heat oil in wok or heavy skillet. Add chicken, mushrooms, celery, green onions, and snow peas. Cook 10–15 minutes, stirring constantly, until chicken is tender and vegetables are still crisp.

4. Stir in water chestnuts.

5.   In small bowl, combine cornstarch and water and add to remaining half of marinade; add to chicken, stirring until thickened.

Yield: 4 servings

1¼ cups contains:

Cal	Carb g	Fat g	Sat Fat g	Chol mg	Sod mg	Fib g
253	16	5	1	77	375	3

Exchanges: 1¼ cups = 4 meats, 3 vegetables

CHICKEN WITH SWEET AND-SOUR SAUCE

nonstick cooking spray

2 tablespoons sesame seeds

½ cup sweet-and-sour sauce, divided

4 deboned chicken breast halves, skin and fat removed

1.   Preheat oven to 400°F. Spray baking dish with nonstick spray.

2.   Place sesame seeds on baking sheet and toast about 5 minutes or until golden brown.

3.   Place half of sweet-and-sour sauce (¼ cup) in shallow bowl. Dip chicken in sauce and sprinkle with sesame seeds.

4.   Arrange chicken pieces in dish so they do not touch.

5.   Bake 15–20 minutes or until chicken is lightly browned.

6.   Serve with remaining sweet-and-sour sauce.

FOR CONVECTION OVEN

1.   Place rack at lowest level (without extender ring). Preheat oven to 400°F.

2.   See Step 2 above.

3.   See Step 3 above.

4.   Place chicken on cooking rack.

5.   Cook at high speed for 10–12 minutes or until lightly browned.

6.   See Step 6 above.

Yield: 4 servings

1 serving contains:

Cal	Carb g	Fat g	Sat Fat g	Chol mg	Sod mg	Fib g
226	9	6	1	77	170	1

Exchanges: Not applicable for this recipe

ORIENTAL MARINATED CHICKEN

1 pound deboned chicken, skin and fat removed

1 recipe Oriental Dressing (page 231)

1.   Place chicken in plastic or glass container with lid.

2.   Pour Oriental Dressing over chicken. Cover and refrigerate overnight.

3.   Drain and discard marinade.

4.   Grill chicken until well done.

Yield: 4 servings

1 serving contains:

Cal	Carb g	Fat g	Sat Fat g	Chol mg	Sod mg	Fib g
164	4	5	1	62	207	0

Exchanges: 1 serving = 3 meats

CRISPY CORNY BAKED CHICKEN

nonstick cooking spray

1 chicken (2–3 pounds), cut up, skin and fat removed

½ teaspoon salt

⅛ teaspoon pepper

½ cup skim milk

1 cup corn flake crumbs

1. Preheat oven to 400°F. Spray 9 × 13-inch baking dish with nonstick spray.

2. Season chicken with salt and pepper.

3. Dip into milk and roll in crumbs.

4. Place chicken in dish so that pieces do not touch.

5. Bake 45 minutes or until tender.

Yield: 6 servings

1 serving contains:

Cal	Carb g	Fat g	Sat Fat g	Chol mg	Sod mg	Fib g
241	18	6	2	74	452	0

Exchanges: 1 serving = 1 starch/bread, 3 meats

FAT-FREE FRIED CHICKEN

1 teaspoon seasoned salt

½ teaspoon pepper

4 deboned chicken breast halves, skin and fat removed

1. Sprinkle seasoned salt and pepper on both sides of chicken.

2. Place in nonstick skillet and cover.

3. Cook over medium heat 10 minutes.

4. Turn chicken and continue cooking over medium heat about 10 minutes.

5. Remove lid to allow moisture to evaporate and chicken to brown.

Yield: 4 servings

1 serving contains:

Cal	Carb g	Fat g	Sat Fat g	Chol mg	Sod mg	Fib g
168	0	4	1	77	413	0

Exchanges: 1 serving = 4 meats

GREEN CHILI ENCHILADAS

2 deboned chicken breast halves, skin and fat removed

nonstick cooking spray

¼ teaspoon pepper

1 can (4½ ounces) mild green chilies, chopped, divided

12 corn tortillas

1 can (10 ounces) green enchilada sauce

½ cup skim milk

8 ounces low-fat sour cream

¼ cup shredded part-skim mozzarella cheese

¼ cup shredded Cheddar cheese (no more than 5 grams fat per ounce)

1. Boil chicken until tender. Cool; use fork to shred.

2. Preheat oven to 400°F. Spray 11 × 7-inch baking dish with nonstick spray.

3. Combine chicken, pepper, and ¾ of green chilies.

4. Heat tortillas in moist paper towels in conventional oven or microwave or place in steamer to soften (this will make them easier to roll).

5. In saucepan, mix enchilada sauce and milk and warm over low heat until simmering. Dip tortillas one at a time into sauce. Place each tortilla in baking dish and fill with $\frac{1}{12}$ of chicken mixture. Roll tortillas tightly and arrange seam side down in baking dish.

6. Spread sour cream evenly over enchiladas. Sprinkle remaining $\frac{1}{4}$ of chilies over sour cream. Pour remainder of enchilada sauce over enchiladas. Sprinkle cheeses evenly on top.

7. Bake 15 minutes or until hot and cheese melts.

Yield: 6 servings

2 enchiladas contain:

Cal	Carb g	Fat g	Sat Fat g	Chol mg	Sod mg	Fib g
253	30	7	3	42	942	3

Exchanges: 2 enchiladas = 2 starch/breads, 2 meats

VARIATION

Low-Sodium Green Chili Enchiladas: Omit green enchilada sauce and replace with following sauce in Step 5. Remove husks from 1 pound green tomatillos; rinse tomatillos and place in saucepan with 4 cups water. Bring to a boil; reduce heat and simmer until tomatillos turn pale green and start to burst (about 15 minutes). Drain tomatillos; combine with $\frac{1}{2}$ teaspoon ground cumin, $\frac{1}{2}$ teaspoon garlic powder, and $\frac{1}{2}$ teaspoon onion powder in blender or food processor and process until smooth.

2 enchiladas have same analysis as above, except 451 mg sodium.

LEMON CHICKEN BREASTS WITH MUSHROOMS

1 tablespoon tub margarine

4 deboned chicken breast halves, skin and fat removed

$\frac{1}{4}$ pound fresh mushrooms, sliced

2 green onions, sliced

1 lemon

2 tablespoons sherry or white wine

1. Heat margarine in skillet, add chicken and cook until browned. Remove from skillet.

2. Add mushrooms and green onions to skillet and cook until tender.

3. Cut half of lemon into slices and add to mushroom mixture.

4. Squeeze juice from other lemon half.

5. Add juice and wine to mushroom mixture.

6. Return chicken breasts to skillet, spooning mixture over them while heating. Be careful not to overcook.

Yield: 4 servings

1 serving contains:

Cal	Carb g	Fat g	Sat Fat g	Chol mg	Sod mg	Fib g
210	4	7	2	77	107	1

Exchanges: 1 serving = 4 meats

SPICY ORANGE CHICKEN*

½ teaspoon garlic salt

¼ teaspoon ground ginger

½ teaspoon crushed red pepper

4 deboned chicken breast halves, skin and fat removed

1 tablespoon cornstarch

¼ cup reduced-sodium soy sauce

1 can (6 ounces) frozen orange juice concentrate, thawed

¼ cup balsamic vinegar

⅛ teaspoon Tabasco

½ cup water

1 teaspoon orange zest or grated orange peel

2 teaspoons sesame oil

4 cups cooked white or brown rice, prepared without salt or fat (optional)

4 thin slices fresh orange

1. Combine garlic salt, ginger, and red pepper; sprinkle mixture lightly over chicken.

2. In small saucepan, mix cornstarch and soy sauce until smooth.

3. Add orange juice concentrate, vinegar, Tabasco, water, and orange zest or peel to soy sauce mixture. Bring mixture to a boil over medium heat; simmer over low heat, stirring constantly, until thickened. Remove from heat, cover, and set aside.

4. In large nonstick skillet, heat oil; add chicken and cook until brown and well done.

5. Add sauce to chicken and heat thoroughly while stirring.

6. Serve chicken with rice if desired; garnish with orange slices.

Yield: 4 servings

1 serving without rice contains:

Cal	Carb g	Fat g	Sat Fat g	Chol mg	Sod mg	Fib g
275	21	6	2	77	794	1

Exchanges: 1 serving without rice = 4 meats, 1 fruit

1 serving with 1 cup rice contains:

Cal	Carb g	Fat g	Sat Fat g	Chol mg	Sod mg	Fib g
487	67	7	2	77	798	1

Exchanges: 1 serving with 1 cup rice = 3 starch/breads, 4 meats, 1 fruit

*This recipe is high in sodium; select other foods throughout the day that are very low in sodium.

SPAGHETTI SAUCE WITH TURKEY

1 pound ground turkey breast

1 medium onion, chopped

1 green bell pepper, finely chopped

1 clove garlic, minced

¼ cup chopped fresh parsley

½ teaspoon dried oregano

1 teaspoon dried basil

1 can (16 ounces) tomatoes, chopped, undrained

1 can (6 ounces) tomato paste

1½ cups water

1 bay leaf

2 tablespoons sugar

½ teaspoon salt

¼ teaspoon pepper

1. In large pan, bring about 1 quart water to a boil. Crumble ground turkey into water and stir constantly. When water starts to boil again, pour water and meat into large strainer in sink.

2.   Place meat in skillet; add onion, bell pepper, and garlic; cook until onion is soft.

3.   Add remaining ingredients. Cover and simmer 2 hours, stirring occasionally.

Yield: 6 servings

1 serving contains:

Cal	Carb g	Fat g	Sat Fat g	Chol mg	Sod mg	Fib g
164	16	3	1	45	568	3

Exchanges: 1 serving = 2 meats, 3 vegetables

VARIATION

Low-Sodium Spaghetti Sauce with Turkey: Omit salt and substitute 1 can (6 ounces) low-sodium tomato paste for regular tomato paste.

1 serving has same analysis as above, except 185 mg sodium.

CAPELLINI WITH RED CLAM SAUCE

nonstick cooking spray

1 teaspoon olive oil

1 medium onion, chopped

2 cloves garlic, minced

1 can (14½ ounces) tomatoes, chopped, undrained

1 can (15 ounces) tomato sauce

1 teaspoon dried oregano, crushed

¼ cup chopped fresh parsley

¼ cup dry red or white wine

¼ teaspoon salt

¼ teaspoon pepper

2 cans (6½ ounces each) minced clams, drained

1 package (12 ounces) capellini or spaghetti, uncooked

¼ cup grated Parmesan cheese (optional)

1.   Coat medium saucepan with nonstick spray; add oil and heat. Add onion and garlic; cook until soft.

2.   Add tomatoes, tomato sauce, oregano, parsley, wine, salt, and pepper. Cover and simmer 15 minutes, stirring occasionally. Stir in clams and heat thoroughly.

3.   Cook capellini according to package directions, omitting salt and fat; drain and place in serving dish.

4.   Pour sauce over capellini and serve. Sprinkle with Parmesan cheese if desired.

Yield: 6 servings

1½ cups without Parmesan cheese contains:

Cal	Carb g	Fat g	Sat Fat g	Chol mg	Sod mg	Fib g
329	58	3	0	22	671	4

Exchanges: 1½ cups without Parmesan cheese = 3 starch/breads, 1 meat, 2 vegetables

1½ cups with Parmesan cheese contains:

Cal	Carb g	Fat g	Sat Fat g	Chol mg	Sod mg	Fib g
344	58	4	1	25	733	4

Exchanges: 1½ cups with Parmesan cheese = 3 starch/breads, 1 meat, 2 vegetables

VARIATION

Low-Sodium Capellini with Red Clam Sauce: Substitute 2 fresh tomatoes, diced, for canned tomatoes. Substitute 1 can (15 ounces) no-salt-added tomato sauce for regular tomato sauce.

1½ cups without Parmesan cheese has same analysis as above, except 157 mg sodium.

TACO BAKED CHICKEN*

nonstick cooking spray
⅓ cup dry bread crumbs
1 package (1¼ ounces) or about ¼ cup dry
   taco seasoning
4 deboned chicken breast halves, skin and fat
   removed

1.   Preheat oven to 400°F. Spray 8 × 8-inch baking dish with nonstick spray.

2.   Combine bread crumbs and taco seasoning in plastic bag. Rinse chicken breasts and leave damp; place 2 chicken breasts in bag at a time and shake until chicken is well coated.

3.   Arrange chicken in dish so pieces do not touch.

4.   Bake 15–20 minutes or until browned and crisp.

FOR CONVECTION OVEN

1.   Follow Steps 1 and 2 above.

2.   Place chicken on rack and cook at 400°F on high speed 10–12 minutes or until browned and crisp.

Yield: 4 servings

1 serving contains:

Cal	Carb g	Fat g	Sat Fat g	Chol mg	Sod mg	Fib g
237	14	5	1	78	598	1

Exchanges: 1 serving = 4 meats

This recipe is moderately high in sodium; select other foods throughout the day that are very low in sodium.

STIR-FRIED CHICKEN

2 deboned chicken breast halves, skin and
   fat removed
¼ teaspoon salt
2 tablespoons cornstarch, divided
nonstick cooking spray
1 clove garlic, finely chopped
1 tablespoon finely grated fresh ginger
1 can (8 ounces) pineapple chunks packed
   in juice, drained, with juice reserved
2 teaspoons reduced-sodium soy sauce
1 cup water
1 medium tomato, cut into wedges
½ green bell pepper, cut into strips
½ red bell pepper, cut into strips
1 can (8 ounces) sliced water chestnuts,
   drained
2 cups cooked rice, prepared without salt
   or fat

1.   Cut chicken into strips.

2.   Combine salt and half of cornstarch (1 tablespoon). Coat chicken with cornstarch mixture.

3.   Spray nonstick skillet with nonstick spray. Cook garlic 1 minute.

4.   Add chicken and stir continuously over high heat 2 minutes. Add ginger, juice from pineapple, and soy sauce. Bring to a boil.

5.   Stir remaining cornstarch (1 tablespoon) into water until dissolved; add to chicken mixture. Add tomato, pineapple, peppers, and water chestnuts. Cook 2 minutes, stirring constantly.

6.   Serve over rice.

Yield: 4 servings

1½ cups contains:

Cal	Carb g	Fat g	Sat Fat g	Chol mg	Sod mg	Fib g
272	44	2	1	39	280	3

Exchanges: 1½ cups = 2 starch/breads, 2 meats, 1 fruit

FANCY FILLETS WITH WINE

nonstick cooking spray

¼ cup chopped onion

½ cup sliced fresh mushrooms

1 pound fish fillets

½ teaspoon salt

⅛ teaspoon pepper

¼ cup white wine

¼ cup water

¼ cup chopped fresh parsley

1. Preheat oven to 350°F. Spray baking dish with nonstick spray.

2. Sprinkle onion and mushrooms over bottom of baking dish.

3. Place fillets on top of onion–mushroom mixture.

4. Sprinkle with salt and pepper.

5. Combine wine and water and pour over fish.

6. Sprinkle with parsley.

7. Bake 20 minutes or until fish flakes easily with a fork.

Yield: 4 servings

1 serving contains:

Cal	Carb g	Fat g	Sat Fat g	Chol mg	Sod mg	Fib g
115	2	1	0	60	363	<1

Exchanges: 1 serving = 3 meats

FANCY PARISIAN FILLETS

1 tablespoon olive oil

1 onion, chopped

1 tablespoon chopped fresh parsley

2 pounds fish fillets

1 clove garlic, minced

½ cup white wine

1 can (16 ounces) tomatoes, chopped, undrained

2 tablespoons lemon juice

1. Preheat oven to 350°F.

2. Place oil, half of onion, and parsley in baking dish. Place fillets on top.

3. Combine remaining ingredients and pour over fish.

4. Bake 25–30 minutes or until fish flakes easily with a fork.

Yield: 8 servings

1 serving contains:

Cal	Carb g	Fat g	Sat Fat g	Chol mg	Sod mg	Fib g
141	5	3	1	60	188	1

Exchanges: 1 serving = 3 meats

FISH FILLETS IN CREOLE SAUCE

1 tablespoon olive oil

1 onion, sliced into rings

1 green bell pepper, cut into strips

1 clove garlic, minced

1 can (14 ounces) chopped tomatoes, undrained

1 can (8 ounces) tomato sauce

2 tablespoons dry red wine

1 teaspoon dried basil

½ teaspoon salt

1 pound fish fillets

1.   Heat oil in large skillet. Add onion, bell pepper, and garlic; cook until onion is soft.

2.   Stir in tomatoes, tomato sauce, wine, basil, and salt. Heat to boiling; reduce heat and cook, uncovered, about 15 minutes, stirring occasionally.

3.   Place fish in tomato mixture.

4.   Cover and simmer about 10–15 minutes or until fish flakes easily with a fork.

Yield: 7 servings

1 cup contains:

Cal	Carb g	Fat g	Sat Fat g	Chol mg	Sod mg	Fib g
109	7	3	<1	34	495	2

Exchanges: 1 cup = 1 meat, 2 vegetables

FISH RAGOUT

2 tablespoons olive oil

¾ cup chopped onion

¼ teaspoon garlic powder

¼ cup chopped green bell pepper

3 stalks celery, sliced diagonally

3 carrots, sliced diagonally

1 cup water

1 can (28 ounces) tomatoes, chopped, undrained

2 chicken bouillon cubes

1 teaspoon salt

⅛ teaspoon pepper

¼ teaspoon dried thyme

¼ teaspoon dried basil

2 tablespoons chopped fresh parsley or
    1 tablespoon dried parsley flakes

2 pounds fish fillets, cut into 1-inch pieces

1.   In large saucepan, heat oil. Add onion, garlic powder, bell pepper, celery, and carrots; cook until onion is soft.

2.   Add remaining ingredients except fish. Cover and simmer 20 minutes.

3.   Add fish; cover and simmer 10 minutes or until fish flakes easily with a fork.

Yield: 10 servings

1 cup contains:

Cal	Carb g	Fat g	Sat Fat g	Chol mg	Sod mg	Fib g
144	8	4	1	48	614	2

Exchanges: 1 cup = 2 meats, 2 vegetables

VARIATION

Low-Sodium Fish Ragout: Omit salt.

1 cup has same analysis as above, except 401 mg sodium.

FLOUNDER ROLL-UPS

nonstick cooking spray

¼ cup chopped onion

1 tablespoon tub margarine

1 can (4 ounces) chopped mushrooms, drained, with liquid reserved (for sauce)

1 package (8 ounces) frozen crabmeat

½ cup coarse saltine cracker crumbs

2 tablespoons chopped fresh parsley

¼ teaspoon salt

¼ teaspoon pepper

8 thinly sliced flounder fillets (about 2 pounds)

SAUCE

3 tablespoons tub margarine

3 tablespoons all-purpose flour

¼ teaspoon salt

1 cup skim milk (approximately)

⅓ cup dry white wine

1 cup shredded part-skim mozzarella cheese

½ teaspoon paprika

1. Preheat oven to 400°F. Spray 12 × 7½ × 2-inch baking dish with nonstick spray.

2. In skillet, cook onion in margarine until soft. Stir in mushrooms, crabmeat, cracker crumbs, parsley, salt, and pepper.

3. Spread over flounder fillets. Roll fillets and place in baking dish, seam side down.

4. To prepare sauce, in saucepan over low heat, melt margarine. Blend in flour and salt.

5. Add enough milk to mushroom liquid to make 1½ cups; stir into flour mixture. Add wine and continue stirring and cooking until thickened and bubbly. Pour over fillets.

6. Bake 25 minutes. Remove from oven; sprinkle with cheese and paprika. Return to oven and bake 10 minutes longer or until fish flakes easily with fork.

Yield: 8 servings

1 roll contains:

Cal	Carb g	Fat g	Sat Fat g	Chol mg	Sod mg	Fib g
265	9	11	3	90	625	1

Exchanges: 1 roll = 1 starch/bread, 3 meats

VARIATION

Low-Sodium Flounder Roll-Ups: Omit salt in filling and sauce.

1 roll has same analysis as above, except 491 mg sodium.

SO GOOD POACHED FILLETS

¾ cup water

1 tablespoon lemon juice

½ onion, sliced

1 tablespoon vinegar

3 peppercorns

1 teaspoon salt

1 pound fish fillets or fish steaks

1. Place all ingredients except fish in saucepan and heat 5 minutes.

2. Cut fish in serving-size pieces; add to saucepan.

3. Simmer 10–15 minutes or until fish flakes easily with a fork.

Yield: 4 servings

1 serving contains:

Cal	Carb g	Fat g	Sat Fat g	Chol mg	Sod mg	Fib g
110	2	1	0	60	360	0

Exchanges: 1 serving = 3 meats

QUICK AND EASY FISH WITH ONIONS

1 pound fish fillets

½ teaspoon lemon pepper, Creole seasoning, or seasoned salt, divided

1 teaspoon olive oil

1 medium onion, cut into thin rings

½ cup chopped fresh parsley

juice of 1 lemon

1. Sprinkle 1 side of fish fillets with half (¼ teaspoon) of lemon pepper or other seasoning. Set aside.

2. In large nonstick skillet with lid, heat oil over low to medium heat.

3. Add onion rings and cover skillet (keep heat on low to medium). Stir occasionally; when onions are soft, remove lid and continue cooking until onions start to turn brown.

4. Lay fish on top of onions with the side sprinkled with seasoning down. Cover and cook 3 minutes or until fish just starts to cook.

5. Sprinkle fish with remaining seasoning (¼ teaspoon). With large spatula, turn onions and fish so that uncooked side of fish is against skillet.

6. Sprinkle with parsley and lemon juice.

7. Cover and cook 3 minutes. Remove cover and cook until fish is done (when pricked with a fork, it will flake easily).

8. Carefully move from skillet to serving platter so parsley stays on top. Serve immediately.

Yield: 4 servings

1 serving contains:

Cal	Carb g	Fat g	Sat Fat g	Chol mg	Sod mg	Fib g
131	4	3	<1	60	141	1

Exchanges: 1 serving = 3 meats

SEAFOOD FETTUCCINE ALFREDO

2 tablespoons tub margarine

1 pound crabmeat or scallops

1 tablespoon all-purpose flour

3 large cloves garlic, minced

1 can (12 ounces) evaporated skim milk

½ pound fresh mushrooms, sliced

¾ cup grated reduced-fat Parmesan cheese

¼ cup white wine

1 teaspoon chopped fresh basil or ½ teaspoon dried basil

1 teaspoon chopped fresh parsley

1 package (9 ounces) fettuccine, prepared according to package directions, omitting salt and fat

1. In nonstick skillet, melt margarine; add seafood and cook. Remove seafood from skillet and set aside.

2. Add flour to margarine and cook over low heat, stirring constantly, until it stops bubbling and becomes a golden paste.

3. Add garlic and continue stirring until garlic softens.

4. Add evaporated milk and simmer over medium heat, stirring constantly, until milk thickens.

5. Add mushrooms and continue cooking over low heat until mushrooms soften.

6. Add Parmesan cheese and stir well. Simmer, stirring often, until cheese melts and is blended thoroughly. Remove from heat.

7. Stir in wine, basil, parsley, and seafood; stir until hot. Toss with hot fettuccine and serve immediately.

Yield: 8 cups

1 cup contains:

Cal	Carb g	Fat g	Sat Fat g	Chol mg	Sod mg	Fib g
265	29	7	2	87	436	2

Exchanges: 1 cup = 2 starch/breads, 2 meats

SWISSED VENISON STEAK

1½ pounds venison round steak, ½ inch thick, well trimmed

½ teaspoon salt

¼ teaspoon pepper

¼ cup all-purpose flour

1 tablespoon olive oil

3 onions, sliced

1 stalk celery, chopped

1 can (8 ounces) tomatoes, undrained

2 tablespoons Worcestershire sauce

1. Preheat oven to 300°F.

2. Season venison with salt and pepper; coat with flour.

3. Heat oil in skillet that can be placed in oven. Add venison and cook until brown.

4. Place other ingredients over meat.

5. Cover and bake 1½ hours or until tender.

Yield: 6 servings

1 serving contains:

Cal	Carb g	Fat g	Sat Fat g	Chol mg	Sod mg	Fib g
204	12	5	1	94	341	2

Exchanges: 1 serving = 3 meats, 2 vegetables

MARINATED PORK TENDERLOIN

¾ cup balsamic vinegar

¼ cup liquefied butter substitute, reconstituted from dry mix

½ cup catsup

1 teaspoon pepper

1 teaspoon dry mustard

1 teaspoon celery salt

½ teaspoon minced garlic

¼ teaspoon dried thyme

¼ teaspoon ground cloves

4 pounds pork tenderloin, fat trimmed off

1.   In large glass or plastic container with lid, combine all ingredients except meat; mix well. Add meat and spoon marinade on top. Cover and refrigerate overnight, turning several times and spooning marinade over meat.

2.   Preheat oven to 350°F. If pork is to be served with Madeira Sauce (see following recipe), drain off ½ cup marinade and reserve. Place meat and remaining marinade in Dutch oven or heavy roasting pan with cover; roast approximately 2½ hours or until done.

3.   Serve pork with cooked marinade from pan or drain off excess marinade and serve with Madeira Sauce.

Yield: 12 servings

1 serving pork with marinade contains:

Cal	Carb g	Fat g	Sat Fat g	Chol mg	Sod mg	Fib g
199	4	5	2	103	322	0

Exchanges: 1 serving pork with marinade = 4 meats

PORK TENDERLOIN WITH MADEIRA SAUCE

1 recipe Marinated Pork Tenderloin (opposite column)

3 tablespoons cornstarch

1 can (14½ ounces) beef broth, divided

½ cup marinade, reserved from Marinated Pork Tenderloin recipe

1 green onion, finely chopped

1 teaspoon Dijon mustard

½ cup Madeira wine

1.   Prepare Marinated Pork Tenderloin recipe and set aside.

2.   In saucepan, combine cornstarch with ½ cup broth and mix until smooth.

3.   Add remaining broth, marinade, green onion, and mustard; heat, stirring, until mixture begins to thicken.

4.   Lower heat and cook sauce about 5 minutes; stir in wine and cook 1 minute.

5.   Serve over Marinated Pork Tenderloin.

Yield: 12 servings

1 serving contains:

Cal	Carb g	Fat g	Sat Fat g	Chol mg	Sod mg	Fib g
208	5	5	2	103	254	0

Exchanges: 1 serving = 4 meats

QUICK AND EASY PORK CHOPS IN SPANISH RICE

1 teaspoon olive oil

1 pound lean pork chops, fat trimmed off

¼ cup chopped onion

¼ cup chopped green bell pepper

1 can (16 ounces) tomatoes, chopped, undrained

1 can (8 ounces) tomato sauce

½ teaspoon salt

1 cup water

1 cup rice, uncooked

1. In large skillet, heat oil; add pork chops and brown. Drain off fat.

2. Add remaining ingredients.

3. Cover and simmer 30 minutes, adding more water if needed, until rice is tender.

Yield: 4 servings

1 serving contains.

Cal	Carb g	Fat g	Sat Fat g	Chol mg	Sod mg	Fib g
365	51	9	3	46	834	3

Exchanges: 1 serving = 3 starch/breads, 2 meats, 1 vegetable

VARIATION

Low-Sodium Quick and Easy Pork Chops in Spanish Rice: Substitute no-salt-added canned tomatoes for regular canned tomatoes. Omit salt.

1 serving has same analysis as above, except 397 mg sodium.

BLACK BEANS AND RICE WITH SAUSAGE

3 cups cooked rice, prepared without salt or fat

1 teaspoon olive oil

1 medium onion, chopped

2 cloves garlic, minced

½ green bell pepper, chopped

1 teaspoon cumin seed

¼ teaspoon salt

1 can (15 ounces) black beans, undrained

1 link (8 ounces) low-fat sausage (10% or less fat), thinly sliced

1 tablespoon balsamic vinegar

fresh cilantro, chopped

1. Heat oil in skillet. Add onion, garlic, and bell pepper. Stir and cook until onion is tender.

2. Stir in cumin, salt, beans, and sausage; bring to a boil. Reduce heat and simmer 10 minutes, stirring occasionally.

3. Remove from heat and stir in vinegar. Serve over rice. Garnish with chopped cilantro.

Yield: 8 servings

¾ cup contains:

Cal	Carb g	Fat g	Sat Fat g	Chol mg	Sod mg	Fib g
184	28	3	1	16	448	3

Exchanges: ¾ cup = 2 starch/breads, 1 meat

VEAL SCALOPPINE

2 tablespoons all-purpose flour

½ teaspoon salt

¼ teaspoon pepper

¼ teaspoon dried basil

¼ teaspoon dried oregano

1 pound veal cutlets, well trimmed

2 teaspoons olive oil

1 medium onion, chopped

1 clove garlic, minced

½ cup white wine

½ pound fresh mushrooms, sliced

2 tablespoons chopped fresh parsley

paprika (optional)

1. Combine flour, salt, pepper, basil, and oregano in plastic bag.

2. Add veal and shake to coat.

3. Heat oil in large nonstick skillet. Add veal and cook until browned.

4. Add onion, garlic, and wine. Cover and simmer about 20 minutes.

5. Add mushrooms and parsley.

6. Cover and cook 5–10 minutes longer or until meat and mushrooms are tender.

7. Sprinkle with paprika if desired.

Yield: 4 servings

1 serving contains:

Cal	Carb g	Fat g	Sat Fat g	Chol mg	Sod mg	Fib g
177	9	7	2	74	333	2

Exchanges: 1 serving = 2 meats, 2 vegetables

HOMEMADE SAUSAGE

1 pound very lean ground beef

½ teaspoon ground sage

¼ teaspoon dried thyme

1 teaspoon salt

1 teaspoon pepper

1 teaspoon Liquid Smoke

1. Mix all ingredients thoroughly and shape into patties.

2. Cook on broiler pan or in skillet. Pour off any fat that cooks out of meat.

3. Drain patties on paper towels.

Yield: 6 servings

VARIATION

Hot Sausage: Add 1 teaspoon crushed red pepper.

1 serving contains:

Cal	Carb g	Fat g	Sat Fat g	Chol mg	Sod mg	Fib g
119	0	5	2	43	394	0

Exchanges: 1 serving = 2 meats

ITALIAN SAUSAGE CALZONES

DOUGH

1 package (¼ ounce) active dry yeast

1⅔ cups lukewarm water (95°–105°F)

3 tablespoons corn oil

4½ cups all-purpose flour

1 teaspoon salt

ITALIAN SAUSAGE FILLING

1 pound very lean ground beef

2 teaspoons fennel seed

1 teaspoon dried oregano

1 teaspoon salt

1 teaspoon pepper

1 medium green bell pepper, cut into
    14 slices

1 small onion, sliced

1 jar (14 ounces) commercial low-fat pizza
    sauce

8 ounces part-skim mozzarella cheese,
    shredded

cornmeal

DOUGH

1. In large bowl, dissolve yeast in lukewarm water. Add oil and stir in flour and salt.

2. Turn onto lightly floured surface and knead until smooth.

3. Place dough back in bowl. Cover and let rise until doubled in bulk, 1½–2 hours.

SAUSAGE FILLING

4. In small bowl, mix ground beef, herbs, and seasonings.

5. Drop in big pieces into hot skillet. Turn pieces to cook on all sides. After all sides are cooked, break into smaller pieces about the size of large marbles. If meat starts to stick, add a little water and cover until thoroughly cooked. Set aside until ready to assemble or refrigerate if not being used promptly.

ASSEMBLY

6. Preheat oven to 425°F.

7. Punch dough down and knead 2–3 minutes. Divide dough into 14 portions.

8. On lightly floured surface, use rolling pin to roll out each portion of dough into a circle about 5 inches in diameter.

9. Spread 3 tablespoons meat, 1 bell pepper slice, onion slices, 3 tablespoons pizza sauce, and 2 tablespoons cheese on half of each circle.

10. Fold over and seal by pressing edges with tines of fork.

11. Sprinkle cornmeal on bottom of baking sheet to keep calzones crisp on bottom.

12. Use a spatula to move calzones to baking sheet. Use fork to poke holes in top of each calzone for steam to evaporate. Bake 25 minutes. Serve with additional pizza sauce on top.

Yield: 14 servings

1 calzone contains:

Cal	Carb g	Fat g	Sat Fat g	Chol mg	Sod mg	Fib g
293	35	9	3	27	528	2

Exchanges: 1 calzone = 2 starch/breads, 1 meat, 1 fat

VARIATION

Low-Sodium Italian Sausage Calzones: Omit salt in filling.

1 calzone has same analysis as above, except 376 mg sodium.

Breakfast Entrées

EGG AND SAUSAGE BURRITOS

12 corn tortillas

½ link (3½ ounces) low-fat sausage, sliced very thin or chopped

2 green onions, chopped

1 cup egg substitute

4 egg whites

1 can (4½ ounces) green chilies, chopped

¼ teaspoon crushed red pepper (optional)

½ teaspoon pepper

1 medium tomato, chopped

3 tablespoons chopped fresh cilantro

Mexican salsa (optional)

1. Preheat oven to 350°F. Wrap tortillas in moist paper towels and warm in oven 5–7 minutes or in microwave 1–2 minutes, or place tortillas in top of steamer (over boiling water) 2 minutes.

2. In nonstick skillet, cook sausage and green onions until onions are soft.

3. Combine egg substitute and egg whites; whisk until frothy.

4. Add egg mixture, chilies, and peppers to sausage; cook.

5. Add tomato and cilantro and cook until hot.

6. Spoon 3 tablespoons of filling into each warm tortilla; fold tortilla around filling and place seam side down on serving plate; serve hot.

7. Add salsa if desired.

Yield: 6 servings

2 burritos contain:

Cal	Carb g	Fat g	Sat Fat g	Chol mg	Sod mg	Fib g
164	22	3	1	10	592	3

Exchanges: 2 burritos = 1 starch/bread, 1 meat, 1 vegetable

VARIATION

Low-Sodium Egg and Sausage Burritos: Substitute 1 fresh jalapeño pepper (seeded and chopped) for canned chilies. Cook jalapeño pepper with sausage and green onions.

2 burritos have same analysis as above, except 343 mg sodium.

Abbreviations: Cal = Calories; Carb = Carbohydrates; Sat Fat = Saturated Fat; Chol = Cholesterol; Sod = Sodium; Fib = Fiber; < = less than.

RICE CRUST FOR QUICHE

nonstick cooking spray

1½ cups cooked rice, prepared without salt or fat

2 tablespoons grated Parmesan cheese

½ teaspoon salt

¼ teaspoon pepper

⅓ cup egg substitute

1. Preheat oven to 375°F. Spray 9-inch pie plate with nonstick spray.

2. Place hot rice in medium bowl; add remaining ingredients. Stir until rice sticks together.

3. Pour into pie plate and press against sides and bottom with back of tablespoon sprayed with nonstick spray.

4. Bake about 25 minutes or until just slightly browned. Remove from oven and set aside to cool before filling.

Yield: 8 servings

⅛ of recipe contains:

Cal	Carb g	Fat g	Sat Fat g	Chol mg	Sod mg	Fib g
50	9	<1	0	1	177	0

Exchanges: ⅛ of recipe = 1 starch/bread

GRANOLA

1 cup uncooked oats

⅓ cup wheat germ

2 tablespoons firmly packed brown sugar

½ teaspoon ground cinnamon

1 tablespoon slivered almonds

3 tablespoons frozen apple juice concentrate, undiluted

1 tablespoon honey

2 teaspoons vanilla extract

⅓ cup chopped dried mixed fruit

1. Preheat oven to 200°F

2. In medium bowl, mix oats, wheat germ, brown sugar, cinnamon, and almonds. Set aside.

3. In small microwave-safe bowl, combine apple juice concentrate, honey, and vanilla. Microwave 45 seconds on high. Stir.

4. Pour apple juice mixture over oat mixture and stir until oats are thoroughly coated.

5. Spread on cookie sheet or jelly roll pan. Bake 1 hour, stirring every 15 minutes.

6. Remove from oven and allow to cool about 15 minutes. Stir in mixed fruit.

Yield: 6 servings

⅓ cup contains:

Cal	Carb g	Fat g	Sat Fat g	Chol mg	Sod mg	Fib g
146	29	2	0	0	5	3

Exchanges: Not applicable for this recipe

BREAKFAST CASSEROLE

nonstick cooking spray

1 recipe Homemade Sausage (see page 284;
    for spicy dish, use variation for
    Hot Sausage)

3 slices day-old bread

1½ cups egg substitute

1 large can (12 ounces) plus 1 small can
    (5 ounces) evaporated skim milk

1½ teaspoons dry mustard

½ cup shredded part-skim mozzarella cheese

Mexican salsa (optional)

1.   Spray 9 × 13-inch baking dish with nonstick
spray.

2.   In mixing bowl, combine ingredients for
sausage. Cook sausage in skillet and stir to break
meat into small pieces. Cook until well done.

3.   Drain meat in colander, then spread on paper
towels until cool.

4.   Cut bread into cubes and arrange in bottom
of casserole dish. Spread sausage on top of bread.

5.   In separate dish, combine egg substitute,
milk, and mustard. Pour over sausage and bread.

6.   Cover and refrigerate overnight. (Can be
frozen. To defrost, set in refrigerator overnight.)

7.   Set oven to 350°F and place uncovered baking dish in oven while it is heating. Cook 45 minutes or until light brown around edges and knife
inserted in center comes out clean.

8.   Top with cheese and return to oven until
cheese melts. Serve hot with salsa if desired.

Yield: 6 servings

1 serving contains:

Cal	Carb g	Fat g	Sat Fat g	Chol mg	Sod mg	Fib g
243	13	8	3	50	677	1

Exchanges: 1 serving = 1 starch/bread, 3 meats

VARIATION

Low-Sodium Breakfast Casserole: Omit salt in
sausage.

1 serving has same analysis as above, except 322
mg sodium.

SPINACH QUICHE

**Rice Crust for Quiche (see recipe page 287),
    prepared without cheese (see Step 2,
    below)**

1 package (10 ounces) frozen chopped
    spinach, thawed

1 teaspoon tub margarine

¼ cup chopped onion

¼ cup shredded part-skim mozzarella cheese

1½ cups skim milk

1 tablespoon all-purpose flour

1 tablespoon grated reduced-fat Parmesan
    cheese

¾ cup egg substitute

⅛ teaspoon salt

¼ teaspoon pepper

1.   Preheat oven to 375°F.

2.   Prepare Rice Crust for Quiche, but omit
Parmesan cheese and bake only 5 minutes. Set
aside. Increase oven temperature to 450°F.

3. Drain spinach and squeeze to remove excess moisture. Set aside.

4. In skillet, heat margarine, add onion, and cook until soft. Add spinach and heat until warm.

5. Spread spinach and onion mixture over bottom of crust; sprinkle with mozzarella cheese.

6. In mixing bowl, whisk together milk, flour, Parmesan cheese, and egg substitute with wire whisk; add salt and pepper.

7. Pour egg mixture over spinach and cheese.

8. Bake 10 minutes. Reduce temperature to 325°F and bake an additional 30–35 minutes.

Yield: 8 servings

1 serving of Spinach or Broccoli or Mushroom and Ham Quiche contains:

Cal	Carb g	Fat g	Sat Fat g	Chol mg	Sod mg	Fib g
100	14	1	1	3	314	1

Exchanges: 1 serving of Spinach or Broccoli or Mushroom and Ham Quiche = 1 starch/bread, 1 meat

VARIATIONS

Broccoli Quiche: Substitute 1 package (10 ounces) chopped broccoli for spinach.

Mushroom and Ham Quiche: Substitute 8 ounces sliced mushrooms and 1 ounce ham for spinach. In Step 4, cook mushrooms and ham (with onion) in margarine until all moisture evaporates.

OMELET*

nonstick cooking spray

1 cup egg substitute

2 tablespoons fat-free cream cheese

¼ cup skim milk

¼ teaspoon salt

¼ teaspoon pepper

¼ cup chopped onion

1½ ounces extra-lean cooked ham, chopped

¼ cup sliced mushrooms

½ cup shredded part-skim mozzarella cheese

1. Spray nonstick skillet with nonstick spray.

2. In medium bowl, beat egg substitute until frothy. Add cream cheese, milk, salt, and pepper; beat well. Set aside.

3. In skillet, cook onion and ham over medium heat until browned.

4. Add mushrooms and cook until mushrooms shrink to half their original size.

5. Pour egg mixture over onion, ham, and mushrooms; without stirring, cook over low to medium heat until eggs are set in center.

6. Sprinkle cheese in center and fold in half.

7. When omelet is cooked, serve immediately on warm plates.

Note: Two egg whites may be added for each additional person to be served.

Yield: 2 servings

1 serving contains:

Cal	Carb g	Fat g	Sat Fat g	Chol mg	Sod mg	Fib g
198	7	6	4	28	1,010	1

Exchanges: 1 serving = 3 meats

This recipe is high in sodium; select other foods throughout the day that are very low in sodium.

Vegetables

FRESH GREEN BEANS AND TOMATOES

1½ pounds fresh green beans

nonstick cooking spray

1 teaspoon olive oil

1 medium onion, chopped

2 cloves garlic, finely chopped

3 ripe medium tomatoes, chopped

¼ cup chopped Italian parsley

1 teaspoon dried Italian seasoning

¼ cup white wine

1 tablespoon balsamic vinegar

½ teaspoon salt

¼ teaspoon freshly ground pepper

1. Snap tips off green beans and pull off strings.

2. Steam beans until crisp-tender and place in serving dish. Set aside.

3. Spray skillet with nonstick spray and add oil. Over medium heat, cook onion and garlic until soft.

4. Add remaining ingredients. Cook, uncovered, over medium heat, stirring occasionally, until sauce is slightly reduced, approximately 5 minutes.

5. Pour tomato mixture over beans and toss gently. Serve warm.

Yield: 7 servings

1 serving contains:

Cal	Carb g	Fat g	Sat Fat g	Chol mg	Sod mg	Fib g
49	10	1	0	0	170	4

Exchanges: 1 serving = 2 vegetables

VARIATION

Low-Sodium Fresh Green Beans and Tomatoes: Omit salt.

1 serving has same analysis as above, except 18 mg sodium.

BROCCOLI SOUFFLÉ

nonstick cooking spray

2 teaspoons tub margarine

2 tablespoons all-purpose flour

½ teaspoon salt

¼ teaspoon pepper

½ cup skim milk

½ of 10-ounce package frozen broccoli, cooked according to package directions, drained, and puréed (⅔ cup)

Abbreviations: Cal = Calories; Carb = Carbohydrates; Sat Fat = Saturated Fat; Chol = Cholesterol; Sod = Sodium; Fib = Fiber; < = less than.

1 tablespoon finely chopped onion

¾ cup egg substitute

4 egg whites

1. Preheat oven to 350°F. Spray 6-inch casserole dish with nonstick spray.

2. Melt margarine in saucepan and blend in flour, salt, and pepper. Mixture will be thick.

3. Use a whisk to stir in milk. Cook mixture over low heat until it begins to simmer. Remove from heat.

4. Stir in broccoli and onion.

5. Whip egg substitute at high speed until frothy.

6. In separate bowl, beat egg whites until stiff peaks form. Set aside.

7. Fold broccoli mixture into beaten egg substitute.

8. Fold broccoli and egg substitute mixture into egg whites.

9. Pour into casserole dish and place in pan of hot water. Bake 50–55 minutes. Serve immediately (soufflé will fall as it cools).

Yield: 4 servings

1 serving contains:

Cal	Carb g	Fat g	Sat Fat g	Chol mg	Sod mg	Fib g
90	8	2	<1	1	456	1

Exchanges: 1 serving = 1 meat, 1 vegetable

VARIATION

Low-Sodium Broccoli Soufflé: Omit salt.

1 serving has same analysis as above, except 190 mg sodium.

GREEN BEAN CASSEROLE

nonstick cooking spray

1 tablespoon oil

1 onion, chopped

½ green bell pepper, chopped

1 package (10 ounces) frozen green beans, cooked until almost tender

½ of 16-ounce can tomatoes, chopped, drained

¼ teaspoon salt

⅛ teaspoon crushed red pepper

⅛ teaspoon garlic powder

1 tablespoon mayonnaise

¼ cup dry bread crumbs

1. Preheat oven to 375°F. Spray casserole dish with nonstick spray.

2. Heat oil in skillet. Add onion and bell pepper; cook until onion is soft.

3. Add remaining ingredients except bread crumbs and stir until heated through.

4. Pour into casserole dish and sprinkle with crumbs. Bake 30 minutes.

Yield: 8 servings

1 serving contains:

Cal	Carb g	Fat g	Sat Fat g	Chol mg	Sod mg	Fib g
53	7	3	0	1	151	2

Exchanges: 1 serving = 1 vegetable, 1 fat

SPICY BEETS

2 teaspoons cornstarch

¾ cup orange juice

1 teaspoon grated orange peel

¼ teaspoon ground allspice

¼ teaspoon salt

1 can (16 ounces) sliced beets, drained

1. Stir cornstarch into orange juice over medium heat until juice is thickened.

2. Stir in remaining ingredients and heat through.

Yield: 4 servings

1 serving contains:

Cal	Carb g	Fat g	Sat Fat g	Chol mg	Sod mg	Fib g
49	12	0	0	0	230	2

Exchanges: 1 serving = 2 vegetables

CABBAGE MEDLEY

½ cup water

¼ cup cider vinegar

½ medium head green cabbage, cut into 1-inch-wide wedges

4 medium carrots, cut into thin strips about 3 inches long

1 medium green bell pepper, cut into thin strips

½ medium onion, chopped

1 tablespoon sugar

1 tablespoon caraway seed

½ teaspoon ground nutmeg

1 teaspoon salt

½ teaspoon coarsely ground pepper

¾ cup raisins

1 tablespoon tub margarine

1. Combine all ingredients in large pot or Dutch oven.

2. Bring to a boil, stirring to mix ingredients.

3. Reduce heat and cover; simmer 10 minutes or until vegetables are crisp-tender.

Yield: 6 servings

1 cup contains:

Cal	Carb g	Fat g	Sat Fat g	Chol mg	Sod mg	Fib g
127	28	2	1	0	427	3

Exchanges: 1 cup = 2 vegetables, 1 fruit

VARIATION

Low-Sodium Cabbage Medley: Omit salt.

1 cup has same analysis as above, except 71 mg sodium.

SWEET-AND-SOUR CABBAGE WITH APPLES

¼ cup balsamic vinegar

2 tablespoons firmly packed brown sugar

1 tablespoon red currant jelly

1 teaspoon caraway seed

⅛ teaspoon ground cloves

2 teaspoons cornstarch

1 teaspoon olive oil

½ medium onion, thinly sliced

½ head red cabbage, cut into thin wedges

1 medium apple with peel, cored, cut into
    ½-inch cubes

1. In small mixing bowl, combine vinegar, brown sugar, jelly, caraway seed, cloves, and cornstarch.

2. In large nonstick pan or Dutch oven, heat oil and cook onion until just tender.

3. Add vinegar mixture, cabbage, and apple to cooked onion and stir. Heat to boiling, then reduce heat, cover, and cook about 10 minutes.

4. Serve alone or as an accompaniment to meat, such as pork tenderloin.

Yield: 8 servings

¾ cup contains:

Cal	Carb g	Fat g	Sat Fat g	Chol mg	Sod mg	Fib g
49	11	1	0	0	14	2

Exchanges: ¾ cup = 1 fruit

CREAMED CARROTS AND CELERY

2 cups sliced carrots

1 cup thinly sliced celery

¼ cup finely chopped onion

1 cup skim milk (cold)

1 tablespoon cornstarch

1 teaspoon chopped fresh parsley

¼ teaspoon salt

⅛ teaspoon pepper

1. Place vegetables in saucepan and cover with water.

2. Cover and simmer 10 minutes or until tender but not soft. Drain.

3. In separate dish, mix cold milk and cornstarch together. Stir into vegetables and cook, stirring constantly, until sauce is thick.

4. Add remaining ingredients.

Yield: 4 servings

1 serving contains:

Cal	Carb g	Fat g	Sat Fat g	Chol mg	Sod mg	Fib g
64	13	0	0	1	213	3

Exchanges: 1 serving = 2 vegetables

BUTTER BEANS

1 ham hock

2 bay leaves

16 cups water

5 cups dried butter beans

½ teaspoon coarsely ground pepper

1 medium onion, chopped

3 cloves garlic, chopped

½ teaspoon garlic salt

1 teaspoon salt

1 teaspoon dried basil

1.   The night before cooking beans, place ham bone and bay leaves in large pot with water. Bring to a boil; simmer about 1½–2 hours or until meat falls from bone. Discard bone and place broth in refrigerator overnight.

2.   Clean beans; rinse and soak overnight.

3.   Skim fat from broth; strain through large strainer to catch pieces of meat and fat.

4.   Drain beans and place in broth with pepper, onion, garlic, and garlic salt.

5.   Bring to a boil, cover, reduce heat, and simmer 1½ hours, stirring frequently.

6.   Add salt and basil and continue simmering about 30 minutes or until beans are tender but not mushy.

Yield: 17 servings

1 cup contains:

Cal	Carb g	Fat g	Sat Fat g	Chol mg	Sod mg	Fib g
153	28	<1	0	0	232	9

Exchanges: 1 cup = 2 starch/breads

GINGER CARROTS

4 large carrots

juice of 1 lemon

¾ teaspoon grated fresh ginger

1 tablespoon firmly packed brown sugar

1 tablespoon tub margarine

¼ teaspoon ground cinnamon

⅛ teaspoon salt

⅛ teaspoon freshly ground pepper

1 tablespoon minced fresh parsley

1.   Peel carrots and slice thinly. Cook in water 5–6 minutes or until tender. Drain carrots in colander.

2.   In saucepan used for cooking carrots, combine lemon juice, ginger, brown sugar, and margarine. Heat and stir until mixed.

3.   Add carrots and cook 1 minute.

4.   Season with cinnamon, salt, and pepper; toss lightly.

5.   Sprinkle with parsley just before serving.

Yield: 4 servings

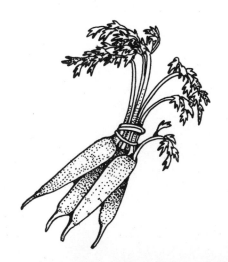

½ cup contains:

Cal	Carb g	Fat g	Sat Fat g	Chol mg	Sod mg	Fib g
89	16	3	1	0	169	3

Exchanges: ½ cup = 3 vegetables

GLAZED CARROTS

2 packages (10 ounces each) frozen carrots
   or 1 pound fresh carrots, sliced or
   julienne cut

1 cup orange juice

2 teaspoons lemon juice

⅛ teaspoon lemon zest or grated lemon peel

½ teaspoon salt

⅛ teaspoon pepper

1. Combine all ingredients in saucepan. Cover and simmer 15 minutes, stirring occasionally.

2. Uncover and continue to simmer, stirring frequently, until most of liquid is evaporated and carrots are tender and glazed. If thicker glaze is desired, add 2 teaspoons cornstarch to ¼ cup water (stir until thoroughly combined) and add to carrots.

3. Continue cooking until sauce is desired thickness.

Yield: 4 servings

1 serving contains:

Cal	Carb g	Fat g	Sat Fat g	Chol mg	Sod mg	Fib g
91	21	0	0	0	359	4

Exchanges: 1 serving = 1 vegetable, 1 fruit

TANGY BUTTERED CORN

1 can (16 ounces) whole-kernel corn,
   undrained

1 tablespoon prepared mustard

2 teaspoons tub margarine

1. Heat corn. Drain most of liquid off corn.

2. Stir in remaining ingredients and heat through.

Yield: 4 servings

1 serving contains:

Cal	Carb g	Fat g	Sat Fat g	Chol mg	Sod mg	Fib g
79	14	3	1	0	304	1

Exchanges: 1 serving = 1 starch/bread

CORN PUDDING

nonstick cooking spray

½ cup egg substitute

1 can (16 ounces) cream-style corn

1 tablespoon cornstarch

½ cup skim milk

1½ tablespoons sugar

1.   Preheat oven to 375°F. Spray 2-quart baking dish with nonstick spray.

2.   Combine egg substitute and corn.

3.   In separate bowl, dissolve cornstarch in milk; add sugar.

4.   Combine all ingredients; pour into baking dish. Bake 1 hour or until golden brown and knife inserted in center comes out clean.

Yield: 8 servings

1 serving contains:

Cal	Carb g	Fat g	Sat Fat g	Chol mg	Sod mg	Fib g
71	15	1	0	0	221	1

Exchanges: 1 serving = 1 starch/bread

GLAZED CARROTS WITH MINT

4 medium carrots, cut diagonally into 1-inch pieces

2 teaspoons tub margarine

1 tablespoon honey

1 tablespoon lightly packed brown sugar

¼ teaspoon white pepper

2 teaspoons chopped fresh mint

1.   In medium saucepan, simmer carrots until tender.

2.   Drain excess water; add margarine, honey, and brown sugar; toss until well coated.

3.   Add pepper and mint; toss lightly. Serve warm.

Yield: 4 servings

1 serving contains:

Cal	Carb g	Fat g	Sat Fat g	Chol mg	Sod mg	Fib g
77	15	2	<1	0	49	2

Exchanges: Not applicable for this recipe

VARIATION

Glazed Carrots with Parsley: Substitute 2 teaspoons chopped fresh parsley for mint.

EGGPLANT AND TOMATOES

1 eggplant, peeled and cut into ½-inch slices

¼ teaspoon garlic powder

¾ teaspoon salt

2 teaspoons olive oil

1 can (16 ounces) tomatoes, chopped, undrained

1½ tablespoons chopped fresh parsley

½ teaspoon pepper

½ teaspoon dried basil

½ teaspoon dried oregano

1.   Sprinkle both sides of eggplant slices with garlic powder and salt. Cook in oil until soft.

2. Add remaining ingredients.

3. Heat thoroughly.

Yield: 6 servings

1 serving contains:

Cal	Carb g	Fat g	Sat Fat g	Chol mg	Sod mg	Fib g
55	10	2	0	0	393	3

Exchanges: 1 serving = 2 vegetables

SOUTHERN CORN

2 teaspoons oil

¼ cup imitation bacon bits

½ green bell pepper, chopped

¼ cup chopped onion

1 can (16 ounces) cream-style corn

¼ teaspoon salt

⅛ teaspoon pepper

1. Heat oil in skillet. Add bacon bits, bell pepper, and onion; cook until onion is tender.

2. Stir in remaining ingredients and heat through.

Yield: 4 servings

1 serving contains:

Cal	Carb g	Fat g	Sat Fat g	Chol mg	Sod mg	Fib g
152	25	5	1	0	631	3

Exchanges: 1 serving = 2 starch/breads, 1 fat

VARIATION

Low-Sodium Southern Corn: Omit bacon bits and salt.

1 serving contains:

Cal	Carb g	Fat g	Sat Fat g	Chol mg	Sod mg	Fib g
120	23	3	<1	0	367	2

Exchanges: 1 serving = 2 starch/breads

EGGPLANT VEGETABLE MEDLEY

2 teaspoons olive oil

1 eggplant, peeled and chopped

2 cloves garlic, minced

1 green bell pepper, chopped

3 tomatoes, chopped

1 onion, chopped

½ pound fresh mushrooms, sliced

¾ teaspoon salt

2 tablespoons chopped fresh parsley or basil

1. Heat oil in nonstick skillet; add eggplant and garlic and cook until lightly browned.

2. Add remaining ingredients. Simmer 8 minutes or until tender.

Yield: 6 servings

1 serving contains:

Cal	Carb g	Fat g	Sat Fat g	Chol mg	Sod mg	Fib g
74	13	2	0	0	278	3

Exchanges: 1 serving = 3 vegetables

VARIATION

Eggplant Vegetable Medley with Cheese: Top with 2 ounces shredded cheese (no more than 5 grams fat per ounce) and broil until cheese melts.

continued

1 serving contains:

Cal	Carb g	Fat g	Sat Fat g	Chol mg	Sod mg	Fib g
100	14	4	1	5	328	3

Exchanges: 1 serving = 3 vegetables, 1 fat

BROILED ONIONS

2 sweet Spanish onions, peeled and halved

¾ cup reduced-sodium chicken broth

¾ cup dry white wine

2 teaspoons tub margarine

¼ cup fine dry bread crumbs

½ teaspoon celery salt

½ teaspoon dried summer savory

1.   Simmer onion halves in broth and wine for 30–40 minutes or until tender. Drain.

2.   Preheat broiler.

3.   Remove center from each onion and chop. Place halves on a baking sheet.

4.   Combine chopped onion centers and remaining ingredients. Stuff ¼ of mixture into each onion half.

5.   Brown lightly under broiler.

Yield: 4 servings

1 serving contains:

Cal	Carb g	Fat g	Sat Fat g	Chol mg	Sod mg	Fib g
62	9	2	1	0	334	1

Exchanges: 1 serving = 2 vegetables

BAKED OKRA AND TOMATOES

nonstick cooking spray

1 pound whole okra, fresh or frozen

1 tablespoon olive oil

1 onion, chopped

3 tomatoes, chopped

½ teaspoon salt

¼ teaspoon pepper

¼ teaspoon garlic powder

1.   Preheat oven to 400°F. Spray casserole dish with nonstick spray.

2.   Wash okra and cut off tips.

3.   In saucepan, heat oil; add okra and remaining ingredients. Cover and simmer until okra is tender, about 15 minutes.

4.   Turn into casserole dish and bake 30 minutes.

Yield: 6 servings

1 serving contains:

Cal	Carb g	Fat g	Sat Fat g	Chol mg	Sod mg	Fib g
67	10	3	0	0	186	4

Exchanges: 1 serving = 1 vegetable, 1 fat

VARIATION

Baked Okra and Tomatoes with Topping: Before baking, top with ¼ cup fine dry bread crumbs.

1 serving contains:

Cal	Carb g	Fat g	Sat Fat mg	Chol mg	Sod g	Fib
83	13	3	<1	0	217	4

Exchanges: 1 serving = 2 vegetables, 1 fat

FLUFFY STUFFED BAKED POTATOES

2 medium potatoes, baked

½ teaspoon salt

⅛ teaspoon pepper

½ teaspoon instant minced onion

½ teaspoon chopped fresh chives

4–6 tablespoons skim milk

1 egg white

2 tablespoons shredded yellow cheese (no more than 5 grams fat per ounce)

paprika

1. Preheat oven to 425°F.

2. Cut potatoes in half lengthwise and scoop out pulp.

3. Whip potatoes, salt, pepper, onion, and chives with electric mixer, adding milk a little at a time, until fluffy. Set aside.

4. In separate bowl, beat egg white until stiff peaks form.

5. Fold egg white into potatoes. Put mixture back into potato skins.

6. Sprinkle with cheese and paprika.

7. Bake until cheese is melted and potatoes are hot.

Yield: 4 servings

1 serving contains:

Cal	Carb g	Fat g	Sat Fat g	Chol mg	Sod mg	Fib g
89	17	1	0	2	316	1

Exchanges: 1 serving = 1 starch/bread

COTTAGE CHEESE–STUFFED BAKED POTATOES

2 potatoes, baked

1 cup low-fat cottage cheese

2 teaspoons chopped fresh chives

1 teaspoon onion powder

paprika

1. Preheat oven to 425°F.

2. Cut potatoes in half lengthwise and scoop out pulp.

3. Place skins in oven and bake until crisp.

4. With an electric mixer, whip potato pulp with cottage cheese, chives, and onion powder.

5. Stuff mixture into potato skins. Sprinkle with paprika.

6. Bake until heated through.

Yield: 4 servings

1 serving contains:

Cal	Carb g	Fat g	Sat Fat g	Chol mg	Sod mg	Fib* g
119	18	1	1	5	235	1

Exchanges: 1 serving = 1 starch/bread

*Analysis includes skin on potatoes.

NEW YEAR'S BLACK-EYED PEAS

1 pound frozen black-eyed peas

2 cups water

1 clove garlic, minced

¼ cup balsamic vinegar

2 teaspoons dry mustard

continued

1 teaspoon sugar

½ teaspoon salt

2 tablespoons chopped fresh parsley

1. Cook peas in 2 cups water according to package directions, omitting salt.

2. Drain cooked peas, reserving ½ cup of liquid.

3. Add garlic, vinegar, mustard, sugar, and salt to reserved liquid in pan. Stir well.

4. Add peas to liquid. Heat, uncovered, 5 minutes or until heated through.

5. Peas can be served hot or cold. Top with parsley before serving.

Yield: 6 servings

½ cup contains:

Cal	Carb g	Fat g	Sat Fat g	Chol mg	Sod mg	Fib g
76	16	<1	0	0	182	3

Exchanges: ½ cup = 1 starch/bread

SPICED PEAS

1 package (10 ounces) frozen green peas

½ cup water

¼ cup chopped celery

3 tablespoons chopped onion

2 tablespoons chopped pimiento

¼ teaspoon dried marjoram

⅛ teaspoon salt

⅛ teaspoon pepper

1. Cook peas in water until tender.

2. Add remaining ingredients. Simmer a few more minutes.

Yield: 4 servings

1 serving contains:

Cal	Carb g	Fat g	Sat Fat g	Chol mg	Sod mg	Fib g
54	10	0	0	0	131	4

Exchanges: 1 serving = 1 starch/bread

CHINESE SPINACH

1 package (10 ounces) frozen chopped spinach, cooked, undrained

1 cup bean sprouts

⅓ cup sliced water chestnuts

1 cup sliced fresh mushrooms or 1 can (2 ounces) mushrooms, drained

1 tablespoon reduced-sodium soy sauce

1. To cooked spinach, add remaining vegetables and heat.

2. Drain and toss with soy sauce.

Yield: 4 servings

1 serving contains:

Cal	Carb g	Fat g	Sat Fat g	Chol mg	Sod mg	Fib g
48	7	1	0	0	196	2

Exchanges: 1 serving = 1 vegetable

SPINACH SOUFFLÉ

1 package (10 ounces) frozen chopped spinach, cooked and drained

3 tablespoons chopped onion

½ cup low-fat cottage cheese

1 teaspoon lemon juice

¼ teaspoon salt

⅛ teaspoon pepper

1 egg white, beaten stiff

1.   Preheat oven to 350°F.

2.   Combine all ingredients except egg white; purée in blender.

3.   Fold in egg white. Place in ungreased small casserole or in muffin tins.

4.   Bake 20–25 minutes or until lightly browned around edges. Serve immediately.

Yield: 3 servings

1 serving contains:

Cal	Carb g	Fat g	Sat Fat g	Chol mg	Sod mg	Fib g
63	6	1	<1	3	404	1

Exchanges: 1 serving = 1 meat, 1 vegetable

BAKED ZUCCHINI

1 pound zucchini, unpeeled, sliced

¼ cup sliced green onion

1 tablespoon olive oil

3 tomatoes, chopped

½ teaspoon salt

⅛ teaspoon pepper

1 clove garlic, minced

½ green bell pepper, chopped

1.   Preheat oven to 350°F.

2.   Cook zucchini and green onion in oil.

3.   Place in casserole dish and top with remaining ingredients.

4.   Cover and bake 30 minutes.

Yield: 6 servings

1 serving contains:

Cal	Carb g	Fat g	Sat Fat g	Chol mg	Sod mg	Fib g
47	6	3	0	0	186	2

Exchanges: 1 serving = 1 vegetable, 1 fat

ITALIANO ZUCCHINI

3 medium zucchini

1 teaspoon olive oil

1 medium onion, thinly sliced

⅛ teaspoon salt

¼ teaspoon pepper

1 teaspoon dried oregano

1 can (8 ounces) tomato sauce

4 ounces part-skim mozzarella cheese, shredded

1.   Cut zucchini in half lengthwise.

2.   Heat oil in nonstick skillet. Add onion and cook until brown.

3.   Add zucchini, cut sides up.

4.   Stir salt, pepper, and oregano into tomato sauce and pour over zucchini. Cover and cook 8–10 minutes or until barely tender.

5.   Just before serving, add cheese to zucchini and heat until melted. Serve immediately.

Yield: 6 servings

1 serving contains:

Cal	Carb g	Fat g	Sat Fat g	Chol mg	Sod mg	Fib g
92	8	4	2	10	376	2

Exchanges: 1 serving = 1 meat, 1 vegetable

SQUASH CASSEROLE

nonstick cooking spray

1 package (16 ounces) frozen yellow crook-
   neck squash

1 can (12 ounces) evaporated skim milk

1 egg

2 teaspoons Worcestershire sauce

½ teaspoon garlic powder

½ teaspoon pepper

1 tablespoon cornstarch

4 ounces shredded Cheddar cheese
   (no more than 5 grams fat per ounce)

1 small green bell pepper, chopped

1 small onion, chopped

¾ cup bread crumbs

1.   Preheat oven to 350°F. Spray 1-quart casserole with nonstick spray.

2.   Thaw squash; squeeze out excess water and
set aside.

3.   In separate bowl, combine milk, egg, Worcestershire sauce, garlic powder, pepper, cornstarch, and cheese. Mix well with wire whisk. Stir
in bell pepper and onion.

4.   In casserole, spread squash; pour egg mixture
on top. Bake 45 minutes.

5.   Remove from oven and sprinkle with bread
crumbs. Bake additional 15 minutes.

Yield: 8 servings

½ cup contains:

Cal	Carb g	Fat g	Sat Fat g	Chol mg	Sod mg	Fib g
141	17	4	2	36	220	1

Exchanges: ½ cup = 1 starch/bread, 1 meat

SPINACH TOMATOES

3 tomatoes, cut in half

2 tablespoons finely chopped onion

¼ cup chopped fresh parsley

1 tablespoon tub margarine

½ of 10-ounce package frozen chopped
   spinach, cooked and drained

2 tablespoons fine dry bread crumbs

1.   Preheat oven to 350°F.

2.   Place tomatoes in shallow baking pan, cut
sides up.

3.   Mix onion, parsley, margarine, and spinach.
Spread on tomatoes and sprinkle with crumbs.

4.   Bake 20 minutes.

Yield: 6 servings

1 tomato half contains:

Cal	Carb g	Fat g	Sat Fat g	Chol mg	Sod mg	Fib g
47	6	2	<1	0	59	2

Exchanges: 1 tomato half = 1 vegetable

ORANGE ACORN SQUASH

nonstick cooking spray

2 acorn squash, cut in half and seeded

1 tablespoon butter flavoring

1 cup orange juice

½ teaspoon salt

¾ teaspoon ground allspice

1.   Preheat oven to 350°F. Spray casserole dish
with nonstick spray.

2. Place squash halves in casserole dish, cut sides up.

3. Combine remaining ingredients and pour into squash cavities.

4. Cover and bake 1 hour or until squash is tender.

Yield: 4 servings

1 serving contains:

Cal	Carb g	Fat g	Sat Fat g	Chol mg	Sod mg	Fib g
113	26	1	0	0	269	6

Exchanges: 1 serving = 1 starch/bread, 1 fruit

SPICY SWEET POTATOES

5 medium sweet potatoes

nonstick cooking spray

¾ cup orange juice

½ teaspoon ground cinnamon

¼ teaspoon ground nutmeg

3 tablespoons firmly packed brown sugar

¾ teaspoon orange zest or grated orange peel

1. Peel potatoes, cut into thick slices, and boil until tender.

2. Preheat oven to 350°F. Spray 1-quart casserole (with lid) with nonstick spray and set aside.

3. Mash potatoes and add remaining ingredients.

4. Place potatoes in casserole dish. Cover and bake about 30 minutes or until heated through. Serve hot.

Yield: 8 servings

1 serving contains:

Cal	Carb g	Fat g	Sat Fat g	Chol mg	Sod mg	Fib g
104	25	0	0	0	9	2

Exchanges: Not applicable for this recipe

SEASONED SQUASH

1 clove garlic, minced

1 tablespoon tub margarine

1¼ pounds yellow squash or zucchini, sliced ¼ inch thick

½ teaspoon seasoned salt

¼ cup chopped green onion

¼ cup water

1 can (8 ounces) tomatoes, chopped, undrained

2 tablespoons chopped fresh parsley

1. Cook garlic in margarine 3 minutes.

2. Add squash, salt, green onion, and water.

3. Cover and simmer, stirring occasionally, until squash is tender.

4. Add tomatoes and parsley.

5. Heat through.

Yield: 6 servings

1 serving contains:

Cal	Carb g	Fat g	Sat Fat g	Chol mg	Sod mg	Fib g
40	5	2	<1	0	202	2

Exchanges: 1 serving = 1 vegetable

SPAGHETTI SQUASH WITH THREE-HERB PESTO

½ medium spaghetti squash (2½–3 pounds), cut lengthwise

¼ cup packed chopped Italian parsley

¼ cup packed chopped fresh dill

¼ cup packed chopped fresh basil

¼ cup grated Parmesan cheese

2 teaspoons pine nuts

⅛ teaspoon pepper

⅛ teaspoon salt

2 cloves garlic

1 tablespoon olive oil

1 tablespoon water

1. Place squash, cut side down, in microwave-safe baking dish and add ¼ cup water. Cover with plastic wrap, leaving one corner open to vent. Microwave on high 12 minutes, rotating dish half a turn after 6 minutes, or until squash can easily be pierced with a fork

2. Let squash stand, covered, 10 minutes.

3. In food processor, add all remaining ingredients except oil and water; process until smooth, pouring oil and water through feed tube while processing. Continue processing until well combined. Set aside.

4. Using a fork, scrape pulp of squash into strands.

5. Place squash strands on serving platter; add pesto and toss to combine.

Yield: 6 servings

½ cup contains:

Cal	Carb g	Fat g	Sat Fat g	Chol mg	Sod mg	Fib g
72	7	4	1	3	114	3

Exchanges: ½ cup = 1 vegetable, 1 fat

STIR-FRIED VEGETABLE MEDLEY

1 tablespoon olive oil

1 onion, sliced and separated into rings

1 clove garlic, minced

2 large carrots, sliced diagonally

1 zucchini, sliced

2 yellow squash, sliced

1 green bell pepper, cut into strips

8 fresh mushrooms, sliced

½ cup bamboo shoots

3 water chestnuts, sliced

1 tablespoon reduced-sodium soy sauce

1. Heat large skillet or wok until a drop of water dances on the surface.

2. Add oil and heat.

3. Cook onion rings and garlic until just tender.

4. Add carrots, stirring with wooden spoon until lightly coated with oil. Cover and cook 3–4 minutes.

5. Add zucchini and yellow squash, stirring lightly. Cover and allow vegetables to steam in their own juices 2–3 minutes.

6. Add remaining vegetables and stir another 1–2 minutes or until tender but crisp.

7. Add soy sauce, cover, and steam 1 additional minute. Serve immediately.

Yield: 8 servings

1 serving contains:

Cal	Carb g	Fat g	Sat Fat g	Chol mg	Sod mg	Fib g
47	7	2	0	0	88	2

Exchanges: 1 serving = 1 vegetable

Stuffings and Dressings

POTATO CARROT STUFFING

1 tablespoon olive oil

3 cups (3–4 medium) red potatoes, peeled and coarsely grated (as if for hash browns)

½ cup grated carrots

1 medium onion, finely chopped

4 stalks celery, chopped

½ cup chopped fresh parsley

⅛ teaspoon ground nutmeg

¼ teaspoon ground sage

1 teaspoon (or to taste) Creole seasoning

¼ cup seasoned bread crumbs

½ cup beef broth

¼ cup egg substitute

1. Heat oil in large skillet, add potatoes, and stir; cook about 6 minutes.

2. Add carrots and cook an additional 4 minutes.

3. Add onion, celery, and parsley; cook until tender.

4. Add nutmeg, sage, Creole seasoning, bread crumbs, and broth; stir well. Add egg substitute and stir thoroughly to ensure even cooking.

5. Can be served with beef roast or pork tenderloin.

Yield: 9 servings

⅔ cup contains:

Cal	Carb g	Fat g	Sat Fat g	Chol mg	Sod mg	Fib g
86	15	2	0	0	249	2

Exchanges: ⅔ cup = 1 starch/bread

Abbreviations: Cal = Calories; Carb = Carbohydrates; Sat Fat = Saturated Fat; Chol = Cholesterol; Sod = Sodium; Fib = Fiber; < = less than.

CORNBREAD DRESSING

2 recipes Cornbread (page 310), modified as
   instructed below

¼ teaspoon ground sage

1 medium onion, chopped

3–4 celery stalks and leaves, chopped

¼ cup chopped fresh parsley

⅔ cup chopped pecans (optional)

nonstick cooking spray

cooked meat from 1 turkey neck or 1 cup
   cooked turkey or chicken, torn into small
   pieces

2–3 cans (14½ ounces each) reduced-sodium
   chicken broth or 4–5 cups fresh turkey
   broth, fat removed (use enough to make
   dressing moist)

½ cup egg substitute

¼ teaspoon salt

pepper to taste

1.   Preheat oven to 400°F.

2.   Prepare cornbread recipe (doubled) according to recipe directions, adding sage, onion, celery, parsley, and pecans if desired.

3.   Divide margarine between two 8-inch iron skillets and melt.

4.   Pour batter into skillets.

5.   Bake 20–25 minutes or until golden brown. Remove from oven and cool slightly. Reduce oven temperature to 350°F. Spray 9 × 13-inch baking dish with nonstick spray.

6.   Tear cornbread into small pieces and put into large mixing bowl.

7.   Add turkey meat, broth, egg substitute, salt, and pepper. Mix thoroughly. (For moister dressing, add more broth.)

8.   Spoon into baking dish; bake 25–30 minutes or until golden brown.

Yield: 24 servings

1 serving without pecans contains:

Cal	Carb g	Fat g	Sat Fat g	Chol mg	Sod mg	Fib g
123	18	3	1	6	329	1

Exchanges: 1 serving without pecans =
1 starch/bread, 1 fat

1 serving with pecans contains:

Cal	Carb g	Fat g	Sat Fat g	Chol mg	Sod mg	Fib g
145	19	5	1	6	329	1

Exchanges: 1 serving with pecans = 1 starch/bread, 1 fat

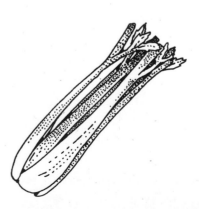

Sauces and Gravies

FAT-FREE CHEESE SAUCE

2 tablespoons all-purpose flour

1 cup skim milk

3 ounces fat-free yellow cheese

¼ teaspoon white pepper

1. In microwave-safe container, blend flour with milk until smooth (2-cup glass measuring cup works well).

2. Heat mixture in microwave at 80% power 3–5 minutes or until thickened, stirring thoroughly at 1-minute intervals while cooking. Watch mixture carefully during the last 1–2 minutes of cooking; it can boil over quickly once thickened.

3. Add cheese and pepper; stir until cheese melts completely.

Yields 5 servings

¼ cup contains:

Cal	Carb g	Fat g	Sat Fat g	Chol mg	Sod mg	Fib g
53	7	0	0	2	289	0

Exchanges: ¼ cup = 1 milk

VARIATION

Low-Fat Cheese Sauce: Substitute processed yellow cheese (no more than 5 grams fat per ounce) for fat-free cheese.

¼ cup contains:

Cal	Carb g	Fat g	Sat Fat g	Chol mg	Sod mg	Fib g
73	6	3	2	10	274	0

Exchanges: ¼ cup = 1 milk, 1 fat

Abbreviations: Cal = Calories; Carb = Carbohydrates; Sat Fat = Saturated Fat; Chol = Cholesterol; Sod = Sodium; Fib = Fiber; < = less than.

GIBLET-STYLE GRAVY

1 turkey neck

4 cups water

¼ teaspoon salt

¼ teaspoon pepper

1 can (14 ounces) reduced-sodium chicken broth

¼ cup cornstarch

1 hard-boiled egg, chopped (optional)

1.   Place turkey neck in covered saucepan with water; simmer 1–1½ hours.

2.   Remove neck from water and set broth aside. When cool, place broth in refrigerator to allow fat to harden. Discard fat.

3.   Remove meat from bone; tear or chop into small pieces. Add meat to broth.

4.   Add salt, pepper, and canned broth to broth from refrigerator. Heat to boiling.

5.   To thicken gravy, mix cornstarch with small amount of cold water; add mixture to broth and stir.

6.   Cook, stirring constantly, until slightly thickened. Add egg if desired and stir.

Yield: 16 servings

¼ cup without egg contains:

Cal	Carb g	Fat g	Sat Fat g	Chol mg	Sod mg	Fib g
29	2	1	0	8	47	0

Exchanges: ¼ cup without egg = Free

¼ cup with egg contains:

Cal	Carb g	Fat g	Sat Fat g	Chol mg	Sod mg	Fib g
33	2	1	0	22	51	0

MUSHROOMS IN RED WINE SAUCE

1 teaspoon tub margarine

2 cloves garlic, minced

1 shallot, minced

1 pound fresh mushrooms, quartered

½ cup red wine

½ tablespoon cornstarch

½ cup reduced-sodium chicken broth

1.   Melt margarine in medium saucepan. Cook garlic and shallot in margarine over low heat 2 minutes.

2.   Add mushrooms and continue to cook over low heat 2 minutes

3.   Add wine. Increase heat; boil 8 minutes to reduce wine.

4.   Mix cornstarch with broth until smooth. Add to mushroom mixture, stirring constantly until sauce thickens. Boil 3 minutes, stirring occasionally.

5.   Serve warm.

Yield: 4 servings

½ cup contains:

Cal	Carb g	Fat g	Sat Fat g	Chol mg	Sod mg	Fib g
56	8	2	0	0	105	1

Exchanges: ½ cup = 2 vegetables

VARIATION

Mushrooms in White Wine Sauce: Substitute white wine for red wine.

Breads and Muffins

BANANA NUT BREAD

nonstick cooking spray

3 ripe bananas

½ cup egg substitute

1 tablespoon corn oil

¼ cup applesauce

1½ tablespoons low-fat buttermilk

1 teaspoon lemon juice

½ cup sugar

2 cups all-purpose flour

1½ teaspoons baking powder

½ teaspoon baking soda

½ cup chopped pecans (optional)

1. Preheat oven to 350°F. Spray 9 × 5-inch loaf pan with nonstick spray.

2. In large mixing bowl, mash bananas. Add egg substitute and beat with mixer on high about 2 minutes.

3. Add oil, applesauce, buttermilk, lemon juice, and sugar. Mix until smooth.

4. In separate bowl, combine flour, baking powder, and soda. Stir with whisk to distribute baking powder and soda into flour.

5. Pour banana mixture into flour mixture. Stir until dry ingredients are moistened. Stir in nuts if desired, being careful not to overmix.

6. Bake 60–75 minutes or until toothpick inserted in center comes out clean. Allow to cool 5 minutes before turning out on wire rack.

Yield: 12 slices

1 slice without nuts contains:

Cal	Carb g	Fat g	Sat Fat g	Chol mg	Sod mg	Fib g
154	32	2	0	0	104	1

Exchanges: Not applicable for this recipe

1 slice with nuts contains:

Cal	Carb g	Fat g	Sat Fat g	Chol mg	Sod mg	Fib g
187	33	5	<1	0	105	2

Abbreviations: Cal = Calories; Carb = Carbohydrates; Sat Fat = Saturated Fat; Chol = Cholesterol; Sod = Sodium; Fib = Fiber; < = less than.

BASIC CRÊPES

⅔ cup all-purpose flour

½ cup egg substitute, divided

¾ teaspoon lemon zest or grated lemon peel

4 teaspoons low-sodium tub margarine, melted

1 cup skim milk

1. Combine flour and ½ of egg substitute (¼ cup) and beat well at low speed.

2. Add remaining egg substitute (¼ cup) and beat 3–5 minutes.

3. Add lemon zest or peel and margarine.

4. Gradually stir in enough milk until batter has consistency of thin cream.

5. Allow batter to sit 2 hours.

6. Brush 6-inch skillet with oil and heat.

7. Pour ¼ cup batter in skillet, tilting skillet so that batter coats surface evenly. Pour any excess batter back into bowl.

8. Cook crêpe until lightly browned on bottom, about 1 minute.

9. Turn and brown other side.

Yield: 9 crêpes

1 crêpe contains:

Cal	Carb g	Fat g	Sat Fat g	Chol mg	Sod mg	Fib g
65	9	2	<1	<1	60	0

Exchanges: 1 crêpe = 1 starch/bread

CORNBREAD

2 tablespoons tub margarine

¾ cup cornmeal

1 cup all-purpose flour

1 tablespoon sugar

1 tablespoon baking powder

¾ teaspoon salt

¼ cup egg substitute

1 cup skim milk

1. Preheat oven to 425°F. Melt margarine in ovenproof skillet; remove from heat.

2. In medium bowl, mix together dry ingredients.

3. In small bowl, whisk egg substitute and milk together. Add to dry ingredients. Mix just until combined.

4. Pour batter into skillet with melted margarine.

5. Bake 20–25 minutes or until golden brown.

Yield: 8 servings

1 serving contains:

Cal	Carb g	Fat g	Sat Fat g	Chol mg	Sod mg	Fib g
151	26	3	1	1	407	1

Exchanges: 1 serving = 2 starch/breads

VARIATION

Low-Sodium Cornbread: Omit salt.

1 serving has same analysis as above, except 207 mg sodium.

ONION BREAD SQUARES

1 tablespoon tub margarine

1 onion, sliced

2 cups all-purpose flour

2 teaspoons baking powder

½ teaspoon salt

2 tablespoons oil

2 tablespoons chopped fresh parsley

1 cup skim milk

8 ounces fat-free sour cream

1.   Preheat oven to 425°F. Oil and flour 8 × 8-inch baking pan.

2.   Heat margarine in skillet; cook onion until tender. Set aside.

3.   Combine flour, baking powder, and salt.

4.   Cut in oil with fork until mixture resembles coarse meal.

5.   Add parsley and milk, mixing just until dry ingredients are moistened.

6.   Pour into pan. Spread onions over top and cover with sour cream.

7.   Bake 20 minutes. Cut into squares and serve hot.

Yield: 16 servings

1 serving contains:

Cal	Carb g	Fat g	Sat Fat g	Chol mg	Sod mg	Fib g
95	15	3	<1	<1	142	1

Exchanges: 1 serving = 1 starch/bread

PUMPKIN BREAD

3 cups all-purpose flour

2 cups sugar

1 cup firmly packed brown sugar

2 teaspoons baking soda

1½ teaspoons salt

1 teaspoon ground cinnamon

½ teaspoon ground nutmeg

⅓ cup oil

1 can (16 ounces) pumpkin

⅔ cup water

½ cup chopped walnuts

1.   Preheat oven to 350°F. Oil and flour two 9 × 5-inch loaf pans.

2.   In large bowl, combine dry ingredients; make a well in center.

3.   In separate bowl, combine oil, pumpkin, and water. Add to well in dry ingredients and mix together; stir in walnuts.

4.   Pour into pans. Bake 1 hour.

Yield: 20 slices per loaf

1 slice contains:

Cal	Carb g	Fat g	Sat Fat g	Chol mg	Sod mg	Fib g
123	24	3	0	0	124	1

Exchanges: Not applicable for this recipe

BRAN MUFFINS

¼ cup egg substitute

1 cup skim milk

2 tablespoons oil

1½ tablespoons molasses

1½ cups bran cereal (bud type)

1 cup all-purpose flour

2½ teaspoons baking powder

½ teaspoon salt

¼ cup firmly packed brown sugar

1.   Preheat oven to 400°F. Oil muffin tins.

2.   In large bowl, beat together egg substitute, milk, oil, and molasses.

3.   Stir in bran and let stand 5 minutes.

4.   In separate bowl, blend flour, baking powder, salt, and brown sugar.

5.   Add flour mixture to bran mixture and fold together very gently, just until moistened. Do *not* overmix, as this will make muffins tough.

6.   Fill muffin tins ⅔ full.

7.   Bake 20 minutes or until done.

Yield: 12 muffins

1 Bran or Spice Bran Muffin contains:

Cal	Carb g	Fat g	Sat Fat g	Chol mg	Sod mg	Fib g
110	21	3	0	0	238	3

Exchanges: 1 Bran or Spice Bran Muffin = 1 starch/bread

VARIATIONS

Spice Bran Muffins: Add 1¼ teaspoons ground cinnamon and ¾ teaspoon ground nutmeg to dry ingredients.

Date Bran Muffins: Add ½ cup chopped dates to bran mixture.

Raisin Bran Muffins: Add ½ cup raisins to mixture.

1 Date Bran or Raisin Bran Muffin contains:

Cal	Carb g	Fat g	Sat Fat g	Chol mg	Sod mg	Fib g
130	26	3	0	0	238	3

Exchanges: 1 Date Bran or Raisin Bran Muffin = 1 starch/bread, 1 fruit

JALAPEÑO CORNBREAD

3 medium jalapeño peppers

2 tablespoons tub margarine

¼ cup chopped onion

¾ cup cornmeal

1 cup all-purpose flour

1 tablespoon sugar

1 tablespoon baking powder

¾ teaspoon salt

¾ cup skim milk

¼ cup egg substitute

1 can (4 ounces) whole-kernel corn

1 jar (2 ounces) chopped pimientos, drained

1.   Preheat oven to 400°F.

2.   To prepare jalapeños, heat iron skillet over medium heat. Sear the whole jalapeños on all sides by gently turning them in the skillet. (Skins will pop.) Remove jalapeños from heat. Gently scrape off loosened skins (as much as possible). Remove stems, slice peppers lengthwise, and remove seeds. Chop peppers to equal ⅓ cup.

3. Heat margarine in skillet; add onion and jalapeños and cook while preparing cornbread batter.

4. In medium bowl, mix together dry ingredients.

5. Stir in milk and egg substitute only until dry ingredients are moistened. Do not overmix.

6. With slotted spoon, remove onion and jalapeños from margarine and add to batter. Discard remaining margarine in skillet.

7. Add corn and pimientos to batter. Stir all ingredients together, mixing just until combined.

8. Pour batter into skillet. Bake 20–25 minutes or until golden brown.

Yield: 8 servings

1 serving contains:

Cal	Carb g	Fat g	Sat Fat g	Chol mg	Sod mg	Fib g
146	29	1	0	0	406	2

Exchanges: 1 serving = 2 starch/breads

VARIATION

Low-Sodium Jalapeño Cornbread: Omit salt.

1 serving has same analysis as above, except 206 mg sodium.

CASSEROLE CHEESE BREAD

4½ cups all-purpose flour, divided

2 packages (¼ ounce each) active dry yeast

3 tablespoons sugar

2 teaspoons salt

⅓ cup nonfat dry milk powder

2 tablespoons tub margarine

1¾ cups hot water (120°–130°F)

¼ cup egg substitute

1 cup shredded yellow cheese (no more than 5 grams fat per ounce)

1 cup oatmeal, uncooked

nonstick cooking spray

1. In large bowl, combine 2 cups flour, yeast, sugar, salt, and milk powder.

2. Add margarine and water, mixing well with electric mixer about 2 minutes.

3. Add egg substitute, cheese, and ½ cup flour, mixing at high speed 2 minutes.

4. Stir in oatmeal and remaining flour to make a stiff dough.

5. Cover and let rise in warm place 45 minutes.

6. Preheat oven to 325°F. Spray casserole with cooking spray.

7. Stir dough down, beating vigorously 30 seconds, and turn into casserole.

8. Bake 50–55 minutes or until lightly browned.

Yield: 20 slices

1 slice contains:

Cal	Carb g	Fat g	Sat Fat g	Chol mg	Sod mg	Fib g
159	27	3	1	3	270	2

Exchanges: 1 slice = 2 starch/breads

QUICK AND EASY HONEY WHEAT BREAD

2½ cups whole-wheat flour

1½ cups wheat germ

⅓ cup firmly packed brown sugar

½ teaspoon salt

1 cup raisins

2 teaspoons baking soda

1¾ cups low-fat buttermilk

⅓ cup honey

1. Preheat oven to 350°F. Oil 9 × 5-inch loaf pan.

2. In large bowl, combine flour, wheat germ, brown sugar, salt, and raisins.

3. In separate bowl, combine soda, buttermilk, and honey.

4. When liquid mixture begins to bubble, stir into dry ingredients quickly. Dough will be stiff.

5. Spoon into pan. Bake 1 hour or until lightly browned.

Yield: 20 slices

1 slice contains:

Cal	Carb g	Fat g	Sat Fat g	Chol mg	Sod mg	Fib g
146	30	1	0	1	163	3

Exchanges: Not applicable for this recipe

DILLY BREAD

1 package (¼ ounce) active dry yeast

¼ cup warm water (105°–115°F)

1 cup fat-free cottage cheese, slightly heated

2 tablespoons sugar

¼ cup egg substitute

1 tablespoon instant minced onion

2 teaspoons dill seed

1 teaspoon salt

¼ teaspoon baking soda

1 tablespoon tub margarine

2¼–2½ cups all-purpose flour

1. Dissolve yeast in warm water.

2. Mix yeast with remaining ingredients. Add enough flour to make a stiff dough. Beat mixture well and cover.

3. Let dough rise in warm place until it doubles in size (about 1 hour).

4. Stir dough down and turn into a well-oiled loaf pan. Let dough rise until doubled in size again (30–40 minutes).

5. Preheat oven to 350°F. Bake 45 minutes or until golden brown.

6. Remove bread from pan and cool on rack.

Yield: 14 slices

1 slice contains:

Cal	Carb g	Fat g	Sat Fat g	Chol mg	Sod mg	Fib g
109	20	1	0	1	187	1

Exchanges: 1 slice = 1 starch/bread

FRENCH BREAD

1¼ cups warm water (105°–115°F)

1 package (¼ ounce) active dry yeast

1 tablespoon sugar

1 teaspoon salt

1 teaspoon tub margarine, melted

3½ cups bread flour, divided

2 tablespoons cornmeal

1. Mix water, yeast, and sugar in mixing bowl until dissolved.

2. Add salt and margarine.

3. Stir in 2 cups flour.

4. Work in remaining flour until well blended, using hands if necessary. Dough will be sticky.

5. Turn onto lightly floured board and knead 8–10 minutes.

6. Place dough in large oiled bowl. Turn once to oil surface.

7. Cover and let rise in a warm place until doubled in volume, about 1 hour.

8. Roll on lightly floured board into rectangle about 10 × 15 inches.

9. Roll up like jelly roll and tuck in ends.

10. Sprinkle cornmeal on oiled baking sheet.

11. Place dough on baking sheet and let rise until doubled, about 30 minutes.

12. Preheat oven to 375°F.

13. Bake for 30 minutes or until lightly browned. Remove from pan and serve immediately or cool on rack.

Yield: 12 slices

1 slice contains:

Cal	Carb g	Fat g	Sat Fat g	Chol mg	Sod mg	Fib g
159	33	1	0	0	182	2

Exchanges: 1 slice = 2 starch/breads

Desserts

AMARETTO CHEESECAKE

nonstick cooking spray

3 graham cracker rectangles ($4\frac{3}{4} \times 2\frac{1}{2}$ inches each), finely crushed, or $\frac{1}{2}$ cup graham cracker crumbs

8 ounces fat-free cream cheese

8 ounces low-fat cream cheese

8 ounces fat-free sour cream

2 tablespoons cornstarch

1 cup sugar

$\frac{1}{2}$ teaspoon imitation butter flavoring

1 teaspoon almond extract

4 tablespoons sliced almonds

1.   Preheat oven to 350°F.

2.   Remove bottom from 9-inch springform pan. Cut square of foil 1 inch larger than bottom of pan. Line pan bottom with foil and reassemble. (Excess foil will hang from bottom of pan. Fold it up and out of the way.) Spray sides and bottom of pan with nonstick spray.

3.   Pour crumbs into pan and tilt to cover bottom of pan evenly. Use fingertips to distribute loose crumbs evenly.

4.   In large bowl, mix together cream cheeses, sour cream, cornstarch, sugar, butter flavoring, and almond extract. Mix just until smooth; do not overmix.

5.   Pour filling into center of crust and spread evenly over crust. (This keeps loose crumbs from getting into filling.)

6.   Sprinkle almond slices around outside edge on top of cake. Lightly push almond slices into top of cheesecake so they will adhere to surface.

7.   Bake 1 hour (decrease time if using larger pan). Top will be firm and brown, but a toothpick inserted into cake will *not* come out clean.

8.   Cool 1 hour.

9.   Cover cheesecake with plastic wrap. Freeze at least 8 hours or overnight.

10. About 1 hour before serving, take cheesecake out of freezer and immediately remove pan and foil. (Crumbs will stick if allowed to thaw.)

Yield: 12 servings

$\frac{1}{12}$ of cake contains:

Cal	Carb g	Fat g	Sat Fat g	Chol mg	Sod mg	Fib g
165	24	5	3	13	256	0

Exchanges: Not applicable for this recipe

Abbreviations: Cal = Calories; Carb = Carbohydrates; Sat Fat = Saturated Fat; Chol = Cholesterol; Sod = Sodium; Fib = Fiber; < = less than.

BASIC WHITE CAKE

2 cups sifted all-purpose flour

1 teaspoon salt

1 tablespoon baking powder

1¼ cups sugar, divided

⅓ cup oil

1 cup skim milk

1 teaspoon vanilla extract

¼ teaspoon imitation butter flavoring

¼ teaspoon almond extract

4 egg whites

1. Preheat oven to 350°F. Oil and flour 10-inch tube pan or sides of two 9-inch round pans and line bottoms with wax paper.

2. In large mixing bowl, sift together flour, salt, baking powder, and 1 cup of sugar.

3. Add oil, milk, vanilla, butter flavoring, and almond extract.

4. Mix with electric mixer on low speed 30 seconds, scraping sides of bowl. Beat on high speed 1 minute.

5. In medium bowl, beat egg whites until frothy. Gradually add remaining ¼ cup sugar. Beat at high speed about 4–5 minutes or until stiff peaks form.

6. Gently fold egg whites into batter, about 30–35 strokes.

7. Bake 35–40 minutes in tube pan or 25–30 minutes in round pans.

8. Cool 5 minutes before removing from pan.

Yield: 24 servings

¼₄ of Basic White Cake or Lemon Cake without frosting contains:

Cal	Carb g	Fat g	Sat Fat g	Chol mg	Sod mg	Fib g
112	19	3	0	0	151	0

Exchanges: Not applicable for this recipe

VARIATIONS

Lemon Cake: Substitute 2 teaspoons lemon extract, 2 tablespoons lemon zest or grated lemon peel, and ¼ teaspoon yellow food coloring for flavorings.

Chocolate Cake: Decrease flour to 1¾ cups. Add ½ cup cocoa powder with dry ingredients.

¼₄ of Chocolate Cake with Mexicali Chocolate Frosting (page 325) contains:

Cal	Carb g	Fat g	Sat Fat g	Chol mg	Sod mg	Fib g
171	32	4	1	0	175	1

Buttermilk Cake: Decrease baking powder to 1 teaspoon. Add ½ teaspoon baking soda with dry ingredients. Substitute 1 cup low-fat buttermilk for skim milk.

¼₄ of Buttermilk Cake without frosting contains:

Cal	Carb g	Fat g	Sat Fat g	Chol mg	Sod mg	Fib g
112	19	3	<1	0	142	0

APPLE CINNAMON CHEESECAKE

nonstick cooking spray

3 graham cracker rectangles (4¾ × 2½ inches each), finely crushed, or ½ cup graham cracker crumbs

2 medium apples, peeled, cored, and chopped

1 cup plus 1 tablespoon sugar, divided

1 teaspoon ground cinnamon

8 ounces fat-free cream cheese

8 ounces low-fat cream cheese

8 ounces fat-free sour cream

2 tablespoons cornstarch

½ teaspoon butter extract

1 teaspoon vanilla extract

1. Preheat oven to 350°F.

2. Remove bottom from 9-inch springform pan. Cut square of foil 1 inch larger than bottom of pan. Line pan bottom with foil and reassemble. (Excess foil will hang from bottom of pan. Fold it up and out of the way.) Spray sides and bottom of pan with nonstick spray.

3. Pour crumbs into pan and tilt to cover bottom of pan evenly. Use fingertips to distribute loose crumbs evenly.

4. In small microwave-safe dish, combine apples, 1 tablespoon sugar, and cinnamon. Microwave about 3 minutes or until apples are soft. Cool.

5. In large bowl, combine cream cheeses, sour cream, cornstarch, 1 cup sugar, and extracts. Mix just until smooth; do not overmix.

6. Fold in apple mixture.

7. Pour filling into center of crust and spread evenly over crust. (This keeps loose crumbs from getting into filling.)

8. Bake 1 hour (decrease time if using larger pan). When cooked, top of cheesecake will be firm and brown, but a toothpick inserted into cake will *not* come out clean.

9. Cool 1 hour.

10. Cover cheesecake with plastic wrap. Freeze at least 8 hours or overnight.

11. About 1 hour before serving, take cheesecake out of freezer and immediately remove pan and foil. (Crumbs will stick if allowed to thaw.)

Yield: 12 servings

¹⁄₁₂ of cake contains:

Cal	Carb g	Fat g	Sat Fat g	Chol mg	Sod mg	Fib g
170	28	4	2	13	256	1

Exchanges: Not applicable for this recipe

CHEESECAKE

nonstick cooking spray

3 graham cracker rectangles (4¾ × 2½ inches each), finely crushed, or ½ cup graham cracker crumbs

8 ounces fat-free cream cheese

8 ounces low-fat cream cheese

16 ounces fat-free sour cream, divided

2 tablespoons cornstarch

1 cup sugar

½ teaspoon imitation butter flavoring

1 teaspoon vanilla extract

¼ cup powdered (confectioners') sugar

1. Preheat oven to 350°F.

2. Remove bottom from 9-inch springform pan. Cut a square of foil 1 inch larger than bottom of pan. Line pan bottom with foil and reassemble.

(Excess foil will hang from bottom of pan. Fold it up and out of the way.) Spray sides and bottom of pan with nonstick spray.

3. Pour crumbs into pan and tilt to cover bottom of pan evenly. Use fingertips to distribute loose crumbs evenly.

4. In large bowl, mix together cream cheeses, ½ of sour cream (1 cup), cornstarch, sugar, butter flavoring, and vanilla. Mix just until smooth; do not overmix.

5. Pour filling into center of crust and spread evenly over crust. (This keeps loose crumbs from getting into filling.)

6. Bake 1 hour (decrease time if using larger pan). Top will be firm and brown, but a toothpick inserted into cake will *not* come out clean.

7. Cool 1 hour.

8. Mix together remaining sour cream (1 cup) and powdered sugar; spread over top of cheesecake.

9. Cover cheesecake with plastic wrap. Freeze at least 8 hours or overnight.

10. About 1 hour before serving, take cheesecake out of freezer and immediately remove pan and foil. (Crumbs will stick if allowed to thaw.)

Yield: 12 servings

1⁄12 of cake contains:

Cal	Carb g	Fat g	Sat Fat g	Chol mg	Sod mg	Fib g
173	27	4	2	13	270	0

Exchanges: Not applicable for this recipe

ANGEL FOOD CAKE ROLL

1 box (16 ounces) angel food cake mix

1 package (3.4 ounces) instant pudding and pie filling mix (any flavor)

1¾ cups skim milk

1 tablespoon powdered (confectioners') sugar

1. Line 15½ × 11½ × ¾-inch jelly roll pan or 13 × 9 × 2-inch sheet cake pan with wax paper.

2. Preheat oven according to directions on cake mix box.

3. Prepare cake mix according to directions on box.

4. Pour batter into jelly roll pan and spread evenly until ⅔ filled. If using sheet cake pan, fill to ½ inch thick. Pour any excess into small loaf pan. Bake for about 30–35 minutes if using jelly roll pan. If using only part of cake, bake about 25 minutes.

5. Meanwhile, prepare filling according to package directions for pie filling and using skim milk. Chill in refrigerator until time to spread on cake.

6. Remove cake from oven and allow to cool about 2 minutes. Dust with powdered sugar using a small mesh strainer or a sifter.

7. Lay clean dish towel over cake and, starting at narrow end, roll it up. As you roll, peel off wax paper.

8. Cool cake on rack about 5 minutes before unrolling and removing dish towel. Reroll cake and cool on rack at least 30 minutes.

9. Unroll cake but do not press it flat because it may crack. Spread filling evenly across cake and reroll.

10. Dust outside of cake with powdered sugar. Refrigerate until ready to serve. Cut into ¾-inch slices.

Yield: 12 servings

1⁄12 of roll contains:

Cal	Carb g	Fat g	Sat Fat g	Chol mg	Sod mg	Fib g
192	43	0	0	1	307	0

Exchanges: Not applicable for this recipe

CHOCOLATE CHEESECAKE

nonstick cooking spray

44 chocolate graham cracker animals, finely crushed, or ½ cup crumbs

8 ounces fat-free cream cheese

8 ounces low-fat cream cheese

8 ounces fat-free sour cream

2 tablespoons cornstarch

1⅛ cups sugar

½ teaspoon imitation butter flavoring

1 teaspoon vanilla extract

3 tablespoons cocoa powder

1. Preheat oven to 350°F.

2. Remove bottom from 9-inch springform pan. Cut square of foil 1 inch larger than bottom of pan. Line pan bottom with foil and reassemble. (Excess foil will hang from bottom of pan. Fold it up and out of the way.) Spray sides and bottom of pan with nonstick spray.

3. Pour crumbs into pan and tilt pan to cover bottom of pan evenly. Use fingertips to distribute loose crumbs evenly.

4. In large bowl, mix together cream cheeses, sour cream, cornstarch, sugar, butter flavoring, vanilla, and cocoa. Mix just until smooth; do not overmix.

5. Pour filling into center of crust and spread evenly over crust. (This keeps loose crumbs from getting into filling.)

6. Bake 1 hour or until top is firm (decrease time if using larger pan). A toothpick inserted into cake will *not* come out clean.

7. Cool 1 hour.

8. Cover cheesecake with plastic wrap. Freeze at least 8 hours or overnight.

9. About 1 hour before serving, take cheesecake out of freezer and immediately remove pan and foil. (Crumbs will stick if allowed to thaw.)

Yield: 12 servings

¹⁄₁₂ of cake contains:

Cal	Carb g	Fat g	Sat Fat g	Chol mg	Sod mg	Fib g
164	26	4	2	13	252	1

Exchanges: Not applicable for this recipe

BANANA PUDDING CAKE ROLL

1 box (16 ounces) angel food cake mix

1 package (3.4 ounces) banana instant pudding and pie filling mix

1¾ cups skim milk

1½ tablespoons powdered (confectioners') sugar

2 medium bananas, thinly sliced

1. Line 15½ × 11¼ × ¾-inch jelly roll pan or 13 × 9 × 2-inch sheet cake pan with wax paper.

2. Preheat oven according to directions on cake mix box.

3. Prepare cake mix according to directions on box.

4. Pour batter into jelly roll pan and spread evenly. If using sheet cake pan, fill to ½ inch thick. Pour any excess into small loaf pan. Bake 30–35 minutes or until golden brown if using jelly roll pan. If using only part of cake, bake about 25 minutes.

5. Meanwhile, prepare filling according to package directions for pie filling and using skim milk. Chill in refrigerator until time to spread on cake.

6. Remove cake from oven and allow to cool about 2 minutes. Dust with powdered sugar using a small mesh strainer or a sifter.

7. Lay clean dish towel over cake and, starting at narrow end, roll it up. As you roll, peel off wax paper.

8. Let cake stand about 5 minutes before unrolling and removing dish towel. Reroll cake and cool at least 30 minutes.

9. Unroll cake but do not try to press it flat because it will crack. Spread banana filling evenly over cake. Scatter banana slices over cake. Reroll.

10. Dust outside of cake with powdered sugar. Refrigerate until ready to serve. Cut into ¾-inch slices.

Yield: 12 servings

1/12 of roll contains:

Cal	Carb g	Fat g	Sat Fat g	Chol mg	Sod mg	Fib g
211	47	0	0	1	307	1

Exchanges: Not applicable for this recipe

BLACK FOREST CAKE ROLL

1 box (16 ounces) angel food cake mix

¼ cup cocoa powder

1 package (3.9 ounces) chocolate instant pudding and pie filling mix

1¾ cups skim milk

1 tablespoon powdered (confectioners') sugar

1 can (20 ounces) cherry pie filling

1. Line 15½ × 11½ × ¾-inch jelly roll pan or 13 × 9 × 2-inch sheet cake pan with wax paper.

2. Preheat oven according to directions on cake mix box.

3. Combine dry cake mix and cocoa powder in bowl and continue according to directions on box.

4. Pour batter into jelly roll pan and spread evenly. If using sheet cake pan, fill to ½ inch thick. Pour any excess into small loaf pan. Bake for 30–35 minutes or until golden brown if using jelly roll pan. If using only part of cake, bake about 25 minutes.

5. Meanwhile, prepare chocolate filling according to package directions for pie filling and using skim milk. Chill in refrigerator until time to spread on cake.

6. Remove cake from oven and cool about 2 minutes. Dust with powdered sugar using a small mesh strainer or a sifter.

7. Lay clean dish towel over cake and, starting at narrow end, roll it up. As you roll, peel off wax paper.

8. Let cake stand about 5 minutes before unrolling and removing dish towel. Reroll cake and cool at least 30 minutes.

9. Unroll cake but do not try to press it flat because it will crack.

10. Spread chocolate filling thinly and evenly over cake.

11. Dollop cherry pie filling randomly over cake. Reroll.

12. Dust outside of cake with cocoa powder. Refrigerate until ready to serve. Cut into ¾-inch slices.

Yield: 12 servings

1/12 of roll contains:

Cal	Carb g	Fat g	Sat Fat g	Chol mg	Sod mg	Fib g
239	54	1	0	1	307	2

Exchanges: Not applicable for this recipe

CARROT RAISIN PINEAPPLE CAKE

CAKE

nonstick cooking spray

2 cups sugar

2 cups all-purpose flour

1 teaspoon baking soda

1 teaspoon baking powder

⅛ teaspoon ground nutmeg

1 teaspoon ground cinnamon

¼ cup oil

4 egg whites, slightly beaten

¾ cup sweetened applesauce

¾ cup raisins

1 can (10 ounces) crushed pineapple packed in juice, drained

3 cups grated carrots

GLAZE (OPTIONAL)

3 ounces fat-free cream cheese

1½ cups powdered (confectioners') sugar

1. Preheat oven to 350°F. Spray 10-inch Bundt cake pan with nonstick spray.

2. Mix sugar, flour, soda, baking powder, nutmeg, and cinnamon. Make a well in center of dry ingredients.

3. Add oil, egg whites, and applesauce to well and stir to combine with dry ingredients.

4. Add raisins, pineapple, and carrots and stir gently. Pour into Bundt pan.

5. Bake 60 minutes or until toothpick inserted in center comes out clean.

6. Let cake cool about 10 minutes. Remove cake from pan and cool completely. Add glaze if desired.

7. For glaze, stir cream cheese gently to soften.

8. Gradually add powdered sugar, stirring until smooth. Spread evenly over top of cake.

Yield: 16 servings

1/16 of cake without glaze contains:

Cal	Carb g	Fat g	Sat Fat g	Chol mg	Sod mg	Fib g
239	50	4	<1	0	99	2

Exchanges: Not applicable for this recipe

1/16 of cake with glaze contains:

Cal	Carb g	Fat g	Sat Fat g	Chol mg	Sod mg	Fib g
287	62	4	<1	0	131	2

CRANBERRY BUNDT CAKE

CAKE

¾ cup sugar

¼ cup tub margarine, softened

¼ teaspoon lemon extract

¼ teaspoon ground nutmeg

½ cup egg substitute

2 cups all-purpose flour

1 tablespoon baking powder

½ cup skim milk

2 cups cranberries, chopped

GLAZE (OPTIONAL)

2–3 tablespoons lemon juice

1½ cups powdered (confectioners') sugar

1. Preheat oven to 325°F. Oil and flour Bundt cake pan.

2. Cream sugar, margarine, lemon extract, and nutmeg. Add egg substitute and beat on high with electric mixer 2 minutes.

3. In separate bowl, combine flour and baking powder.

4. By hand, stir ⅓ of flour mixture into margarine mixture; add ½ of milk and stir. Stir in ⅓ of flour mixture and remaining milk. Gently stir in remaining ⅓ of flour.

5. Stir in cranberries.

6. Pour batter into pan and bake about 30 minutes or until toothpick inserted in center comes out clean.

7. Cool in pan 10 minutes before removing. Cool completely on wire rack.

8. To prepare glaze, add small amount of lemon juice to powdered sugar and stir; continue adding lemon juice until desired consistency is reached. Drizzle over cake.

Yield: 14 servings

¼₄ of cake without glaze contains:

Cal	Carb g	Fat g	Sat Fat g	Chol mg	Sod mg	Fib g
150	27	3	1	0	141	1

Exchanges: Not applicable for this recipe

¼₄ of cake with glaze contains:

Cal	Carb g	Fat g	Sat Fat g	Chol mg	Sod mg	Fib g
201	40	3	1	0	142	1

SOUPER RAISIN CAKE

1 can (10¾ ounces) condensed tomato soup, undiluted

1 cup sugar

1½ cups all-purpose flour

1 teaspoon baking soda

½ teaspoon ground cloves

1 teaspoon ground cinnamon

1 cup raisins

½ cup chopped nuts (optional)

1. Preheat oven to 350°F. Oil and flour 9 × 5-inch loaf pan.

2. By hand, combine soup and sugar; thoroughly mix in flour, soda, cloves, and cinnamon.

3. Stir in raisins and nuts if desired. Turn into pan.

4. Bake 45–50 minutes.

Yield: 14 servings

¼₄ of cake without nuts contains:

Cal	Carb g	Fat g	Sat Fat g	Chol mg	Sod mg	Fib g
152	36	<1	0	0	214	1

Exchanges: Not applicable for this recipe

¼₄ of cake with nuts contains:

Cal	Carb g	Fat g	Sat Fat g	Chol mg	Sod mg	Fib g
181	37	3	0	0	214	1

EXCELLENT DOUBLE BOILER FROSTING

2 egg whites (unbeaten)

1½ cups white or light brown sugar

⅓ cup cold water

1 tablespoon light corn syrup or ¼ teaspoon cream of tartar

1 teaspoon vanilla extract

1.   Put all ingredients except vanilla in top part of double boiler and beat thoroughly.

2.   Place over boiling water and beat steadily 7–10 minutes.

3.   Remove from heat; add vanilla and beat until thick enough to spread on cake.

Yield: 16 servings (enough frosting for 2-layer cake)

1 serving contains:

| Cal | Carb | Fat | Sat Fat | Chol | Sod | Fib |
	g	g	g	mg	mg	g
79	20	0	0	0	9	0

Exchanges: Not applicable for this recipe

COCOA FUDGE

3 cups sugar

⅔ cup cocoa powder

⅛ teaspoon salt

⅛ teaspoon cream of tartar

1 can (12 ounces) evaporated skim milk

¼ cup tub margarine

1 teaspoon vanilla extract

¼ cup chopped pecans (optional)

1.   Oil 8 × 8-inch pan.

2.   In large saucepan, combine sugar, cocoa, salt, and cream of tartar; mix thoroughly. Add milk and mix until smooth.

3.   Insert candy thermometer into mixture and bring to a rolling boil over medium heat, stirring constantly.

4.   When mixture reaches rolling boil, reduce heat and stop stirring. Continue cooking without stirring until mixture reaches soft-ball stage (234°F).

5.   When mixture reaches 234°F, turn off heat. Add margarine and vanilla but do not stir.

6.   When mixture cools to approximately 120°F, add nuts and stir until fudge loses its shiny appearance. The warmer the fudge, the longer it will have to be stirred. If fudge cools too much, it may be too stiff to stir; reheat carefully to avoid burning.

7.   Pour fudge into pan to cool.

Yield: 16 servings

1 serving without pecans contains:

| Cal | Carb | Fat | Sat Fat | Chol | Sod | Fib |
	g	g	g	mg	mg	g
196	42	3	1	1	78	1

Exchanges: Not applicable for this recipe

1 serving with pecans contains:

| Cal | Carb | Fat | Sat Fat | Chol | Sod | Fib |
	g	g	g	mg	mg	g
208	42	5	1	1	78	1

MEXICALI CHOCOLATE FROSTING

2 tablespoons cocoa powder

2 tablespoons tub margarine, melted

1½ teaspoons vanilla extract

⅛ teaspoon salt

½ teaspoon ground cinnamon

¼ teaspoon imitation butter flavoring

2½ cups powdered (confectioners') sugar

2–3 tablespoons skim milk

1.   Combine cocoa, margarine, vanilla, salt, cinnamon, and butter flavoring.

2.   Gradually stir in powdered sugar and enough milk to make a good spreading consistency.

Yield: 24 servings

2½ teaspoons contains:

Cal	Carb g	Fat g	Sat Fat g	Chol mg	Sod mg	Fib g
59	13	1	0	0	29	0

Exchanges: Not applicable for this recipe

MOLASSES SPICE COOKIES

nonstick cooking spray

2 cups whole-wheat flour

1 cup oatmeal, uncooked

2 teaspoons ground cinnamon

1 teaspoon ground ginger

⅛ teaspoon ground cloves

1½ teaspoons baking soda

2 tablespoons tub margarine

¼ cup firmly packed brown sugar

⅔ cup molasses

¼ cup egg substitute

¼ cup canned evaporated skim milk

3 tablespoons powdered (confectioners') sugar

1.   Preheat oven to 350°F. Spray cookie sheet lightly with nonstick spray.

2.   In medium bowl, combine flour, oatmeal, cinnamon, ginger, cloves, and soda.

3.   In large bowl, cream margarine and sugar. Add molasses, egg substitute, and milk; mix well.

4.   Add dry ingredients to sugar mixture, stirring only enough to mix. Do *not* overstir or cookies will be tough.

5.   Form dough into balls approximately 1 inch in diameter; roll in powdered sugar and place on cookie sheet about 2 inches apart. Mash slightly to flatten.

6.   Bake 12–13 minutes or until browned on bottom.

Yield: 30 cookies

1 cookie contains:

Cal	Carb g	Fat g	Sat Fat g	Chol mg	Sod mg	Fib g
76	15	1	0	0	59	1

Exchanges: Not applicable for this recipe

BANANA OATMEAL COOKIES

1½ cups all-purpose flour

1 cup sugar

½ teaspoon baking soda

1 teaspoon salt

¼ teaspoon ground nutmeg

¾ teaspoon ground cinnamon

⅓ cup tub margarine

¼ cup egg substitute

1 cup mashed ripe bananas (2 medium)

1¾ cups oatmeal, uncooked

½ cup chopped walnuts

1.   Preheat oven to 400°F.

2.   In large mixing bowl, combine flour, sugar, soda, salt, nutmeg, and cinnamon.

3.   Add margarine, egg substitute, and bananas, beating well.

4.   Mix in oatmeal and walnuts until thoroughly blended.

5.   Drop from teaspoon onto ungreased baking sheet.

6.   Bake 12–13 minutes. Remove from pan immediately.

Yield: 52 cookies

1 cookie contains:

Cal	Carb g	Fat g	Sat Fat g	Chol mg	Sod mg	Fib g
61	10	2	0	0	65	<1

Exchanges: Not applicable for this recipe

CHOCOLATE CHIP COOKIES

½ cup firmly packed brown sugar

¼ cup sugar

¼ cup tub margarine

1½ teaspoons vanilla extract

2 tablespoons egg substitute

½ cup whole-wheat flour

½ cup all-purpose flour

½ teaspoon baking soda

¼ teaspoon salt

½ cup miniature semisweet chocolate chips

1.   Preheat oven to 400°F.

2.   In large bowl, combine sugars, margarine, vanilla, and egg substitute.

3.   Stir flours, soda, and salt into sugar mixture; stir in chocolate chips.

4.   For each cookie, drop about 1 heaping teaspoon of dough onto ungreased nonstick cookie sheet, spacing cookies approximately 2 inches apart.

5.   Bake about 9 minutes or until lightly browned on bottom.

Yield: 30 cookies

1 cookie contains:

Cal	Carb g	Fat g	Sat Fat g	Chol mg	Sod mg	Fib g
62	10	2	1	0	53	1

Exchanges: Not applicable for this recipe

WALNUT CRISPIES

3 egg whites

⅛ teaspoon salt

1 teaspoon vanilla extract

1 cup sugar

½ cup chopped walnuts

1.   Preheat oven to 350°F. Oil baking sheet.

2.   Beat egg whites until stiff.

3.   Add salt and vanilla; gradually add sugar.

4.   Fold in nuts. Drop batter from teaspoon onto baking sheet.

5.   Bake 2–3 minutes.

6.   Turn off oven and leave cookies in oven 1 hour.

Yield: 72 cookies

1 cookie contains:

Cal	Carb g	Fat g	Sat Fat g	Chol mg	Sod mg	Fib g
17	3	<1	0	0	6	0

Exchanges: Not applicable for this recipe

PUMPKIN SPICE BARS

⅓ cup tub margarine

½ cup firmly packed brown sugar

½ cup egg substitute

¾ cup buttermilk

½ cup canned pumpkin

½ cup light molasses

2½ cups all-purpose flour

2 teaspoons orange zest or grated orange peel

1 teaspoon baking soda

½ teaspoon salt

1 teaspoon ground cinnamon

½ teaspoon ground nutmeg

powdered (confectioners') sugar (optional)

1.   Preheat oven to 350°F. Oil and flour 9 × 13-inch baking pan.

2.   In large bowl, cream margarine and brown sugar.

3.   Add egg substitute and beat 5 minutes.

4.   In separate bowl, combine buttermilk, pumpkin, and molasses.

5.   In third bowl, combine remaining ingredients except powdered sugar.

6.   Add liquid mixture and dry mixture alternately to creamed mixture, beating well after each addition. Pour into pan.

7.   Bake 30–35 minutes.

8.   Sprinkle with powdered sugar if desired.

Yield: 24 servings

1 serving contains:

Cal	Carb g	Fat g	Sat Fat g	Chol mg	Sod mg	Fib g
113	20	3	1	0	131	1

Exchanges: Not applicable for this recipe

CHUNKY PEANUT BUTTER COOKIES

nonstick cooking spray

1¼ cups all-purpose flour

1 teaspoon baking soda

2 tablespoons tub margarine

¼ cup firmly packed brown sugar

¼ cup sugar

½ cup crunchy peanut butter, fat reduced by 25%

¾ teaspoon vanilla extract

¼ cup skim milk

1. Preheat oven to 350°F. Spray cookie sheet lightly with nonstick spray.

2. In medium bowl, combine flour and soda.

3. In large bowl, cream margarine with sugars; add peanut butter, vanilla, and milk and mix well.

4. Add dry ingredients to peanut butter mixture, stirring only enough to mix. Do *not* overstir or cookies will be tough.

5. For each cookie, drop about 1 rounded tablespoon of dough onto cookie sheet, spacing cookies approximately 2 inches apart.

6. Bake 12–14 minutes or until lightly browned on the bottom.

Yield: 24 cookies

1 cookie contains:

Cal	Carb g	Fat g	Sat Fat g	Chol mg	Sod mg	Fib g
81	12	3	1	0	51	<1

Exchanges: Not applicable for this recipe

PEPPERMINT PUFFS

nonstick cooking spray

2 egg whites

½ cup sugar

¾ teaspoon peppermint extract

6–8 drops red food coloring

1. Preheat oven to 200°F. Spray cookie sheet with nonstick spray.

2. In large bowl, beat egg whites on high speed until foamy.

3. Gradually add sugar about 1 teaspoon at a time. Continue to beat, scraping bowl occasionally, until mixture holds stiff, glossy peaks.

4. Fold in peppermint extract and food coloring.

5. Drop by rounded teaspoons onto cookie sheet, spacing cookies 1 inch apart.

6. Bake until outside of cookies is dry and set (about 1 hour). Cookies should not turn brown. Let cool on cookie sheet about 5 minutes, then transfer to wire rack and cool completely. Store in airtight container.

Yield: 24 puffs

1 puff contains:

Cal	Carb g	Fat g	Sat Fat g	Chol mg	Sod mg	Fib g
18	4	0	0	0	5	0

Exchanges: Not applicable for this recipe

COCOA NUT BROWNIES

nonstick cooking spray

1 cup all-purpose flour

½ teaspoon baking soda

½ cup cocoa powder

⅓ cup sugar

⅓ cup firmly packed brown sugar

⅓ cup low-fat mayonnaise

⅓ cup egg substitute

2 teaspoons vanilla extract

⅔ cup skim milk

⅓ cup chopped pecans

1. Preheat oven to 350°F. Lightly spray 8 × 8-inch nonstick pan with nonstick spray.

2. In medium mixing bowl, combine flour, soda, and cocoa; set aside.

3. In large mixing bowl, cream sugars and mayonnaise. Add egg substitute, vanilla, and skim milk; mix well.

4. Add dry ingredients to liquid mixture, stirring until smooth; stir in pecans.

5. Pour batter into pan and bake 30–35 minutes or until a toothpick inserted in center comes out clean.

Yield: 16 servings

1 brownie contains:

Cal	Carb g	Fat g	Sat Fat g	Chol mg	Sod mg	Fib g
119	21	4	<1	0	81	1

Exchanges: Not applicable for this recipe

RASPBERRY BARS

½ cup tub margarine

1 cup firmly packed brown sugar

1¾ cups all-purpose flour

1 teaspoon salt

½ teaspoon baking soda

1½ cups oatmeal, uncooked

1 package (12 ounces) frozen unsweetened raspberries, thawed and drained

1. Preheat oven to 400°F. Oil 9 × 13-inch baking pan.

2. Cream margarine and sugar.

3. Mix in flour, salt, and soda; blend well.

4. Stir in oatmeal.

5. Press half of mixture into pan; bake 10 minutes. Cool 10 minutes.

6. Spread raspberries over cooled mixture and sprinkle with remaining oatmeal mixture.

7. Bake 20–25 minutes. Cool 5 minutes before cutting into bars.

Yield: 24 servings

1 serving contains:

Cal	Carb g	Fat g	Sat Fat g	Chol mg	Sod mg	Fib g
128	21	4	1	0	154	1

Exchanges: Not applicable for this recipe

FROZEN PUMPKIN PIE

nonstick cooking spray

24 gingersnaps (2-inch diameter), divided

1 quart vanilla ice milk, softened

⅔ cup canned pumpkin

¼ cup sugar

¾ teaspoon ground cinnamon

⅛ teaspoon ground ginger

¼ teaspoon ground nutmeg

⅛ teaspoon ground cloves

¼ teaspoon salt

1. Remove bottom from 9-inch springform pan. Cut square of foil 1 inch larger than bottom of pan. Line pan bottom with foil and reassemble. (Excess foil will hang from bottom of pan. Fold it up and out of the way.) Spray sides and bottom of pan with nonstick spray.

2. Finely crush 12 gingersnaps. Pour into pan and tilt to cover bottom and sides of pan evenly. Use fingertips to distribute loose crumbs evenly.

3. Combine remaining ingredients; mix well.

4. Pour pumpkin mixture over gingersnap crumbs in springform pan.

5. Cover pie with plastic wrap. Freeze until firm or overnight.

6. About 20 minutes before serving, take pie out of freezer and immediately remove pan and foil. (Crumbs will stick to foil if allowed to thaw.)

7. Transfer to serving dish.

8. Just before serving, cut remaining gingersnaps in half and stand around edge of pie. Serve immediately.

Yield: 12 servings

⅟₁₂ of pie contains:

Cal	Carb g	Fat g	Sat Fat g	Chol mg	Sod mg	Fib g
157	28	4	2	6	178	<1

Exchanges: Not applicable for this recipe

FROZEN RASPBERRY CUPS

8 ounces low-fat raspberry yogurt

½ cup low-fat sour cream

1 cup fresh or frozen unsweetened raspberries (if frozen, thaw and drain)

1 cup banana slices

1 can (11 ounces) mandarin oranges, drained

3 tablespoons chopped pecans

1. Line 8 muffin tins with paper baking cups.

2. In medium bowl, combine yogurt and sour cream until smooth. Gently stir in raspberries, bananas, oranges, and nuts. Pour into baking cups.

3. Freeze until firm.

4. Let stand at room temperature 45 minutes before serving.

Yield: 8 servings

1 serving contains:

Cal	Carb g	Fat g	Sat Fat g	Chol mg	Sod mg	Fib g
102	17	3	1	6	32	1

Exchanges: 1 serving = 1 fruit, 1 fat

FROZEN STRAWBERRY PIE

nonstick cooking spray

66 small chocolate graham cracker animals

1 bag (10 ounces) frozen unsweetened strawberries or 1½ cups fresh strawberries

2 tablespoons sugar

¾ cup strawberry preserves

1 container (15 ounces) part-skim ricotta
cheese

½ cup plain fat-free yogurt

4 fresh strawberries, cut in half

1.   Remove bottom from 9-inch springform pan.
Cut a square of foil 1 inch larger than bottom of
pan. Line pan bottom with foil and reassemble.
(Excess foil will hang from bottom of pan. Fold it
up and out of the way.) Spray sides and bottom of
pan with nonstick spray.

2.   Finely crush chocolate graham crackers to
make ¾ cup. Pour into pan and tilt to cover sides
and bottom of pan evenly. Use fingertips to distribute loose crumbs evenly.

3.   Combine strawberries, sugar, and preserves
in blender or food processor. Cover and process
until smooth.

4.   Add ricotta cheese and yogurt; mix.

5.   Pour over cracker crumbs in pan.

6.   Cover pie with plastic wrap. Freeze at least 8
hours or overnight.

7.   About 20 minutes before serving, take pie
out of freezer and immediately remove pan and
foil. (Crumbs will stick to foil if allowed to thaw.)

8.   Transfer to serving dish.

9.   Just before serving, garnish with strawberry
halves.

Yield: 12 servings

¹⁄₁₂ of pie contains:

Cal	Carb g	Fat g	Sat Fat g	Chol mg	Sod mg	Fib g
139	23	4	2	11	86	1

Exchanges: Not applicable for this recipe

APPLE CRISP

nonstick cooking spray

7 apples, peeled, cored, and sliced

4 teaspoons lemon juice

1 cup firmly packed brown sugar

½ teaspoon ground cinnamon

1 cup oatmeal, uncooked

¼ cup tub margarine

1.   Preheat oven to 400°F. Spray 8 × 8-inch baking dish with nonstick spray.

2.   Layer apples in baking dish and sprinkle with
lemon juice.

3.   In large bowl, combine brown sugar, cinnamon, and oatmeal; cut in margarine with pastry
blender until mixture looks crumbly. Sprinkle
over apples.

4.   Bake 45 minutes or until apples are tender.

Yield: 16 servings

1 serving contains:

Cal	Carb g	Fat g	Sat Fat g	Chol mg	Sod mg	Fib g
129	25	3	1	0	39	2

Exchanges: Not applicable for this recipe

APPLE ORANGE CRUMB

nonstick cooking spray

4 apples, peeled, cored, and sliced

½ cup orange juice

¼ teaspoon ground cinnamon

⅓ cup oatmeal, uncooked

2 tablespoons all-purpose flour

2 tablespoons tub margarine, melted

1.   Preheat oven to 400°F. Spray 9 × 9-inch baking dish with nonstick spray.

2.   Combine apples and orange juice in baking pan.

3.   Mix remaining ingredients until crumbly and sprinkle over apple mixture.

4.   Bake 35–40 minutes or until apples are tender.

Yield: 6 servings

1 serving contains:

Cal	Carb g	Fat g	Sat Fat g	Chol mg	Sod mg	Fib g
119	20	4	1	0	45	2

Exchanges: 1 serving = 1 fruit, 1 fat

SUNSHINE TRIFLE

16 ounces fat-free sour cream

1 teaspoon almond extract

1 can (12 ounces) frozen orange juice concentrate, slightly thawed

½ cup powdered (confectioners') sugar

1 package (3.4 ounces) vanilla instant pudding and pie filling mix

2 cups skim milk

4 kiwifruits

3 star fruits

1 angel food cake

⅓ cup triple sec, divided

1 can (20 ounces) crushed pineapple packed in juice, undrained

1 can (11 ounces) mandarin oranges, drained

1.   In large bowl, whisk together sour cream, almond extract, orange juice concentrate, and powdered sugar. Set aside.

2.   Prepare pudding with skim milk according to package directions. Set aside.

3.   Peel and slice kiwifruits. Cut star fruit into ¾-inch slices. Set aside.

4.   Tear angel food cake into 2-inch pieces. Layer ⅓ of pieces on bottom of glass salad bowl or trifle bowl.

5.   Drizzle ⅓ of triple sec (about 1½ tablespoons) over cake with a spoon.

6.   Spread ⅓ of pudding over angel food cake.

7.   Spread ¼ of pineapple, mandarin oranges, kiwifruit, and star fruit over pudding.

8.   Layer ⅓ of sour cream mixture over fruit.

9.   Repeat layers, ending with fruit. Arrange fruit decoratively on top—pineapple in center and kiwifruits and starfruits alternately around outside of pineapple. Cover with plastic wrap and chill overnight.

Yield: 18 servings

¾ cup contains:

Cal	Carb g	Fat g	Sat Fat g	Chol mg	Sod mg	Fib g
237	52	0	0	1	228	1

Exchanges: Not applicable for this recipe

APPLE CRANBERRY CRISP

nonstick cooking spray

3 cups (about 1 pound) apples, unpeeled, cored and chopped

2 cups fresh or frozen cranberries

¾ cup granulated sugar

1 cup oatmeal, uncooked

½ teaspoon ground cinnamon

1 cup firmly packed brown sugar

¼ cup tub margarine

1. Heat oven to 350°F. Spray 9 × 9 inch baking dish or 9-inch deep-dish pie plate with nonstick spray.

2. In medium bowl, stir together apples, cranberries, and sugar; turn into baking dish. Set aside.

3. In separate bowl, combine oatmeal, cinnamon, and brown sugar; cut in margarine with pastry blender until mixture looks crumbly.

4. Sprinkle over filling.

5. Bake 45 minutes or until topping is browned and filling is bubbling.

Yield: 12 servings

1 serving contains:

Cal	Carb g	Fat g	Sat Fat g	Chol mg	Sod mg	Fib g
201	41	4	1	0	52	2

Exchanges: Not applicable for this recipe

BAKED PEARS

4 pears, peeled, halved, and cored

¾ cup pear nectar

¾ cup water

2 teaspoons lemon juice

1 teaspoon vanilla extract

1 teaspoon rum extract

1 cinnamon stick

¼ teaspoon ground mace

1. Preheat oven to 350°F.

2. Arrange pears in large casserole.

3. Mix remaining ingredients and pour over pears.

4. Cover and bake 30 minutes.

5. Turn pears gently and bake, uncovered, 30 minutes longer or until tender, basting every 10 minutes.

6. Remove from oven, cover, and cool. Baste every few minutes as the pears cool.

Yield: 4 servings

2 pear halves contain:

Cal	Carb g	Fat g	Sat Fat g	Chol mg	Sod mg	Fib g
112	29	0	0	0	8	5

Exchanges: 2 pear halves = 2 fruits

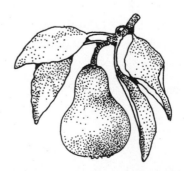

BAKED APPLES

¼ cup firmly packed brown sugar

1 tablespoon tub margarine

2 teaspoons ground cinnamon

4 baking apples, cored

1. Preheat oven to 350°F.

2. Mix brown sugar, margarine, and cinnamon.

3. Place mixture in centers of cored apples.

4. Put apples in casserole and add water to depth of ¼ inch.

5. Cover and bake 30 minutes.

Yield: 4 servings

1 apple contains:

Cal	Carb g	Fat g	Sat Fat g	Chol mg	Sod mg	Fib g
161	35	3	1	0	39	3

Exchanges: Not applicable for this recipe

FRUIT POACHED IN WINE

2 cups red or white wine

¾ cup sugar

sliced peel of ½ fresh lemon

2 tablespoons lemon juice

1 cinnamon stick

4 pieces fresh fruit of choice, such as pears, peaches, or nectarines, peeled and cored

1. Place wine, sugar, lemon peel, lemon juice, and cinnamon stick in saucepan.

2. Stir over medium heat until sugar is dissolved and mixture comes to a boil.

3. Reduce heat and simmer 5 minutes.

4. Add fruit and simmer until tender, occasionally basting with juice. Do not allow liquid to boil.

5. Let sit in juice 20 minutes before serving.

Yield: 4 servings

1 serving contains:

Cal	Carb g	Fat g	Sat Fat g	Chol mg	Sod mg	Fib g
112	29	0	0	0	8	5

Exchanges: Not applicable for this recipe

PINEAPPLE FREEZE

1 can (16 ounces) crushed pineapple packed in juice

1. Open can of pineapple and set in freezer until hard.

2. Hold unopened end of can under hot running water 30 seconds; remove pineapple from can.

3. Place ½ of pineapple in blender or food processor; process until creamy. Repeat with remaining pineapple.

4. Serve immediately.

Yield: 4 servings

1 serving contains:

Cal	Carb g	Fat g	Sat Fat g	Chol mg	Sod mg	Fib g
68	18	0	0	0	1	2

Exchanges: 1 serving = 1 fruit

BERRY CHERRY PIE

1 package (10 ounces) frozen unsweetened raspberries or blackberries, thawed

1 can (16 ounces) pitted red sour cherries

¾ cup sugar

3 tablespoons cornstarch

¼ teaspoon almond extract

4 drops red food coloring

1 recipe Dessert-Type Rice Crust (page 340)

1 recipe Lydia Wyatt's Never-Fail Meringue (page 341)

1. Preheat oven to 350°F.

2. Drain raspberries and cherries, reserving 1¼ cups juice. Set fruit aside.

3. In saucepan, combine sugar and cornstarch; gradually stir in juice.

4. Cook and stir over medium heat until mixture begins to boil; continue cooking and stirring 2 minutes.

5. Remove from heat; stir in almond extract and food coloring.

6. Gently fold in fruit; cool slightly.

7. Pour filling into rice crust and top with meringue.

8. Bake 12–15 minutes or until golden brown.

9. Cool before serving.

Yield: 8 servings

⅛ of pie contains:

Cal	Carb g	Fat g	Sat Fat g	Chol mg	Sod mg	Fib g
237	56	1	0	0	204	2

Exchanges: Not applicable for this recipe

CHERRY PIE

2 cans (16 ounces each) pitted red sour cherries

¾ cup sugar

3 tablespoons cornstarch

1 tablespoon lemon juice

4 drops red food coloring (optional)

1 recipe Dessert-Type Rice Crust (page 340), unbaked

1 recipe Lydia Wyatt's Never-Fail Meringue (page 341)

1. Preheat oven to 350°F.

2. Drain cherries, reserving 1 cup juice. Set cherries and juice aside.

3. In large saucepan, combine sugar and cornstarch; stir in reserved cherry juice.

4. Cook over medium heat, stirring constantly, until mixture comes to a boil; boil 1 minute, stirring constantly.

5. Remove from heat and stir in cherries, lemon juice, and food coloring; cool.

6. Pour cherry mixture into unbaked rice crust.

7. Bake about 25 minutes. Cool.

8. Add meringue and bake 12–15 minutes or until golden brown.

Yield: 8 servings

⅛ of pie contains:

Cal	Carb g	Fat g	Sat Fat g	Chol mg	Sod mg	Fib g
240	56	1	0	0	204	1

Exchanges: Not applicable for this recipe

CREAMY COCOA PIE

2 cups skim milk, divided

¼ cup cocoa powder

¼ cup cornstarch

¾ cup sugar

2 teaspoons oil

1 tablespoon vanilla extract

1 teaspoon imitation butter flavoring

1 recipe Dessert-Type Rice Crust (page 340)

1 recipe Lydia Wyatt's Never-Fail Meringue (page 341)

1. Preheat oven to 350°F.

2. Heat 1½ cups milk in microwave until it boils.

3. In separate bowl, combine cocoa, cornstarch, and sugar; mix well. Add remaining milk (½ cup) to make paste.

4. Stir paste into hot milk; heat in microwave until thick, stirring every minute.

5. Add oil. Set aside to cool.

6. When cooled slightly, add vanilla and butter flavoring.

7. Pour into rice crust and top with meringue.

8. Bake 12–15 minutes or until meringue is golden brown.

Yield: 8 servings

⅛ of pie contains:

Cal	Carb g	Fat g	Sat Fat g	Chol mg	Sod mg	Fib g
243	53	2	<1	1	236	1

Exchanges: Not applicable for this recipe

KEY LIME PIE

1 can (12 ounces) evaporated skim milk

¾ cup sugar

½ cup water

1 package (3 ounces) lime gelatin mix

1 teaspoon lime zest or grated lime peel

½ cup lime juice

¼ cup egg substitute

1 recipe Graham Cracker Crumb Crust (page 339)

1. Heat milk and sugar to boiling, stirring constantly. Set aside to cool.

2. Heat water in small pan until it boils. Remove from heat and add gelatin.

3. Add lime zest or peel and juice. Add egg substitute and milk, stirring constantly.

4. Chill until slightly thickened, stirring occasionally.

5. Pour into graham cracker crust. Refrigerate at least 3 hours. Garnish with lime slices.

Yield: 8 servings

⅛ of pie contains:

Cal	Carb g	Fat g	Sat Fat g	Chol mg	Sod mg	Fib g
231	45	4	1	2	199	0

Exchanges: Not applicable for this recipe

LEMON MERINGUE PIE

¼ cup plus 2 tablespoons cornstarch

1½ cups sugar

¼ teaspoon salt

½ cup fresh lemon juice

½ cup cold water

½ cup egg substitute

1 tablespoon tub margarine

1½ cups boiling water

peel grated from ½ lemon

several drops yellow food coloring (optional)

1 recipe Dessert-Type Rice Crust (page 340)

1 recipe Lydia Wyatt's Never Fail Meringue (page 341)

1. Preheat oven to 350°F.

2. In medium saucepan, thoroughly combine cornstarch, sugar, and salt.

3. Gradually blend in lemon juice and cold water.

4. Stir in egg substitute; add margarine and boiling water.

5. Bring to a boil over medium-high heat, stirring constantly. Reduce heat to medium and boil 1 minute.

6. Remove from heat and stir in lemon peel and food coloring if desired.

7. Pour into rice crust and top with meringue. Bake 12–15 minutes or until golden brown.

8. Cool 2 hours before serving.

Yield: 8 servings

⅛ of pie contains:

Cal	Carb g	Fat g	Sat Fat g	Chol mg	Sod mg	Fib g
306	70	2	0	0	320	0

Exchanges: Not applicable for this recipe

PUMPKIN PIE

½ cup egg substitute

1 can (16 ounces) pumpkin

¾ cup sugar

½ teaspoon salt

1 teaspoon ground cinnamon

½ teaspoon ground ginger

¼ teaspoon ground cloves

1 can (12 ounces) evaporated skim milk

1 9-inch unbaked Margarine Pastry (page 340)

1. Preheat oven to 425°F.

2. Beat egg substitute 5 minutes.

3. Mix in pumpkin, sugar, salt, spices, and milk; pour into pie shell.

4. Bake 15 minutes. Reduce temperature to 350°F and continue baking 45 50 minutes or until knife inserted in center comes out clean.

Yield: 8 servings

⅛ of pie contains:

Cal	Carb g	Fat g	Sat Fat g	Chol mg	Sod mg	Fib g
265	42	8	2	2	448	1

Exchanges: Not applicable for this recipe

PINEAPPLE CREAM PIE

½ cup sugar

2 tablespoons cornstarch

½ teaspoon salt

1 can (20 ounces) crushed pineapple in syrup

1 cup fat-free sour cream

1 tablespoon lemon juice

½ cup egg substitute

1 recipe Dessert-Type Rice Crust, cooled (page 340)

1 recipe Lydia Wyatt's Never-Fail Meringue (page 341)

1.   Preheat oven to 350°F.

2.   In saucepan, combine sugar, cornstarch, and salt. Add pineapple with syrup, sour cream, and lemon juice; mix well. Cook over medium heat, stirring constantly, until mixture thickens and bubbles.

3.   Slowly add egg substitute, stirring constantly; cook 2 minutes longer. Spoon into rice crust.

4.   Spread meringue over pie, sealing to edge of crust.

5.   Bake 12–15 minutes or until peaks of meringue are golden brown. Cool.

Yield: 8 servings

⅛ of pie contains:

Cal	Carb g	Fat g	Sat Fat g	Chol mg	Sod mg	Fib g
233	52	0	0	1	391	1

Exchanges: Not applicable for this recipe

SWIRLED BLUEBERRY PIE

1 can (22 ounces) blueberry pie filling

1 recipe Graham Cracker Crumb Crust (page 339)

4 ounces low-fat cream cheese

2 tablespoons sugar

1 egg white

¼ teaspoon lemon extract

1.   Preheat oven to 300°F.

2.   Pour pie filling into prepared crust.

3.   Beat together cream cheese, sugar, egg white, and lemon extract.

4.   Pour cheese mixture over pie filling in circles; use tip of knife to swirl.

5.   Bake pie 20 minutes.

6.   Cool at room temperature 30 minutes.

7.   Chill in refrigerator at least 3 hours.

Yield: 8 servings

⅛ of pie contains:

Cal	Carb g	Fat g	Sat Fat g	Chol mg	Sod mg	Fib g
313	65	7	3	8	221	1

Exchanges: Not applicable for this recipe

VARIATION

Swirled Cherry Pie: Substitute 1 can (22 ounces) cherry pie filling for blueberry pie filling.

SWIRLED PUMPKIN PIE

8 ounces low-fat cream cheese, softened

½ cup light corn syrup, divided

1 teaspoon vanilla extract

1 recipe Graham Cracker Crumb Crust
   (opposite column)

1 cup canned pumpkin

½ cup egg substitute

½ cup canned evaporated skim milk

¼ cup sugar

1½ teaspoons pumpkin pie spice

¼ teaspoon salt

1. Heat oven to 325°F.

2. In small bowl, beat cream cheese with mixer at medium speed until light and fluffy.

3. Gradually beat in ¼ cup corn syrup and vanilla until smooth.

4. Spread evenly over bottom of pie crust.

5. In same bowl, combine pumpkin, egg substitute, evaporated milk, sugar, pumpkin pie spice, salt, and remaining corn syrup (¼ cup); beat until smooth.

6. Carefully pour pumpkin mixture over cream cheese mixture.

7. With knife or small spatula, swirl mixtures to give marbled effect.

8. Bake 45–50 minutes or until knife inserted halfway between edge and center comes out clean.

9. Cool completely on wire rack. Store in refrigerator.

Yield: 8 servings

⅛ of pie contains:

Cal	Carb g	Fat g	Sat Fat g	Chol mg	Sod mg	Fib g
254	39	9	4	17	403	1

Exchanges: Not applicable for this recipe

GRAHAM CRACKER CRUMB CRUST

1 cup graham cracker crumbs

2 tablespoons tub margarine, melted

2 tablespoons sugar

⅛ teaspoon ground nutmeg

1. Preheat oven to 350°F.

2. Combine all ingredients and mix well.

3. Press into 9-inch pie pan and place in oven 1 minute.

4. Chill in refrigerator until firm.

Yield: 8 servings

⅛ of recipe contains:

Cal	Carb g	Fat g	Sat Fat g	Chol mg	Sod mg	Fib g
78	11	4	1	0	105	0

Exchanges: Not applicable for this recipe

DESSERT-TYPE RICE CRUST

nonstick cooking spray

1½ cups cooked rice, prepared as directed below

2 egg whites (if instant or boil-in-bag rice is used, decrease egg whites to 1)

2 tablespoons sugar

½ teaspoon salt

1 teaspoon vanilla extract

1.   Preheat oven to 375°F. Spray 9-inch pie plate with nonstick spray.

2.   Cook rice according to package directions, but omitting salt and margarine, until very soft (may need to add extra water).

3.   In mixing bowl, mix egg whites, sugar, salt, and vanilla together with whisk.

4.   Add egg mixture to hot rice; stir until rice sticks together.

5.   Place half of rice in pie plate and press against bottom with back of spoon sprayed with nonstick spray. Add remaining rice a little at a time around sides and press with spoon.

FOR CREAM PIE FILLING:

Bake about 20 minutes or until just slightly brown. (To prevent excessive shrinkage of crust, place pie weights or second pie plate sprayed with nonstick spray inside pie crust before baking.) Cool before filling.

FOR FRUIT PIE FILLING:

After adding filling, bake about 20 minutes. Cool and top with meringue.

Yield: 8 servings

⅛ of recipe contains:

Cal	Carb g	Fat g	Sat Fat g	Chol mg	Sod mg	Fib g
57	12	0	0	0	148	0

Exchanges: Not applicable for this recipe

MARGARINE PASTRY

1 cup all-purpose flour

½ teaspoon salt

⅓ cup tub margarine

2–3 tablespoons water

1.   Preheat oven to 425°F.

2.   In mixing bowl, combine flour and salt.

3.   Cut in margarine until mixture has texture of coarse meal.

4.   Sprinkle water over mixture and work in gradually with a fork.

5.   Form dough into ball and chill 10 minutes.

6.   Roll out ball from center to edge until about ⅛ inch thick.

7.   Fit into 9-inch pie pan and flute edges of pastry.

8.   If prebaked shell is needed, prick crust with fork and bake 12–15 minutes.

Yield: 8 servings

⅛ of recipe contains:

Cal	Carb g	Fat g	Sat Fat g	Chol mg	Sod mg	Fib g
124	12	8	2	0	221	1

Exchanges: ⅛ of recipe = 1 starch/bread, 1 fat

LYDIA WYATT'S NEVER-FAIL MERINGUE

½ cup sugar, divided

1 tablespoon cornstarch

½ cup water

3 egg whites

⅛ teaspoon salt

½ teaspoon vanilla extract

1.   Preheat oven to 350°F.

2.   In small saucepan, combine 2 tablespoons sugar and cornstarch.

3.   Add water and cook over medium heat, stirring until thick and clear.

4.   In mixing bowl, beat egg whites with salt and vanilla until soft mounds form.

5.   Add remaining sugar (6 tablespoons) gradually.

6.   Add cornstarch mixture and beat until stiff peaks form.

7.   Spread meringue on pie filling, sealing against pastry.

8.   Bake 12–15 minutes or until peaks are golden brown.

Yield: 8 servings

⅛ of recipe contains:

Cal	Carb g	Fat g	Sat Fat g	Chol mg	Sod mg	Fib g
59	14	0	0	0	55	0

Exchanges: Not applicable for this recipe

BREAD PUDDING

4 cups skim milk

1¼ cups sugar

1 cup egg substitute

1 tablespoon vanilla extract

2 teaspoons ground cinnamon

1 loaf (16 ounces) stale French bread

nonstick cooking spray

1 large baking apple, peeled, cored, and diced

1 cup raisins

1.   In large mixing bowl, combine milk, sugar, egg substitute, vanilla, and cinnamon.

2.   Cut or tear bread into small chunks and add to milk mixture. Let mixture sit 1 hour, stirring twice, so bread becomes soggy.

3.   Preheat oven to 350°F. Spray 9 × 13 × 2-inch baking dish with nonstick spray.

4.   Add apple and raisins to bread mixture and stir gently. Carefully spoon bread mixture into baking pan.

5.   Bake 1 hour or until brown and knife inserted in center comes out clean.

6.   Serve warm and top with warm Whiskey Sauce or Lemon Sauce (page 344 or 343).

Yield: 12 servings

1 serving contains:

Cal	Carb g	Fat g	Sat Fat g	Chol mg	Sod mg	Fib g
273	60	1	0	2	307	2

Exchanges: Not applicable for this recipe

BANANA LEMON PUDDING

5½ ounces vanilla wafers (about 40)

5 medium bananas, cut in ½-inch slices

2 packages (3 ounces each) lemon instant pudding and pie filling mix

3½ cups skim milk

¼ cup lemon juice

¼ cup chopped pecans (optional)

1. Line bottom and sides of 8 × 11-inch glass baking dish with vanilla wafers.

2. Place banana slices over vanilla wafers on bottom of baking dish.

3. In medium mixing bowl, add pudding mix to milk and beat at medium speed 1 minute; add lemon juice and beat until thickened.

4. Pour pudding into baking dish; sprinkle pecans over top of pudding if desired.

5. Chill 2 hours or overnight before serving.

Yield: 12 servings

¾ cup without pecans contains:

Cal	Carb	Fat	Sat Fat	Chol	Sod	Fib
	g	g	g	mg	mg	g
195	39	3	1	6	314	1

Exchanges: Not applicable for this recipe

¾ cup with pecans contains:

Cal	Carb	Fat	Sat Fat	Chol	Sod	Fib
	g	g	g	mg	mg	g
212	39	5	1	6	314	1

OLD-TIME TAPIOCA PUDDING

½ cup egg substitute

⅛ teaspoon salt

2 tablespoons quick-cooking tapioca

⅓ cup sugar, divided

2¼ cups skim milk, divided

1 cup miniature marshmallows

3 egg whites

1 teaspoon vanilla extract

1. In saucepan, combine egg substitute, salt, tapioca, 2½ tablespoons sugar, and ¼ cup milk; blend well.

2. Cook over medium heat, gradually adding remaining milk (2 cups); bring to a gentle boil.

3. Remove from heat; add marshmallows and stir until partially dissolved. Set aside.

4. In mixing bowl, beat egg whites until frothy, gradually adding remaining sugar. Continue beating until stiff.

5. Carefully fold the hot tapioca into beaten egg whites; add vanilla and stir gently.

6. Chill before serving.

Yield: 8 servings

¾ cup contains:

Cal	Carb	Fat	Sat Fat	Chol	Sod	Fib
	g	g	g	mg	mg	g
99	20	0	0	1	122	0

Exchanges: Not applicable for this recipe

RICE PUDDING

nonstick cooking spray

1½ cups skim milk

½ teaspoon imitation butter extract

1 cup egg substitute

⅓ cup sugar

1 teaspoon vanilla extract

1 teaspoon lemon zest or grated lemon peel

½ teaspoon ground cinnamon

¼ teaspoon ground nutmeg

½ cup raisins

2 cups cooked rice, prepared without
   salt or fat

1.   Preheat oven to 325°F. Spray 1½-quart casserole dish with nonstick spray.

2.   In large bowl, mix all ingredients except rice with wire whisk. Stir in rice.

3.   Pour into casserole dish. Bake 15 minutes; stir. Bake about 40 minutes or until knife inserted in center comes out clean.

Yield: 8 servings

½ cup contains:

Cal	Carb g	Fat g	Sat Fat g	Chol mg	Sod mg	Fib g
145	30	0	0	1	87	1

Exchanges: Not applicable for this recipe

LEMON SAUCE

6 tablespoons fresh lemon juice

1 teaspoon lemon zest or finely grated lemon peel

1 cup plus 6 tablespoons water, divided

½ cup sugar

4 teaspoons cornstarch

2 teaspoons vanilla extract

2 drops yellow food coloring (optional)

1.   In medium saucepan, mix lemon juice, lemon zest or peel, 1 cup water, and sugar; bring to a boil.

2.   Dissolve cornstarch in remaining 6 tablespoons water and add to lemon mixture. Add vanilla. Cook 1 minute over high heat, stirring constantly.

3.   Add yellow food coloring for a richer color if desired. Serve warm over Bread Pudding (page 341).

Yield: 12 servings

2 tablespoons contains:

Cal	Carb g	Fat g	Sat Fat g	Chol mg	Sod mg	Fib g
38	10	0	0	0	2	0

Exchanges: Not applicable for this recipe

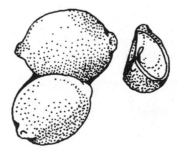

TRADITIONAL MERINGUE

3 egg whites

¼ teaspoon cream of tartar

½ teaspoon vanilla extract

6 tablespoons sugar

1.   Preheat oven to 350°F.

2.   Beat egg whites with cream of tartar and vanilla until soft peaks form. Gradually add sugar while beating until stiff and glossy.

3.   Spread meringue on pie filling, sealing against edge of pastry.

4.   Bake for 12–15 minutes or until peaks are golden brown.

Yield: 8 servings

⅛ of recipe contains:

Cal	Carb g	Fat g	Sat Fat g	Chol mg	Sod mg	Fib g
43	10	0	0	0	27	0

Exchanges: Not applicable for this recipe

PEACHY DESSERT SAUCE

2 cups sliced fresh or frozen peaches or any fresh or frozen fruit

1 tablespoon lemon juice

2 tablespoons sugar

1.   Combine all ingredients in food processor or blender; process until smooth.

2.   Serve chilled or warm over cake or sherbet.

Yield: 7 servings

¼ cup contains:

Cal	Carb g	Fat g	Sat Fat g	Chol mg	Sod mg	Fib g
35	9	0	0	0	0	1

Exchanges: ¼ cup = 1 fruit

VARIATION

Spicy Peachy Dessert Sauce: Add ¼ teaspoon almond extract and ¼ teaspoon ground nutmeg.

WHISKEY SAUCE

5 tablespoons tub margarine

1 cup powdered (confectioners') sugar

½ cup egg substitute

¼ cup whiskey

1.   Stir margarine and powdered sugar together in top of double boiler over simmering water. Heat until sugar is dissolved and mixture is very hot. Remove from heat.

2.   Beat egg substitute well and whisk it into sugar mixture. Remove pan from base of double boiler and continue stirring until sauce has cooled to room temperature.

3.   Add whiskey and serve over warm Bread Pudding (page 341).

Yield: 10 servings

2 tablespoons contains:

Cal	Carb g	Fat g	Sat Fat g	Chol mg	Sod mg	Fib g
116	12	6	1	0	100	0

Exchanges: Not applicable for this recipe

Appendix

Food Groups and Serving Sizes

The food groups are provided for individuals who are interested in

1. Lowering their intake of fat, saturated fat, and cholesterol

2. Keeping their intake of calories, carbohydrate, protein, and fat about the same from day to day

Within each food group three columns are shown: (1) the "choose" column identifies foods that may be selected often; (2) the "serving size" column identifies the amount of each food considered 1 serving; and (3) the "decrease" column identifies foods that are high in fat, saturated fat, or cholesterol and should not be eaten often. For additional information on selection of foods, please see the following sections of this book:

- Chapter 7, page 128, "The Living Heart Guide to Selecting Food in Super-markets"

- Chapter 8, page 152, "The Living Heart Guide to Selecting Food When Eating Out"

- Appendix, page 372, "Nutrient Content of Common Foods"

MEAT, POULTRY, AND FISH

- Choose meat labeled "lean" or "extra lean" that has no more than 3 grams of fat per ounce, or 9 grams of fat per 3 ounces.

- Select beef that is "Choice" or "Select" in grade and trim off any visible fat before cooking the meat.

- Remove skin on chicken before cooking.

- Use cooking methods that require very little or no fat.

- Limit meat, poultry, and fish to 5 to 6 ounces cooked daily.
  Rule of thumb: 3 ounces of meat, poultry, or fish is about the size of a deck of playing cards.

One ounce of cooked meat, poultry, or fish averages:

Cal	Carb g	Fat g	Sat Fat g	Chol mg
60	0	3	1	27

CHOOSE	SERVING SIZE	DECREASE
Lean beef, veal, pork, lamb		Fatty cuts of beef, spare ribs, organ meats, "Prime" beef
Lean ground meat (1 lb raw divided in 4 portions)	3 oz	Regular ground beef
Roast beef slice (3″ × 3″ × ½″)	3 oz	
Chopped cooked meat (½ cup)	3 oz	
Ham slice* (3″ × 3″ × ½″)	3 oz	
Pork chop (½″ thick)	3 oz	
Poultry w/o skin		Poultry w/ skin and fried chicken
1 half of whole chicken breast	3 oz	
Drumstick and thigh	3 oz	
Half of Cornish hen	4 oz	
Fish and shellfish		Fried fish and shellfish
Fillet (3½″ × 3″ × ½″)	3 oz	
Luncheon meat* with no more than 3 g fat per oz	3 oz	Regular luncheon meat, such as bologna, salami, sausage, pepperoni, frankfurters
Meat substitutes (1 serving equals 1 oz meat, poultry, fish)		
Cheese* (no more than 5 g fat per oz)	1 oz	Regular cheese, such as American, blue, Cheddar, Colby, Monterey Jack, Swiss, cream cheese, Neufchâtel cheese
Cottage cheese,* low-fat or fat-free	¼ cup	Cottage cheese, regular
Dried beans and peas,† such as pinto beans, split peas, lentils	½ cup cooked	
Peanut butter	1 tbsp	

*Most varieties are high in sodium.
†Count as 1 oz meat plus 1 serving from bread, cereal, pasta, and starchy vegetable group.
‡Regular canned varieties have salt added.

g = gram; tbsp = tablespoon; tsp = teaspoon.

EGGS

- Limit to 4 egg yolks per week on Step I Diet and to 2 per week on Step II Diet.

- Account for egg yolk used in food preparation (for example, tuna salad, custard, cake).

- Use egg whites as desired (2 egg whites can be substituted for 1 whole egg in most recipes).

One whole egg averages:

Cal	Carb g	Fat g	Sat Fat g	Chol mg
80	1	6	2	213

CHOOSE	SERVING SIZE	DECREASE
Egg yolk (no more than 3 per week)	1 egg	Egg yolk in excess of 3 per week (including egg yolk used in food preparation)
Egg whites	As desired	
Egg substitute,* fat-free, cholesterol-free	As desired	
Egg substitute,* low-fat, cholesterol-free	¼ cup	

*Most varieties are high in sodium.

DAIRY PRODUCTS

- Select 2 to 3 servings of fat-free and low-fat dairy products daily. (They provide at least as much calcium and protein as their high-fat counterparts.)

- Frozen desserts, such as ice milk and frozen yogurt, are in the sweets and alcohol group on page 353.

- Cheese and cottage cheese can be counted as dairy products or as substitutes for meat, poultry, and fish (see page 345).

- Diabetics are usually advised to count cheese and cottage cheese as substitutes for meat because they are low in carbohydrate.

g = gram; tbsp = tablespoon; tsp = teaspoon.

One serving of low-fat dairy products averages:

Cal	Carb g	Fat g	Sat Fat g	Chol mg
90	12	3	2	10

CHOOSE	SERVING SIZE	DECREASE
Milk		
Skim, ½%, or 1%, low-fat buttermilk*	1 cup	Whole milk, 2% low-fat milk
Evaporated skim milk (diluted w/ equal amount of water)	1 cup	Evaporated milk, cream, half-and-half, nondairy creamer, whipping cream
Yogurt, plain, fat-free or low-fat	1 cup	Whole-milk yogurt
Cheese* w/ no more than 5 g fat per oz	1–2 oz or amount equal to about 90 calories	Regular cheese, such as American, blue, Cheddar, Colby, Monterey Jack, Swiss, cream cheese, Neufchâtel cheese
Cottage cheese,* low-fat or fat-free	½ cup	Cottage cheese, regular

Most varieties are high in sodium.

FATS AND OILS

- Meat, poultry, fish, and vegetables prepared away from home usually have fat added during preparation. The following guidelines can be used for estimating the amount:

  Meat, poultry, and fish

Broiled or grilled	2 grams of fat per 3 oz
Pan-fried	2 grams of fat per 3 oz
Breaded and deep-fried	14 grams of fat per 3 oz

  Vegetables

Seasoned with fat	2 grams of fat per ½ cup

- Limit to no more than 6 to 8 servings daily.

g = gram; tbsp = tablespoon; tsp = teaspoon.

One serving of fat or oil averages:

Cal	Carb g	Fat g	Sat Fat g	Chol mg
45	0	5	1	Trace

CHOOSE	SERVING SIZE	DECREASE
Avocado	⅛ medium	
Margarine, regular, diet, tub, squeeze	1–2 tsp or amount equal to about 45 calories	Butter, lard, shortening, bacon fat, stick margarine
Mayonnaise & mayonnaise-type dressing, regular or low-calorie	2 tsp or amount equal to about 45 calories	
Nuts* (chopped) or seeds*	1 tbsp	Coconut, Brazil nuts, macadamia nuts, cashews
Oil, such as safflower, sunflower, corn, soybean, canola, olive, peanut	1 tsp	Coconut oil, palm kernel oil, palm oil
Olives*	10 small or 5 large	
Peanut butter	2 tsp	
Salad dressings,* regular or low-calorie (see page 355 for fat-free)	1 tbsp or amount equal to about 45 calories	Dressings made w/ egg yolk, cheese, sour cream, whole milk

Most varieties are high in sodium.

BREAD, CEREAL, PASTA, AND STARCHY VEGETABLES

- Include daily as a source of complex carbohydrate.

- Include 6 or more servings of bread, cereal, pasta, and starchy vegetables daily.

One serving of bread, cereal, pasta, or starchy vegetables averages:

Cal	Carb g	Fat g	Sat Fat g	Chol mg
80	15	1	Trace	Trace

g = gram; tbsp = tablespoon; tsp = teaspoon.

CHOOSE	SERVING SIZE	DECREASE
Breads		
Bagel	½ of whole	
Biscuit*†	1 small (2½″ diameter)	
Cornbread*†	1 piece (2″ × 2″ × 2″)	
English muffin	½ of whole	
Hamburger or hot dog bun	½ of whole (1 oz)	
Muffin, plain†	1 small	
Pita	½ of whole (6″ diameter)	
Roll, plain	1 small (1 oz)	
White, whole-wheat, rye, pumpernickel	1 slice (1 oz) or 2 slices diet or light	Butter bread, egg bread, croissant
Cereal (unsweetened)		
Cooked	½ cup cooked	
Ready-to-eat*	1 oz	Granola with nuts, sugar, oil
Pancakes*†	2 pancakes (4″ diameter)	
Pasta	½ cup cooked	
Popcorn* (popped without fat)	3 cups popped	Popped in shortening or w/ butter added
Pretzels* & low-fat crackers,* such as animal crackers, graham crackers, soda crackers, bread-sticks, melba toast	Amount equal to about 80 calories	High-fat crackers
Rice	⅓ cup cooked	

(continued)

g = gram; tbsp = tablespoon; tsp = teaspoon.

CHOOSE	SERVING SIZE	DECREASE
Soups* such as chicken or beef noodle, minestrone, tomato, vegetable, cream soups made w/ skim milk	¾–1 cup or amount equal to about 80 calories	Soup containing whole milk, cream, cheese, meat fat, poultry fat, poultry skin
Starchy vegetables		Vegetables fried or prepared w/ butter, bacon, ham hocks, meat fat, cheese, cream sauce
Baked beans‡ (w/o meat)	¼ cup	
Corn†	½ cup	
Dried beans & peas,‡ such as pinto beans, split peas, lentils	⅓ cup cooked	
Peas, green‡	½ cup	
Potato, baked	1 small (3 oz)	
Potato, mashed	½ cup	
Squash, acorn or butternut	1 cup	
Sweet potato or yam‡	⅓ cup	
Tortilla (corn)	1 (6″ diameter)	Flour tortilla
Waffle*†	1 (4½″ square)	

Most varieties are high in sodium.
†*Count as 1 serving from bread, cereal, pasta, and starchy vegetable group plus 1 serving from fat group.*
‡*Regular canned varieties have salt added.*

VEGETABLES

- Vegetables are low in calories except for the starchy vegetables above.

- See page 348 for guidelines on accounting for fat used to season vegetables.

- Include 3 to 5 servings daily.

One serving of vegetables without added fat or sauce averages:

Cal	Carb	Fat	Sat Fat	Chol
	g	g	g	mg
25	5	Trace	Trace	0

g = gram; tbsp = tablespoon; tsp = teaspoon.

CHOOSE	SERVING SIZE	DECREASE
Fresh, frozen, or canned* vegetables w/o added fat or sauce	½ cup cooked or 1 cup raw	Vegetables fried or prepared w/ butter, bacon, ham hocks, meat fat, cheese, cream sauce
Vegetable juice*	½ cup	
Salad greens, such as endive, escarole, lettuce, romaine, spinach	As desired	

Regular canned varieties have salt added.

FRUITS

- Fruits contain only a trace of fat.

- Avocados and olives are listed with fats and oils.

- Include 2 or more servings daily (diabetics should check with their physician or dietitian).

One serving of fruit averages:

Cal	Carb g	Fat g	Sat Fat g	Chol mg
60	15	Trace	Trace	0

CHOOSE	SERVING SIZE	DECREASE
Fresh fruit		Fruit that is fried or prepared w/ butter or cream sauce
Apple, kiwi, nectarine, orange, peach, pear	1 medium	
Banana, grapefruit, mango	½ medium	
Cantaloupe, honeydew melon	1 cup cubes	
Grapes	15 small	
Strawberries (whole), watermelon	1¼ cups	

(continued)

g = gram; tbsp = tablespoon; tsp = teaspoon.

CHOOSE	SERVING SIZE	DECREASE
Canned fruit, unsweetened		
Applesauce, apricots, cherries, fruit cocktail, peaches, pears	½ cup	
Pineapple	⅓ cup	
Fruit juice, unsweetened		
Apple, grapefruit, orange, pineapple	½ cup	
Cranberry, grape, prune	⅓ cup	
Dried fruit		
Dates	2½ medium	
Prunes	3 medium	
Raisins	2 tbsp	

SWEETS AND ALCOHOL

- Sweets and alcoholic beverages may be incorporated in moderate amounts into eating patterns that contain 1,400 calories or more.

- Serving sizes are not listed with this food group because of the wide variation in calories: for example, 1 teaspoon of sugar has 16 calories, 1 serving of the cheesecake on pages 318–19 has 173 calories, and 1 can of beer has 150 calories. The table on page 74 shows the approximate calories (up to 200) that can be incorporated from this food group at various calorie levels.

- Alcohol should be limited to no more than 2 drinks per day (see page 60).

- You can find calories for sweets and alcohol in

  "Nutrient Content of Common Foods," starting on page 372 in the Appendix
  Alcoholic beverages, page 370 in the Appendix
  Recipes in the dessert section, pages 316–44
  Nutrient information on food labels

- Sweets and alcohol are usually limited for individuals with diabetes; check with your physician.

- Examples of sweets that are fat free or low in fat are shown in the following table.

g = gram; tbsp = tablespoon; tsp = teaspoon.

CHOOSE	DECREASE
Beverages such as fruit-flavored drinks, lemonade, fruit punch	Beverages made with cream, whole, or 2% low-fat milk
Cookies, cakes, pies, pudding prepared at home w/ egg whites or egg substitute; skim, ½%, or 1% low-fat milk; oil or margarine	Homemade desserts prepared w/ eggs, whole milk, cream, butter, shortening
Commercial desserts w/ 3 g fat or less per serving, such as gingersnaps, fig & other fruit bar cookies, fat-free cookies, angel food cake	Commercial desserts w/ more than 3 g fat per serving, such as pies, cakes, doughnuts, high-fat cookies, cream pies
Frozen desserts with 3 g fat or less per serving, such as fat-free or low-fat yogurt, ice milk, sherbet, sorbet, fruit ice, fruit juice bars	Ice cream, frozen treats made w/ ice cream
Sweets such as sugar, syrup, honey, jam, candy made w/o fat (candy corn, gumdrops, jelly beans, hard candy), flavored gelatin	Candy made w/ milk chocolate, coconut oil, palm kernel oil, palm oil

FREE FOODS

- Most foods listed below have negligible calories and can be eaten as desired. However, the calories in catsup, picante sauce, fat-free salad dressings, sugar-free jam and jelly, and sugar-free pancake syrup can add up if large amounts are eaten.

- Diabetics should not eat large amounts of catsup, which contains sugar, or sugar-free jam or jelly and sugar-free pancake syrup containing nutritive sweeteners (see page 113).

- Catsup, mustard, and picante sauce can provide too much sodium if eaten in large amounts.

g = gram; tbsp = tablespoon; tsp = teaspoon.

CHOOSE

Beverages & beverage flavorings
  Bitters
  Carbonated drinks (sugar-free), club soda
  Coffee or tea (no sugar or cream)
  Drink mixes & tonic water (sugar-free)

Condiments
  Catsup
  Horseradish
  Mustard
  Picante sauce*
  Pickles, dill (unsweetened)*
  Soy sauce*
  Worcestershire sauce*

Egg whites

Fruits
  Cranberries (sweetened w/ sugar substitute)
  Lemon
  Lime
  Rhubarb (sweetened w/ sugar substitute)

Ingredients
  Cocoa powder (unsweetened)
  Flavoring essence, such as maple, vanilla, butter flavor
  Liquid smoke
  Spices & herbs
  Sugar substitutes†
  Vinegar

Salad dressings,* fat-free

Soups
  Bouillon,* fat-free
  Broth* & consommé,* fat-free

Sweets
  Flavored gelatin, sugar-free
  Jam or jelly, sugar-free
  Pancake syrup, sugar-free

Vegetables (see Vegetables, page 351)

---

*Most varieties are high in sodium.
†Subject to current warnings about sugar substitutes.

g = gram; tbsp = tablespoon; tsp = teaspoon.

Estimating Calorie Needs

This section contains information on two ways to estimate the calories you need each day to maintain your present weight or to lose weight.

METHOD I

To use this method for estimating your calorie needs, keep a food diary of what you actually eat for several days and list the calories in each food. It is important to eat as you usually do or you will not get a true picture of your typical intake. Then add up the calories consumed on all the days and divide the total calories by the number of days to get your average calorie intake.

If you are overweight, you will need to eat fewer calories than the level needed to maintain your desirable weight. It takes a deficit of about 3,500 calories per week to lose 1 pound of body weight per week:

$$500 \text{ calories} \times 7 \text{ days} = 3,500 \text{ calories}$$

To estimate the calories you need to lose 1 pound per week, decrease your daily calorie intake by 500 or increase your calories burned through physical activity each day by 500 (which is a lot of exercise). For most people the best plan is a combination of both decreasing calories from food and increasing calories burned by physical activity.

METHOD II

To use this method, you will need to know your height, frame size, and activity level before using the tables on pages 358–59.

HEIGHT – Measure your height without shoes.

FRAME SIZE – Use one of the following two simple techniques to determine your frame size. The first technique requires no equipment. Place the thumb and index finger of one hand around your other wrist. Be sure your thumb and index finger go around the radius and ulna bones at your wrist (the smallest part, closest to your hand).

- If thumb and index finger *overlap*, you have a *small* frame.
- If thumb and index finger *just touch*, you have a *medium* frame.
- If thumb and index finger *do not meet*, you have a *large* frame.

The second technique for determining frame size is to use a flexible measuring tape to measure around your wrist at the smallest area, nearest your hand. Match your wrist measurement with your height in the following table to get your frame size.

Frame Size Based on Wrist Measurement

Height	Small Frame	Medium Frame	Large Frame
Under 5'3"	Less than 5½"	5½"–5¾"	Greater than 5¾"
5'3"–5'4"	Less than 6"	6"–6¼"	Greater than 6¼"
Over 5'4"	Less than 6¼"	6¼"–6½"	Greater than 6½"

ACTIVITY LEVEL – Consider all your activities for a typical day, including the amount of time you spend resting, walking around your house, sitting at a desk, watching television, and exercising. Many people overestimate their activity level, thereby overestimating the calories they need. Be honest with yourself when choosing the activity level that most closely reflects your predominant lifestyle. For example, very few Americans regularly engage in heavy activity. Use the list below to determine your level of activity.

Activity Level

- Very light activity
  Seated and standing activities, such as working in a laboratory, driving, typing, sewing, ironing, cooking, playing cards, playing a musical instrument

- Light activity
  Walking on a level surface at 2.5–3 mph, garage work, electrical work, restaurant work, carpentry, housecleaning, child care, golf, sailing, table tennis

- Moderate activity
  Walking 3.5–4 mph, weeding, carrying a load, cycling, skiing, tennis, dancing

- Heavy activity
  Walking uphill with a load, heavy manual labor such as digging, climbing, basketball, football, soccer

*Adapted from National Research Council, Recommended Dietary Allowance, 10th ed. National Academy Press, Washington, D.C., 1989.

CALORIE LEVEL – Use your height, frame size, and level of activity with the table either for men (page 358) or women (page 359) to determine the approximate number of calories needed to maintain the "desirable weight" listed in the third column of the table.

Desirable Weights and Calorie Levels for Men

Height Without Shoes*	Frame Size	Desirable Weight (Pounds)	Calorie Level Based on Physical Activity			
			Very Light (Calories)	Light (Calories)	Moderate (Calories)	Heavy (Calories)
5'5"	Small	129 (124–133)	1,700	1,950	2,200	2,600
	Medium	137 (130–143)	1,800	2,050	2,350	2,750
	Large	147 (138–156)	1,900	2,200	2,500	2,950
5'6"	Small	133 (128–137)	1,750	2,000	2,250	2,650
	Medium	141 (134–147)	1,850	2,100	2,400	2,800
	Large	152 (142–161)	2,000	2,300	2,600	3,050
5'7"	Small	137 (132–141)	1,800	2,050	2,350	2,750
	Medium	145 (138–152)	1,900	2,200	2,450	2,900
	Large	157 (147–166)	2,050	2,350	2,650	3,150
5'8"	Small	141 (136–145)	1,850	2,100	2,400	2,850
	Medium	149 (142–156)	1,950	2,250	2,550	3,000
	Large	161 (151–170)	2,100	2,400	2,750	3,200
5'9"	Small	145 (140–150)	1,900	2,200	2,450	2,900
	Medium	153 (146–160)	2,000	2,300	2,600	3,050
	Large	165 (155–174)	2,150	2,500	2,800	3,300
5'10"	Small	149 (144–154)	1,950	2,250	2,550	3,000
	Medium	158 (150–165)	2,050	2,350	2,700	3,150
	Large	169 (159–179)	2,200	2,550	2,850	3,400
5'11"	Small	153 (148–158)	2,000	2,300	2,600	3,050
	Medium	162 (154–170)	2,100	2,450	2,750	3,250
	Large	174 (164–184)	2,250	2,600	2,950	3,500
6'0"	Small	157 (152–162)	2,050	2,350	2,650	3,150
	Medium	167 (158–175)	2,150	2,500	2,850	3,350
	Large	179 (168–189)	2,350	2,700	3,050	3,600
6'1"	Small	162 (156–167)	2,100	2,450	2,750	3,250
	Medium	171 (162–180)	2,200	2,550	2,900	3,400
	Large	184 (173–194)	2,400	2,750	3,150	3,700
6'2"	Small	166 (160–171)	2,150	2,500	2,800	3,300
	Medium	176 (167–185)	2,300	2,650	3,000	3,500
	Large	189 (178–199)	2,450	2,850	3,200	3,800
6'3"	Small	170 (164–175)	2,200	2,550	2,900	3,400
	Medium	181 (172–190)	2,350	2,700	3,100	3,600
	Large	193 (182–204)	2,500	2,900	3,300	3,850

Adapted from 1959 Metropolitan Life Insurance Company, New York City. These tables are based on 1959 rather than 1983 Metropolitan Life Insurance Company height–weight tables because the earlier tables specify lower weights, more appropriate to health-related concerns.
*Table adjusted for measurement of height without shoes.

Desirable Weights and Calorie Levels for Women

Height Without Shoes*	Frame Size	Desirable Weight (Pounds)	Calorie Level Based on Physical Activity			
			Very Light (Calories)	Light (Calories)	Moderate (Calories)	Heavy (Calories)
5'0"	Small	106 (102–110)	1,400	1,600	1,800	2,100
	Medium	113 (107–119)	1,450	1,700	1,900	2,250
	Large	123 (115–131)	1,600	1,850	2,100	2,450
5'1"	Small	109 (105–113)	1,400	1,650	1,850	2,200
	Medium	116 (110–122)	1,500	1,750	1,950	2,300
	Large	126 (118–134)	1,650	1,900	2,150	2,500
5'2"	Small	112 (108–116)	1,450	1,700	1,900	2,250
	Medium	119 (113–126)	1,550	1,800	2,000	2,400
	Large	129 (121–138)	1,700	1,950	2,200	2,600
5'3"	Small	115 (111–119)	1,500	1,750	1,950	2,300
	Medium	123 (116–130)	1,600	1,850	2,100	2,450
	Large	133 (125–142)	1,750	2,000	2,250	2,650
5'4"	Small	118 (114–123)	1,550	1,750	2,000	2,350
	Medium	127 (120–135)	1,650	1,900	2,150	2,550
	Large	137 (129–146)	1,800	2,050	2,350	2,750
5'5"	Small	122 (118–127)	1,600	1,850	2,050	2,450
	Medium	131 (124–139)	1,700	1,950	2,250	2,600
	Large	141 (133–150)	1,850	2,100	2,400	2,800
5'6"	Small	126 (122–131)	1,650	1,900	2,150	2,500
	Medium	135 (128–143)	1,750	2,050	2,300	2,700
	Large	145 (137–154)	1,900	2,200	2,450	2,900
5'7"	Small	130 (126–135)	1,700	1,950	2,200	2,600
	Medium	139 (132–147)	1,800	2,100	2,350	2,800
	Large	149 (141–158)	1,950	2,250	2,550	3,000
5'8"	Small	135 (130–140)	1,750	2,050	2,300	2,700
	Medium	143 (136–151)	1,850	2,150	2,450	2,850
	Large	154 (145–163)	2,000	2,300	2,600	3,100
5'9"	Small	139 (134–144)	1,800	2,100	2,350	2,800
	Medium	147 (140–155)	1,900	2,200	2,500	2,950
	Large	158 (149–168)	2,050	2,350	2,700	3,150
5'10"	Small	143 (138–148)	1,850	2,150	2,450	2,850
	Medium	151 (144–159)	1,950	2,250	2,550	3,000
	Large	163 (153–173)	2,100	2,450	2,750	3,250

Adapted from 1959 Metropolitan Life Insurance Company, New York City. These tables are based on 1959 rather than 1983 Metropolitan Life Insurance Company height–weight tables because the earlier tables specify lower weights, more appropriate to health-related concerns.
*Table adjusted for measurement of height without shoes.

Name _____

Date _____

MEDFICTS: Dietary Assessment Questionnaire

(Meats, Eggs, Dairy, Frying foods, In baked goods, Convenience foods, Table fats, Snacks)

Directions: For each food category for both Group 1 and Group 2 listings: Please check a box in the "Weekly Consumption" column and in the "Serving Size" column. If patient rarely or never eats the food listed, please check only the "Weekly Consumption" box.

FOOD CATEGORY	WEEKLY CONSUMPTION			SERVING SIZE			SCORE
	Rarely/ Never	Less often 3 or less serv/wk	Frequently 4 or more serv/wk	Small	Average	Large	For office use

M Meats

- Recommended amount per day: ≤ 6 oz (equal in size to 2 decks of playing cards).
- Base estimate on foods consumed most often
- Beef and Lamb selections are trimmed to 1/8" fat

per day
<6oz 6 oz >6 oz

Group 1 10 grams or more total fat in 3 oz. cooked portion

Beef	Processed meats	Other Meat, Poultry, Seafood
Ground Beef	1/4 lb. Burger or Larger	Porkchops (Center Loin)
Ribs	Sandwich	Pork Roast (Blade Boston, Sirloin)
Steak (T-bone, Flank	Bacon	Pork Spareribs
Porterhouse, Tenderloin)	Lunchmeat	Ground Pork
Chuck Blade Roast	(Bologna, Salami)	Lamb Chops (Arm, Blade)
Brisket	Sausage/Knockwurst	Lamb (Rib)
Meatloaf (w/ground beef)	Hot Dogs	Organ Meats*
Corned Beef	Ham (Bone-end)	Chicken w/skin (Leg, Thigh, Wing)
	Ground Turkey	Eel, Mackarel, Pompano

Weekly Consumption: Less often 3 pts / Frequently 7 pts
Serving Size: X 1 pt / 2 pts / 3 pts =

< = less than
> = greater than
≤ = equal to or less than
≥ = equal to or greater than

Group 2 Less than 10 g total fat in 3 oz. cooked portion

Lean Beef Cuts	Low-fat Processed Meats	Other Meat, Poultry, Seafood
Round Steak (Eye of Round, Top)	Low-fat Lunchmeat	Chicken, Turkey (without skin§)
Sirloin**	Canadian Bacon	Most Seafood*
Tip & Bottom Round**	"Lean" Fast-food	Lamb (Leg-shank)
Arm Pot Roast**	Sandwich	Pork Tenderloin
Top Loin**	Boneless Ham	Pork Sirloin, Top Loin (Boneless)
		Veal Cutlets, Sirloin, Shoulder,
		Ground Veal
		Venison
		Veal Chops and Ribs**
		Lamb (whole leg, loin, fore-shank sirloin)**

†
6 pts =

E Eggs
- Weekly consumption is expressed as times/week

Check the number of eggs eaten each time
≤1   2   ≥3

Group 1
Whole eggs, Yolks
Less often 3 pts / Frequently 7 pts
X 1 pt / 2 pts / 3 pts =

Group 2
- Egg whites, Egg substitutes (1/2 cup = 2 eggs)

D Dairy

Milk • Average serving: 1 cup
Group 1
Whole milk, 2% Milk, 2% Buttermilk, Yogurt (whole milk)
3 pts / 7 pts
X 1 pt / 2 pts / 3 pts =
Group 2
Skim milk, 1% Milk, Skim milk-buttermilk, Yogurt (nonfat & lowfat)

Cheese • Average serving: 1 oz.
Group 1
Cream cheese, Cheddar, Monterey Jack, Colby, Swiss, American processed, Blue cheese
Regular cottage cheese (1/2 cup) and Ricotta (1/4 cup)
3 pts / 7 pts
X 1 pt / 2 pts / 3 pts =

Group 2
Low fat & fat free cheeses, Skim milk mozzarella, String cheese
Low fat, skim milk & fat free cottage cheese (1/2 cup) and Ricotta (1/4 C)

Frozen Desserts • Average serving: 1/2 cup
Group 1
Ice cream, Milk shakes
3 pts / 7 pts
X 1 pt / 2 pts / 3 pts =
Group 2
Ice milk, Frozen yogurt

*Organ meats, shrimp, abalone, and squid are low in fat but high in cholesterol.   §All parts not listed in Group 1 have <10 g total fat.
Only lean cuts with all visible fat trimmed. If not trimmed of all visible fat, score as if in Group 1.   †Score 6 points if this box is checked. **Total _____

Comments: _____

MEDFICTS

FOOD CATEGORY	WEEKLY CONSUMPTION			SERVING SIZE			SCORE
	Rarely/ Never	Less often 3 or less serv/wk	Frequently 4 or more serv/wk	Small	Average	Large	For office use

F Frying Foods • Average serving: see below
This section refers to method of preparation, for vegetables and meat

Group 1
French fries, Fried vegetables: (1/2 cup)
Fried chicken, Fish, and Meat: (3 oz.)
☐ | 3 pts | 7 pts | X 1 pt | 2 pts | 3 pts = ____

Group 2
Vegetables,- not deep fried: (1/2 cup)
Meat, Poultry, and Fish - prepared by baking, broiling, grilling,
poaching, roasting, stewing: (3 oz)
☐ ☐ ☐ ☐ ☐ ☐

I In Baked Goods • Average serving: 1 serving

Group 1
Doughnuts, Biscuits, Butter rolls, Muffins, Croissants,
Sweet rolls, Danish, Cakes, Pies, Coffee cakes, Cookies
☐ | 3 pts | 7 pts | X 1 pt | 2 pts | 3 pts = ____

Group 2
Fruit bars, Low fat cookies/Cakes/Pastries, Angel food cake,
Homemade baked goods with vegetable oils, Breads, Bagels
☐ ☐ ☐ ☐ ☐ ☐

C Convenience Foods • Average serving: See below

Group 1
Canned, Packaged, or Frozen dinners; e.g., Pizza (1 slice), Macaroni & cheese
(about 1 cup), Pot pie (1), Cream soups (1cup)
Potato, rice, & pasta dishes with cream/cheese sauces (1/2 cup)
☐ | 3 pts | 7 pts | X 1 pt | 2 pts | 3 pts = ____

Group 2
Diet/Reduced calorie or reduced fat dinners (1 dinner), Potato, rice, & pasta
dishes without cream/cheese (1/2 cup)
☐ ☐ ☐ ☐ ☐ ☐

T Table Fats • Average serving: 1 tablespoon

Group 1
Butter, Stick margarine; Regular salad dressing; Mayonnaise
Sour cream (2 tbsp)
☐ | 3 pts | 7 pts | X 1 pt | 2 pts | 3 pts = ____

Group 2
Diet and tub margarine; Low fat & fat free salad dressings
Lowfat & fat free mayonnaise
☐ ☐ ☐ ☐ ☐ ☐

S Snacks • Average serving: See below

Group 1
Chips (potato, corn, taco), Cheese puffs, Snack mix, Nuts. (1 oz)
Regular crackers: (1/2 oz)
Candy (milk chocolate, caramel, coconut): (about 1.5 oz)
Regular popcorn: (3 cups)
☐ | 3 pts | 7 pts | X 1 pt | 2 pts | 3 pts = ____

Group 2
Pretzels, Fat free chips: (1 oz)
Low fat crackers: (1/2 oz)
Fruit, Fruit rolls, Licorice, Hard candy: (1 med. piece)
Bread sticks: (1-2 pc)
Air-popped or low fat popcorn: (3 cups)
☐ ☐ ☐ ☐ ☐ ☐

Directions for scoring:
Multiply Weekly Consumption points (3 or 7) by Serving
Size points (1, 2, or 3) for Group 1 foods only except for
a large serving of Group 2 meats
Example:
3 pts 7 pts ✓   1 pt 2 pts 3 pts ✓
7 x 3 = 21 points
Add score on page 1 and page 2 to get Final Score

Key
≥70 - Need to make dietary changes
40 to 70 - Step I Diet
less than 40 - Step II Diet

☐ = Foods high in fat, saturated fat,
and/or cholesterol

Total ____

Score from page 1 + ____

Final Score ____

Comments: _____
(Note frequent use of foods high in fat or saturated fat, e.g. coffee creamer, whipped topping, cream/cheese based sauces)

RECIPE SUBSTITUTIONS TO LOWER FAT AND/OR CHOLESTEROL*

Instead of Using	Try Substituting
Bacon	Canadian bacon or lean ham
Baking chocolate (1 square)	Cocoa powder (3 tbsp) plus tub margarine (1 tbsp) or oil (1 tsp)
Butter	Tub margarine
Cheese, regular	Low-fat or reduced-fat cheese (3–5 g or less fat per oz)
Coconut	Coconut extract (texture of finished product will be different)
Cottage cheese, regular	Fat-free or low-fat cottage cheese
Cream—whipping cream or half-and-half	Canned evaporated skim milk (can be whipped)
Cream cheese	Reduced-fat or fat-free cream cheese
Eggs, whole	Egg whites (2 equal 1 whole egg) or egg substitute
Fudge sauce	Chocolate syrup
Ground beef or hamburger meat	Extra lean ground beef or turkey (10% or less fat)
Margarine, tub	Reduced amount of tub margarine or equal amount of a reduced-fat margarine or spread may be suitable for some recipes
Milk, evaporated	Canned evaporated skim milk
Milk, whole or 2%	Skim, ½%, or 1% low-fat milk or canned evaporated skim milk
Nuts	Reduce amount in recipe by ½ to ⅓
Oil	Can reduce amount by ¼ to ⅓ in many recipes; may substitute equal amount of applesauce in some quick-bread or muffin recipes
Shortening or lard (½ cup)	Tub margarine (½ cup) or oil (⅓ cup)
Sour cream	Low-fat or fat-free sour cream or plain, fat-free yogurt
Tuna, oil-pack	Tuna, water pack

A similar table that can be used to reduce sodium is on page 99.

tbsp = tablespoon; tsp = teaspoon.

SUBSTITUTES FOR MISSING INGREDIENTS

When You Don't Have	You Can Substitute
Baking powder, double-acting (1 tsp)	Baking soda ($\frac{1}{4}$ tsp) plus cream of tartar ($\frac{1}{2}$ tsp)
Cornstarch, for thickening (1 tbsp)	Flour, all-purpose (2 tbsp) or arrowroot (2 tsp)
Flour, all-purpose, for thickening (1 tbsp)	Cornstarch ($1\frac{1}{2}$ tsp) or arrowroot (2 tsp)
Garlic, fresh (1 clove)	Garlic powder ($\frac{1}{8}$ tsp)
Ginger, fresh, finely chopped (1 tbsp)	Ginger, ground ($\frac{1}{8}$ tsp)
Herbs, fresh (1 tbsp)	Herbs, dried ($1\frac{1}{2}$ tsp)
Onion, whole (1 medium) or chopped ($\frac{2}{3}$ cup)	Onion, instant, minced (1 tbsp) plus 2 tbsp water
Sugar, confectioners' (1 cup)	Granulated sugar ($\frac{1}{2}$ cup plus 1 tbsp)
Sugar, granulated (1 cup)	Powdered (confectioners') sugar ($1\frac{3}{4}$ cups) or light brown sugar (1 cup packed)
Lemon juice (2 tsp)	Vinegar (1 tsp)

tbsp = tablespoon; tsp = teaspoon.

Weights and Approximate Volumes of Selected Foods

BAKING INGREDIENTS
Flour, all-purpose: 1 pound = $3\frac{2}{3}$ cups
Flour, cake: 1 pound = $4\frac{1}{4}$ cups
Flour, whole-wheat: 1 pound = $3\frac{3}{4}$ cups
Sugar, granulated: 1 pound = $2\frac{1}{4}$ cups
Sugar, light brown: 1 pound = 2 cups

CEREALS
Corn grits: $1\frac{1}{2}$ ounces uncooked = $4\frac{1}{2}$ tablespoons uncooked = 1 cup plus $2\frac{1}{2}$ tablespoons cooked
Oat bran: $1\frac{1}{2}$ ounces uncooked = 7 tablespoons uncooked = 1 cup plus $2\frac{1}{2}$ tablespoons cooked
Oatmeal: $1\frac{1}{2}$ ounces uncooked = $\frac{1}{2}$ cup uncooked = $1\frac{1}{8}$ cups cooked

tbsp = tablespoon; tsp = teaspoon.

CHEESE

Cheese, low-fat: 1 pound = 4 cups grated
Cottage cheese, low-fat: 1 pound = 2 cups
Creamed cheese, low-fat: 1 ounce = 2 tablespoons

DRIED BEANS, PEAS, AND LENTILS

Kidney beans: 1 pound uncooked = 6 cups cooked
Lentils: 1 pound uncooked = $6\frac{2}{3}$ cups cooked
Lima beans: 1 pound uncooked = $5\frac{3}{4}$ cups plus 2 tablespoons cooked
Navy beans: 1 pound uncooked = $5\frac{3}{4}$ cups cooked
Split peas: 1 pound uncooked = $6\frac{2}{3}$ cups cooked

EGGS

Egg, white: 1 = 2 tablespoons
Egg, whole: 1 = 3 tablespoons

FRUITS

Apples: 1 pound = 3 medium = $3\frac{1}{2}$ cups peeled slices
Apricots, dried: 1 pound = $3\frac{1}{2}$ cups uncooked = $5\frac{1}{4}$ cups cooked
Apricots, fresh: 1 pound = 12 uncooked = $2\frac{3}{4}$ cups uncooked = 3 cups cooked
Avocado: 1 pound = 2 medium
Bananas: 1 pound = 3 medium = 2 cups slices
Berries: 1 pint = 2 cups
Cranberries: 1 pound = $4\frac{3}{4}$ cups uncooked = $1\frac{2}{3}$ cups cooked
Grapefruit: 1 pound = $\frac{3}{4}$ medium = 1 cup sections
Grapes, seedless: 1 pound = $2\frac{3}{4}$ cups
Lemon: 1 large = $\frac{1}{4}$ cup juice and 1 tablespoon grated rind or zest
Lime: 1 medium = $1\frac{1}{2}$ tablespoons juice and 1 teaspoon grated rind or zest
Oranges: 1 pound = $2\frac{1}{2}$ medium; 1 medium = $\frac{1}{3}$ cup juice and 3 tablespoons grated rind or zest
Peaches: 1 pound = 4 medium = 2 cups slices
Pears: 1 pound = $2\frac{1}{2}$ medium = $2\frac{1}{2}$ cups slices
Pineapple: 1 pound = $1\frac{1}{2}$ cups diced
Prunes, dried, pitted: 1 pound = $2\frac{1}{2}$ cups uncooked = $2\frac{3}{4}$ cups cooked
Raisins: 1 pound = 3 cups
Strawberries: 1 pound = $2\frac{3}{4}$ cups plus 2 tablespoons

MEAT, POULTRY, AND FISH

Chicken (broiler): 1 = 1 pound $1\frac{1}{2}$ ounces cooked meat = $3\frac{1}{2}$ cups cooked meat
Chicken breast: 1 (2 halves) = 7 ounces cooked meat
Fish: 1 pound uncooked = 11 ounces cooked = $2\frac{1}{3}$ cups pieces, cooked
Meat, ground, lean: 1 pound uncooked = 12 ounces cooked

PASTA

Macaroni: 1 pound uncooked = $3\frac{1}{2}$ cups uncooked = 9 cups cooked
Noodles: 1 pound uncooked = $10\frac{3}{4}$ cups uncooked = $7\frac{1}{4}$ cups plus 2 tablespoons cooked
Spaghetti: 1 pound uncooked = 9 cups plus 2 tablespoons cooked

RICE

Brown rice: 2 ounces uncooked = $\frac{1}{3}$ cup uncooked = 1 cup cooked
White rice, instant: 2 ounces uncooked = $\frac{1}{3}$ cup uncooked = 1 cup plus 3 tablespoons cooked
White rice, regular: 2 ounces uncooked = $\frac{1}{2}$ cup plus $1\frac{1}{2}$ tablespoons uncooked = 1 cup plus $1\frac{1}{2}$ tablespoons cooked

VEGETABLES, FRESH

Asparagus: 1 pound = 15 medium spears = $1\frac{3}{4}$ cups cooked
Beans, green or snap: 1 pound uncooked = 3 cups cooked
Broccoli: 1 pound uncooked = $1\frac{1}{2}$ cups chopped, cooked
Cabbage: 1 pound = 5 cups plus 3 tablespoons shredded, uncooked = $2\frac{3}{4}$ cups shredded, cooked
Carrots: 1 pound = $5\frac{1}{2}$ medium = $3\frac{2}{3}$ cups shredded, uncooked = $2\frac{1}{2}$ cups slices, cooked
Cauliflower: 1 pound = $2\frac{1}{2}$ cups uncooked = $1\frac{1}{3}$ cups pieces, cooked
Celery: 1 pound = $2\frac{3}{4}$ cups diced, uncooked = 2 cups cooked
Eggplant: 1 pound = $4\frac{1}{2}$ cups cubed, uncooked = $3\frac{1}{2}$ cups cubed, cooked
Mushrooms: 1 pound = $6\frac{1}{4}$ cups uncooked = $2\frac{2}{3}$ cups pieces, cooked
Onions: 1 pound = $2\frac{1}{2}$ cups chopped, uncooked = $1\frac{2}{3}$ cups chopped, cooked
Peppers, bell: 1 pound = 5 medium = $3\frac{3}{4}$ cups chopped, uncooked or cooked
Potatoes: 1 pound = 3 medium = $2\frac{3}{4}$ cups plus 2 tablespoons cooked
Spinach: 1 pound = 6 cups chopped, uncooked = $1\frac{3}{4}$ cups cooked
Squash, summer: 1 pound = $3\frac{1}{3}$ cups slices, uncooked = 2 cups slices, cooked
Squash, winter: 1 pound = $3\frac{1}{4}$ cups uncooked = $1\frac{2}{3}$ cups cubes, cooked
Sweet potatoes: 1 pound = 3 medium = $1\frac{1}{4}$ cups mashed, cooked
Tomatoes: 1 pound = $3\frac{1}{2}$ medium = $2\frac{1}{4}$ cups chopped = $1\frac{1}{3}$ cups cooked

Conversion Tables

VOLUME

1 teaspoon = $\frac{1}{3}$ tablespoon = $\frac{1}{6}$ fluid ounce = 5 milliliters
1 tablespoon = 3 teaspoons = $\frac{1}{2}$ fluid ounce = 15 milliliters
4 tablespoons = $\frac{1}{4}$ cup = 2 fluid ounces = 60 milliliters
16 tablespoons = 48 teaspoons = 1 cup = 8 fluid ounces = 240 milliliters
1 cup = $\frac{1}{2}$ pint = $\frac{1}{4}$ quart = $\frac{1}{16}$ gallon
2 pints = 1 quart = 32 fluid ounces = 960 milliliters or 0.96 liter
1 quart = 4 cups = 32 fluid ounces = 960 milliliters or 0.96 liter
4 quarts = 1 gallon = 128 fluid ounces = 3,840 milliliters or 3.8 liters
1 liter = 33.3 fluid ounces = 1.057 quarts = 0.264 gallon

WEIGHT

1 ounce = 0.06 pound = 30 grams
16 ounces = 1 pound = 453.59 grams
1 pound = 0.45 kilogram
1 gram = 0.035 ounce
1 kilogram= 2.21 pounds
1,000 grams = 1 kilogram

VOLUME AND WEIGHT

2 tablespoons = 1 ounce = $\frac{1}{8}$ cup = 30 grams
4 tablespoons = 2 ounces = $\frac{1}{4}$ cup = 60 grams
16 tablespoons = 8 ounces = 1 cup = 240 grams

FOOD ENERGY

1 kilojoule = 4.184 kilocalories (calories)
1 kilocalorie = 0.239 kilojoule

CONVERTING BLOOD CHOLESTEROL AND TRIGLYCERIDE VALUES TO MG/DL OR MMOL/L

To convert values in mmol/L to mg/dL, the following formulas can be used:
Cholesterol: mmol/L × 38.7 = mg/dL*
Triglyceride: mmol/L × 88.6 = mg/dL

To convert values in mg/dL to mmol/L the following formula can be used:
Cholesterol: mg/dL ÷ 38.7 = mmol/L*
Triglyceride: mg/dL ÷ 88.6 = mmol/L

mmol/L = millimoles per liter; mg/dL = milligrams per deciliter.
*Formula can be used for total cholesterol, LDL-cholesterol, and HDL-cholesterol.

CORRESPONDING LEVELS FOR CHOLESTEROL AND TRIGLYCERIDE IN MG/DL AND MMOL/L

Cholesterol		Triglyceride	
mg/dL	mmol/L	mg/dL	mmol/L
35	0.9	100	1.1
60	1.6	150	1.7
100	2.6	200	2.3
130	3.4	300	3.4
160	4.1	400	4.5
190	4.9	1,000	11.3
200	5.2		
220	5.7		
240	6.2		
300	7.8		

mmol/L = millimoles per liter; mg/dL = milligrams per deciliter.

Fat Replacers and Sweetening Agents

TYPES AND USES OF SELECTED FAT REPLACERS

Type	Calories per Gram	Common Uses in Food
Carbohydrate-based		
Cellulose (Avicel cellulose gel)	None	Replace some or all fat in dairy-type products, sauces, frozen desserts, & salad dressings
Dextrins (N-Oil)	4	Replace some or all fat in salad dressings, puddings, spreads, frozen desserts, & dairy-type products
Gums (Splendid)*	None	Replace fat in fat-free salad dressings, & reduce fat in desserts and processed meats

Brand names appear in parentheses.
*Gums include xanthan gum, locust bean gum, gum arabic, pectin, and carrageenan.

TYPES AND USES OF SELECTED FAT REPLACERS (cont.)

Type	Calories per Gram	Common Uses in Food
Carbohydrate-based, *continued*		
Maltodextrins (Lycadex, Paselli SA2, STAR-DRI, and Oatrim)	4	Replace fat in baked goods, dairy-type products, salad dressings, spreads, sauces, frostings and fillings, frozen desserts, and processed meat
Modified food starch (STA-SLIM, Stellar, N-Lite, and LEANesse)	1–4	Replace fat in processed meats, salad dressings, baked goods, fillings and frostings, sauces, dairy-type products, condiments, and frozen desserts
Polydextrose (Litesse)	1	Replace fat in baked goods, chewing gums, confections, salad dressings, frozen dairy desserts, gelatins, and puddings
Protein-based		
Microparticulated protein (Simplesse)	1–2	Replace fat in dairy-type products, salad dressings, margarine, mayonnaise-type products, baked goods, soups, and sauces
Others (Lita, Trailblazer, ULTRA-BAKE, and ULTRA-FREEZE)	NA	Reduce fat in frozen desserts and baked goods
Fat-based		
Caprenin	5	Reduce fat in candy and sweet coatings
Emulsifiers (Dur-Lo, EC-25, and Veri-Lo)	9	Replace some or all fat in cake mixes, cookies, icings, and vegetable-based dairy-type products
Lipid Analogues (DDM)[†]	None	Replace fat in snack foods, such as chips, and in mayonnaise and margarine-type products
Esterified propoxylated glycerol (EPG)*	NA	Replace some or all fat used in baking and frying
Sucrose polyester (Olestra)[†]	None	Replace fat in home cooking, in commercial frying, and in snack foods

Brand names appear in parentheses.

Type	Calories per Gram	Common Uses in Food
Fat-based, *continued*		
TACTA*	NA	Replace fat in margarine- & mayonnaise-type products
Salatrim	5	Replace fat in chocolate coatings & bars, sour cream, cheese, margarines, & spreads

NA = not available.
Brand names appear in parentheses.
*Not approved by the FDA at this time.

RELATIVE SWEETNESS OF SELECTED SWEETENING AGENTS

Sugar Substitutes*	Relative Sweetness (Sucrose = 1)
Caloric sugar substitutes	
Aspartame (NutraSweet, Equal, and other brand names)	200
Fructose	1.2–1.7
High-fructose corn syrup (90% fructose & 10% dextrose)	1.5
Sugar alcohols	
Mannitol	0.7
Sorbitol	0.5–0.7
Xylitol	1
Noncaloric sugar substitutes	
Acesulfame-K (Sunette & Sweet One)	200
Cyclamate	30
Saccharin	300

*Brand names appear in parentheses.

Alcoholic Beverages

CALORIE AND ALCOHOL CONTENT OF ALCOHOLIC BEVERAGES

Beverage	Calories	Alcohol g
Beer (12 fl oz)	146	13
"Near" beer (12 fl oz)	65	1
Lite beer (12 fl oz)	100	11
Black Russian (2¼ fl oz)	159	16
Bloody Mary (8 fl oz)	186	22
Bourbon & soda (4 fl oz)	105	15
Brandy (1½ fl oz)	96	14
Champagne (6 fl oz)	124	16
Coffee liqueur (1½ fl oz)	174	11
Crème de menthe (1½ fl oz)	186	15
Daiquiri, frozen (4 fl oz)	62	5
Daiquiri, on the rocks (4 fl oz)	222	28
Gin, rum, vodka, whiskey		
80 proof (1½ fl oz)	97	14
86 proof (1½ fl oz)	105	15
90 proof (1½ fl oz)	110	16
94 proof (1½ fl oz)	116	17
100 proof (1½ fl oz)	124	18
Irish coffee w/alcohol (8 fl oz)	132	15
Long Island iced tea (4 fl oz)	111	11
Manhattan (4 fl oz)	256	35
Margarita w/crushed ice, frozen (12 fl oz)	185	16
Martini (4 fl oz)	250	36
Rum (See Gin)		

CALORIE AND ALCOHOL CONTENT OF ALCOHOLIC BEVERAGES *continued*

Rum & cola (4 fl oz)	91	8
Rum punch (4 fl oz)	128	14
Scotch and soda (4 fl oz)	97	14
Screwdriver (8 fl oz)	199	16
Vodka (See Gin)		
Vodka Collins (4 fl oz)	74	9
Vodka tonic (12 fl oz)	231	19
Whiskey (See Gin)		
White Russian (4 fl oz)	271	22
Wine		
Dessert or sweet (2 fl oz)	90	9
Red or white (6 fl oz)	123	16

fl oz = fluid ounce

ALCOHOLIC BEVERAGES CONTAINING FAT, SATURATED FAT, AND CHOLESTEROL

Beverage	Calories	Alcohol g	Fat g	Saturated Fat g	Cholesterol mg
Brandy Alexander (4 fl oz)	276	16	8	5	26
Eggnog w/ brandy (6 fl oz)	288	14	11	6	84
Grasshopper (4 fl oz)	299	12	8	5	27
Hot buttered rum (4 fl oz)	145	13	6	3	14
Piña colada (12 fl oz)	699	37	7	5	0

fl oz = fluid ounce

NUTRIENT CONTENT OF COMMON FOODS

Food	Calories	Carbohydrate g	Protein g	Fat g	Saturated Fat g	Cholesterol mg	Sodium mg
Alcoholic beverages, see page 370							
Alfalfa sprouts, raw (1 cup)	10	1	1	0.2	0.0	0	2
Almonds, honey-roasted (1 oz, or 26 nuts)	168	8	5	14.2	1.3	0	37
Almonds, salted (1 oz, or 22 nuts)	167	7	5	14.7	1.4	0	50
Anchovies, canned, in oil, drained (5)	42	0	6	1.9	0.4	17	734
Apple, canned, sweetened, sliced (½ cup)	68	17	0	0.5	0.1	0	3
Apple, dried (10 rings)	155	42	1	0.2	0.0	0	56
Apple, fresh, w/ skin, 2¾″ diameter (1)	81	21	0	0.5	0.1	0	1
Apple butter (1 tbsp)	33	9	0	0.1	0.0	0	0
Apple crisp, prepared w/ apples, bread, sugar, margarine, cinnamon, salt (½ cup)	230	46	3	5.1	1.0	0	257
Apple juice (6 fl oz)	90	22	0	0.2	0.0	0	6
Applesauce, sweetened or cinnamon (½ cup)	97	25	0	0.2	0.0	0	4
Applesauce, unsweetened (½ cup)	53	14	0	0.1	0.0	0	2
Apricot nectar (6 fl oz)	108	27	1	0.2	0.0	0	6
Apricots, canned, in heavy syrup (3 halves)	70	18	0	0.7	0.0	0	3
Apricots, canned, in juice (3 halves)	40	10	1	0.0	0.0	0	3
Apricots, canned, in light syrup (3 halves)	54	14	0	0.0	0.0	0	3
Apricots, canned, in water (3 halves)	22	5	1	0.1	0.0	0	2
Apricots, dried (10 halves)	83	22	1	0.2	0.0	0	3
Apricots, fresh (3)	51	12	1	0.4	0.0	0	1
Artichoke, boiled (1 medium)	53	12	3	0.2	0.0	0	79
Artichoke hearts, marinated, in oil (½ cup)	62	9	3	2.4	0.4	0	25
Artichokes, frozen, boiled (3 oz)	36	7	2	0.4	0.1	0	42
Asparagus, boiled, plain (½ cup)	22	4	2	0.3	0.1	0	7
Asparagus, boiled, prepared w/ margarine & salt (½ cup)	42	4	3	2.3	0.5	0	196
Asparagus, canned, drained (½ cup)	24	3	3	0.8	0.2	0	472
Asparagus, canned, drained, no salt added (½ cup)	24	3	3	0.8	0.2	0	5
Asparagus, frozen, boiled (4 spears)	17	3	2	0.3	0.1	0	2
Avocado, California (¼ whole)	77	3	1	7.5	1.1	0	5
Bacon, pan-fried (3 slices)	109	0	6	9.4	3.3	16	303
Bagel, plain, 3½″ diameter (1)	195	38	8	1.1	0.2	0	379
Baking powder (1 tsp)	2	1	0	0.0	0.0	0	488
Baking powder, low-sodium (1 tsp)	5	2	0	0.0	0.0	0	4
Baking soda (1 tsp)	0	0	0	0.0	0.0	0	1,259
Bamboo shoots, canned, sliced, drained (½ cup)	13	2	1	1.0	0.1	0	5
Banana, fresh, 8¾″ long (1)	105	27	1	0.6	0.2	0	1
Banana chips (1 oz)	147	17	1	9.5	8.2	0	2
Barbecue sauce (1 tbsp)	12	2	0	0.3	0.0	0	127
Barbecued beef (1 cup)	163	8	9	10.0	3.7	28	553
Barley, pearled, cooked (½ cup)	97	22	2	0.4	0.1	0	2
Basil, fresh, chopped (2 tbsp)	1	0	0	0.0	0.0	0	0
Bass, freshwater, cooked, dry heat (3 oz)	124	0	21	4.0	0.9	74	87

fl oz = fluid ounce; tbsp = tablespoon; tsp = teaspoon

NUTRIENT CONTENT OF COMMON FOODS (cont.)

Food	Calories	Carbohydrate g	Protein g	Fat g	Saturated Fat g	Cholesterol mg	Sodium mg
Beans, baked w/ pork & tomato sauce, canned (½ cup)	123	24	7	1.3	0.5	9	554
Beans, broad, canned, undrained (½ cup)	91	0	0	0.3	0.0	0	580
Beans, green or snap, boiled, plain (½ cup)	22	5	1	0.2	0.0	0	2
Beans, green or snap, boiled, prepared w/ margarine & salt (½ cup)	33	4	1	2.0	0.4	0	201
Beans, green or snap, canned, drained (½ cup)	13	3	1	0.1	0.0	0	170
Beans, green or snap, canned, drained, no salt added (½ cup)	13	3	1	0.1	0.0	0	1
Beans, green or snap, frozen, boiled (½ cup)	18	4	1	0.1	0.0	0	9
Beans, kidney, boiled (½ cup)	112	20	8	0.4	0.1	0	2
Beans, kidney, canned, undrained (½ cup)	104	19	7	0.4	0.1	0	445
Beans, lima, boiled (½ cup)	104	20	6	0.3	0.1	0	14
Beans, lima, canned, undrained (½ cup)	93	18	6	0.4	0.1	0	309
Beans, navy, boiled (½ cup)	129	24	8	0.5	0.1	0	1
Beans, navy, canned, undrained (½ cup)	148	27	10	0.6	0.1	0	587
Beans, pinto, boiled, plain (½ cup)	117	22	7	0.4	0.1	0	1
Beans, pinto, boiled, prepared w/ bacon (½ cup)	132	22	7	2.0	0.7	1	193
Beans, pinto, canned, undrained (½ cup)	93	17	5	0.4	0.1	0	499
Beans, white, cooked, boiled (½ cup)	123	23	9	0.3	0.1	0	6
Beef, arm pot roast, Choice, lean only, trimmed to ¼" fat, braised (3 oz)	191	0	28	7.9	2.9	86	56
Beef, arm pot roast, Select, lean only, trimmed to ¼" fat, braised (3 oz)	175	0	28	6.1	2.2	86	56
Beef, blade roast, Choice, lean & fat, trimmed to ¼" fat, braised (3 oz)	308	0	22	23.7	9.4	88	54
Beef, blade roast, Choice, lean only, trimmed to ¼" fat, braised (3 oz)	223	0	26	12.2	4.8	90	60
Beef, bottom round, Choice, lean only, trimmed to 0" fat, braised (3 oz)	181	0	27	7.4	2.5	82	43
Beef, bottom round, Select, lean only, trimmed to 0" fat, braised (3 oz)	163	0	25	5.4	1.8	82	43
Beef, bottom round, Choice, lean only, trimmed to ¼" fat, braised (3 oz)	187	0	27	8.0	2.7	82	43
Beef, bottom round, Select, lean only, trimmed to ¼" fat, braised (3 oz)	167	0	27	5.8	2.0	82	43
Beef, brains, simmered (3 oz)	136	0	9	10.7	2.5	1,746	102
Beef, brisket, corned, cooked (3 oz)	213	0	15	16.1	5.4	83	964
Beef, brisket, all grades, flat half, lean only, trimmed to 0" fat, braised (3 oz)	162	0	27	5.3	1.7	81	54
Beef, eye of round, Choice, lean only, trimmed to 0" fat, roasted (3 oz)	149	0	25	4.8	1.8	59	53
Beef, eye of round, Select, lean only, trimmed to 0" fat, roasted (3 oz)	132	0	25	3.0	1.1	59	53

fl oz = fluid ounce; tbsp = tablespoon; tsp = teaspoon

NUTRIENT CONTENT OF COMMON FOODS (cont.)

Food	Calories	Carbohydrate g	Protein g	Fat g	Saturated Fat g	Cholesterol mg	Sodium mg
Beef, flank, Choice, lean only, trimmed to 0″ fat, broiled (3 oz)	176	0	23	8.6	3.7	57	70
Beef, ground, extra-lean, broiled (3 oz)	217	0	22	13.9	5.5	71	59
Beef, ground, lean, broiled (3 oz)	231	0	21	15.7	6.2	74	65
Beef, ground, regular, broiled (3 oz)	246	0	20	17.6	6.9	76	70
Beef, heart, simmered (3 oz)	148	0	24	4.8	1.4	164	54
Beef, jerky, chopped & formed (1 oz)	96	4	11	3.7	1.7	32	815
Beef, kidney, simmered (3 oz)	122	1	22	2.9	0.9	329	114
Beef, liver, braised (3 oz)	137	3	21	4.2	1.6	331	59
Beef, rib, Choice, large end, lean & fat, trimmed to ¼″ fat, roasted (3 oz)	326	0	19	27.2	11.0	73	54
Beef, rib, Choice, large end, lean only, trimmed to ¼″ fat, roasted (3 oz)	213	0	23	12.5	5.0	69	62
Beef, rib, Choice, small end, lean only, trimmed to ¼″ fat, broiled (3 oz)	198	0	24	10.7	4.3	68	59
Beef, rib, Select, small end, lean only, trimmed to ¼″ fat, broiled (3 oz)	176	0	24	8.2	3.3	68	59
Beef, rib, Select, whole, lean only, trimmed to ¼″ fat, broiled (3 oz)	175	0	22	8.9	3.6	66	60
Beef, shank, Choice, crosscuts, lean only, trimmed to ¼″ fat, simmered (3 oz)	171	0	29	5.4	1.9	66	54
Beef, stew, prepared in restaurant (1 cup)	221	20	23	5.3	1.9	60	461
Beef, stroganoff with noodles, prepared in restaurant (¾ cup noodles & ¼ cup sauce)	416	26	23	23.0	9.6	106	507
Beef, sweetbreads, braised (3 oz)	271	0	19	21.2	7.3	250	99
Beef, T-bone steak, Choice, lean only, trimmed to ¼″ fat, broiled (3 oz)	182	0	24	8.8	3.5	68	56
Beef, tenderloin, Choice, lean only, trimmed to 0″ fat, broiled (3 oz)	180	0	24	8.6	3.2	71	54
Beef, tenderloin, Select, lean only, trimmed to ¼″ fat, broiled (3 oz)	169	0	24	7.4	2.8	71	54
Beef, thymus, see Beef, sweetbreads							
Beef, tip round, Choice, lean only, trimmed to 0″ fat, roasted (3 oz)	153	0	24	5.4	1.9	69	55
Beef, tip round, Select, lean only, trimmed to 0″ fat, roasted (3 oz)	145	0	24	4.5	1.6	69	55
Beef, tongue, simmered (3 oz)	241	0	19	17.6	7.6	91	51
Beef, top loin, Choice, lean only, trimmed to 0″ fat, broiled (3 oz)	177	0	24	8.2	3.1	65	58
Beef, top loin, Select, lean only, trimmed to 0″ fat, broiled (3 oz)	157	0	24	5.9	2.2	65	58
Beef, top round, Choice, lean only, trimmed to 0″ fat, braised (3 oz)	176	0	31	4.9	1.7	76	38
Beef, top round, Select, lean only, trimmed to 0″ fat, braised (3 oz)	162	0	31	3.4	1.2	76	38

fl oz = fluid ounce; tbsp = tablespoon; tsp = teaspoon

NUTRIENT CONTENT OF COMMON FOODS (cont.)

Food	Calories	Carbohydrate g	Protein g	Fat g	Saturated Fat g	Cholesterol mg	Sodium mg
Beef, top round, Select, lean only, trimmed to ¼" fat, broiled (3 oz)	143	0	27	3.1	1.1	71	52
Beef, top sirloin, Choice, lean only, trimmed to 0" fat, broiled (3 oz)	170	0	26	6.6	2.6	76	56
Beef, top sirloin, Select, lean only, trimmed to 0" fat, broiled (3 oz)	153	0	26	4.8	1.9	76	56
Beef, tripe, raw (3 oz)	84	0	12	3.4	1.7	81	39
Beefalo, roasted (3 oz)	160	0	26	5.4	2.3	49	70
Beer, see page 370							
Beets, canned, sliced, drained (½ cup)	27	6	1	0.1	0.0	0	116
Beets, canned, sliced, drained, no salt added (½ cup)	27	6	1	0.1	0.0	0	65
Beets, cooked, sliced (½ cup)	26	6	1	0.0	0.0	0	42
Beets, Harvard, canned, undrained (½ cup)	89	22	1	0.1	0.0	0	199
Beets, pickled, canned, sliced, undrained (½ cup)	75	19	1	0.1	0.0	0	301
Beverage, chocolate-flavor milk mix powder, dry (3 tsp)	75	20	1	0.7	0.4	0	45
Beverage, fruit juice drink, citrus (6 fl oz)	84	22	1	0.0	0.0	0	6
Beverage, strawberry-flavor milk mix powder, dry (3 tsp)	84	21	0	0.0	0.0	0	8
Biscuit, prepared w/ 2% milk & shortening, 2½" diameter × 1½" (1)	212	27	4	9.8	2.6	?	348
Biscuit, refrigerated dough, 2½" diameter × 1" (1)	93	13	2	4.0	1.0	0	324
Black-eyed peas, boiled, plain (½ cup)	89	15	7	0.7	0.2	0	4
Black-eyed peas, boiled, prepared w/ bacon (½ cup)	114	18	7	2.0	0.8	1	195
Blackberries, canned, in heavy syrup (½ cup)	118	30	2	0.1	0.0	0	3
Blackberries, fresh (½ cup)	37	9	1	0.3	0.0	0	0
Blueberries, canned, in heavy syrup (½ cup)	112	28	1	0.4	0.0	0	4
Blueberries, fresh (½ cup)	41	20	1	0.6	0.0	0	5
Bologna, beef (1 oz)	88	0	4	8.1	3.4	16	278
Bologna, beef & pork (1 oz)	89	1	3	8.0	3.0	16	288
Bologna, turkey (1 oz)	57	0	4	4.3	1.3	28	249
Boysenberries, canned, in heavy syrup (½ cup)	113	29	1	0.2	0.0	0	4
Boysenberries, frozen, unsweetened (½ cup)	33	8	1	0.2	0.0	0	1
Braunschweiger, pork (3 oz)	306	3	11	27.3	9.3	132	972
Brazil nuts, unsalted (1 oz, or 8 medium nuts)	186	4	4	18.8	4.6	0	0
Bread, banana, prepared w/ margarine, eggs, low-fat milk, 4⅜" × 2½" × ½" (1 slice)	195	33	3	6.3	1.3	26	181
Bread, diet or light (1.2 oz, or 2 slices)	96	20	4	1.2	0.3	0	208
Bread, egg, 5" × 3" × ½" (1 slice)	115	19	4	2.4	0.6	20	197
Bread, French (1 oz)	78	15	3	0.8	0.2	0	172
Bread, Italian (1 oz)	77	16	3	0.2	0.0	0	166
Bread, multigrain or 7-grain (1 oz)	71	13	3	1.1	0.2	0	138

fl oz = fluid ounce; tbsp = tablespoon; tsp = teaspoon

NUTRIENT CONTENT OF COMMON FOODS (cont.)

Food	Calories	Carbohydrate g	Protein g	Fat g	Saturated Fat g	Cholesterol mg	Sodium mg
Bread, oat bran (1 slice)	71	12	3	1.3	0.2	0	122
Bread, pumpernickel (1 oz, or 1 slice)	71	14	3	0.9	0.1	0	190
Bread, raisin (1 oz, or 1 slice)	78	15	2	1.3	0.3	0	111
Bread, rye (1 oz, or 1 slice)	73	14	2	0.9	0.2	0	187
Bread, sourdough (1 oz, or 1 slice)	78	15	3	0.8	0.2	0	172
Bread, wheat bran (1 oz, or 1 slice)	70	14	3	1.0	0.2	0	138
Bread, white (1 oz, or 1 slice)	76	14	2	1.0	0.2	0	153
Bread, whole-wheat (1 oz, or 1 slice)	70	13	3	1.2	0.3	0	149
Breadfruit ($\frac{1}{2}$ cup)	114	30	1	0.6	0.0	0	2
Bread pudding, prepared w/ whole milk, eggs, margarine ($\frac{1}{2}$ cup)	212	31	6	7.4	2.9	83	291
Breadstick, $9\frac{1}{4}'' \times \frac{3}{8}''$ diameter (1)	25	4	1	0.6	0.1	0	39
Broccoli, boiled (1 spear)	53	10	5	0.5	0.1	0	19
Broccoli, boiled, chopped, plain ($\frac{1}{2}$ cup)	23	4	2	0.2	0.0	0	8
Broccoli, boiled, chopped, prepared w/ margarine & salt ($\frac{1}{2}$ cup)	43	5	3	2.0	0.4	0	215
Broccoli, frozen, chopped, boiled ($\frac{1}{2}$ cup)	25	5	3	0.1	0.0	0	22
Broccoli, raw, chopped ($\frac{1}{2}$ cup)	12	2	1	0.2	0.0	0	12
Broccoli, w/ cheese sauce ($\frac{1}{2}$ cup)	124	7	7	8.3	4.3	20	412
Brownie, $2\frac{3}{4}''$ square $\times \frac{7}{8}''$ (1)	227	36	3	9.1	2.4	10	175
Brussels sprouts, boiled, plain ($\frac{1}{2}$ cup)	30	7	2	0.4	0.1	0	17
Brussels sprouts, boiled, prepared w/ margarine & salt ($\frac{1}{2}$ cup)	50	6	3	2.2	0.5	0	211
Brussels sprouts, frozen, boiled ($\frac{1}{2}$ cup)	33	6	3	0.3	0.1	0	18
Bun, hamburger, medium, $3\frac{1}{2}''$ diameter (1)	123	22	4	2.2	0.5	0	241
Bun, hot dog, medium, 6" long (1)	123	22	4	2.2	0.5	0	241
Butter (1 pat)	36	0	0	4.1	2.5	11	41
Cabbage, Chinese, shredded, boiled ($\frac{1}{2}$ cup)	10	2	1	0.1	0.0	0	29
Cabbage, Chinese, shredded, raw ($\frac{1}{2}$ cup)	5	1	1	0.1	0.0	0	23
Cabbage, shredded, raw ($\frac{1}{2}$ cup)	8	2	0	0.1	0.0	0	6
Cake, angel food, plain or flavored ($\frac{1}{12}$ of 9" diameter)	73	16	2	0.2	0.0	0	212
Cake, carrot, w/ cream cheese frosting, prepared w/ oil, eggs, nuts, cream cheese, margarine ($\frac{1}{12}$ of 9" diameter)	484	52	5	29.3	5.4	60	273
Cake, coconut, prepared w/ low-fat milk, egg white, shortening ($\frac{1}{12}$ of 9" diameter)	399	71	5	11.5	4.4	2	318
Cake, coffee, w/ cinnamon & crumb topping, commercial ($\frac{1}{9}$ of 20 oz)	263	29	4	14.7	3.6	20	221
Cake, devil's food, no icing, 2-layer, prepared w/ low-fat milk, eggs, shortening, baking chocolate ($\frac{1}{12}$ of 9" diameter)	198	32	4	7.6	1.7	35	370
Cake, German chocolate, w/ coconut-pecan frosting, prepared w/ mix, oil, eggs ($\frac{1}{12}$ of 9" diameter)	404	55	4	20.6	5.3	53	369

fl oz = fluid ounce; tbsp = tablespoon; tsp = teaspoon

NUTRIENT CONTENT OF COMMON FOODS (cont.)

Food	Calories	Carbohydrate g	Protein g	Fat g	Saturated Fat g	Cholesterol mg	Sodium mg
Cake, gingerbread, prepared w/ mix, water, eggs (1/9 of 9" square)	207	34	3	6.8	1.7	24	307
Cake, pineapple upside-down cake, prepared w/ low-fat milk, vegetable shortening, margarine, eggs (1/9 of 8" square)	367	58	4	13.9	3.4	25	367
Cake, pound, no icing, prepared w/ butter & eggs (1/16 of 9" loaf)	230	25	3	13.1	7.6	91	153
Cake, sponge, prepared w/ eggs (1/12 of 10" diameter)	140	37	3	2.0	0.6	80	107
Cake, white, no icing, 2-layer, prepared w/ mix & egg whites (1/12 of 9" diameter)	190	34	3	4.8	0.7	3	301
Cake, yellow, no icing, 2-layer, prepared w/ mix & eggs (1/12 of 9" diameter)	202	34	3	5.9	1.0	37	299
Canadian bacon, grilled (3 oz)	157	1	21	7.2	2.4	49	1,314
Candy, candy corn (1 oz)	101	26	0	0.0	0.0	0	34
Candy, caramels, plain or chocolate (10 pieces)	306	67	4	6.5	5.3	6	196
Candy, divinity (1 piece)	38	10	0	0.0	0.0	0	5
Candy, fudge, plain (1 oz)	108	23	0	2.4	1.5	4	18
Candy, fudge, w/ nuts, 1" × 1" × 7/8" (1 piece)	81	14	1	3.1	1.1	3	11
Candy, gumdrops (10 small)	135	35	0	0.0	0.0	0	15
Candy, hard (1 oz)	106	28	0	0.0	0.0	0	11
Candy, jelly beans (10 large pieces)	104	26	0	0.1	0.0	0	7
Candy, milk chocolate bar, plain (4 oz)	582	67	8	34.7	20.9	25	93
Candy, milk chocolate bar, w/ almonds (4 oz)	596	60	10	39.0	19.3	22	84
Candy, milk chocolate bar, w/ rice cereal (4 oz)	562	72	7	30.0	18.0	22	164
Candy, mints, uncoated (1 oz)	101	26	0	0.0	0.0	0	34
Candy, peanut brittle (1 oz)	128	20	2	5.4	1.4	4	128
Candy, peanuts, chocolate-coated (30 pieces)	624	60	15	40.2	17.4	12	48
Candy, praline (1 piece)	177	24	1	9.5	0.7	0	24
Candy, raisins, milk-chocolate coated (30 pieces)	117	21	0	4.5	2.7	0	12
Candy, truffles (1 piece)	59	5	1	4.1	2.6	6	8
Carrot, raw, 7½" × 1" diameter (1)	31	7	1	0.1	0.0	0	25
Carrot, raw, baby, 2¾" long (1)	4	1	0	0.1	0.0	0	3
Carrot juice (6 fl oz)	73	17	2	0.3	0.0	0	538
Carrots, boiled, prepared w/ margarine & salt (½ cup)	52	8	1	2.0	0.4	0	244
Carrots, canned, sliced, drained (½ cup)	17	4	0	0.1	0.0	0	176
Carrots, canned, sliced, drained, no salt added (½ cup)	17	4	0	0.1	0.0	0	31
Carrots, frozen, sliced, boiled (½ cup)	26	6	1	0.1	0.0	0	43
Carrots, plain, sliced, boiled (½ cup)	35	8	1	0.1	0.0	0	52
Cashew nuts, salted (1 oz, or 18 medium nuts)	163	9	4	13.2	2.6	0	179
Catfish, breaded, fried (3 oz)	194	7	15	11.3	2.8	69	238

fl oz = fluid ounce; tbsp = tablespoon; tsp = teaspoon

NUTRIENT CONTENT OF COMMON FOODS (cont.)

Food	Calories	Carbohydrate g	Protein g	Fat g	Saturated Fat g	Cholesterol mg	Sodium mg
Catfish, cooked, dry heat (3 oz)	129	0	16	6.8	1.5	54	68
Catsup, low-sodium (1 tbsp)	16	4	0	0.1	0.0	0	3
Catsup, regular (1 tbsp)	16	4	0	0.1	0.0	0	156
Cauliflower, boiled, 1″ pieces (½ cup)	15	3	1	0.1	0.0	0	4
Cauliflower, frozen, 1″ pieces, boiled (½ cup)	17	4	1	0.2	0.0	0	16
Cauliflower, raw, 1″ pieces (½ cup)	12	2	1	0.9	0.0	0	7
Celery, diced, boiled (½ cup)	11	3	0	0.8	0.0	0	48
Celery, raw, 7½″ × 1″ (1 stalk)	6	1	0	0.1	0.0	0	35
Cereal, bran flakes (1 oz, or ⅔ cup)	85	21	3	0.6	0.1	0	210
Cereal, buckwheat groats, roasted, cooked, prepared w/ water (½ cup prepared)	91	20	3	0.6	0.1	0	4
Cereal, cornflakes (1 oz, or 1 cup)	110	25	2	0.4	0.1	0	291
Cereal, cornflakes, presweetened (1 oz, or ¾ cup)	110	26	1	0.2	0.0	0	200
Cereal, corn grits, regular & quick, prepared w/ water (1 cup prepared)	146	31	4	0.5	0.1	0	0
Cereal, Cream of Wheat, regular, prepared w/ water & no salt (1 cup prepared)	105	28	4	0.6	0.1	0	4
Cereal, farina, prepared w/ water & no salt (1 cup prepared)	116	25	3	0.2	0.0	0	1
Cereal, granola, homemade (1 oz)	138	16	4	7.7	1.4	0	3
Cereal, Grapenuts (1 oz)	101	23	3	0.1	0.0	0	197
Cereal, oat bran, prepared w/ water & no salt (½ cup prepared)	44	12	3	1.0	0.2	0	1
Cereal, oatmeal, regular, prepared w/ water & no salt (1 cup prepared)	145	25	6	2.4	0.4	0	1
Cereal, 100% bran (1 oz, or ½ cup)	76	21	4	1.4	0.3	0	196
Cereal, puffed wheat, plain (1 oz)	104	23	4	0.4	0.0	0	2
Cereal, raisin bran (1 oz)	87	21	3	0.5	0.0	0	202
Cereal, shredded wheat (1 large biscuit)	83	19	3	0.3	0.0	0	0
Cereal, wheat germ, plain, toasted (¼ cup)	108	14	8	3.0	0.5	0	1
Cheese, American (1 oz)	106	0	6	8.9	5.6	27	406
Cheese, American processed spread (1 oz)	82	2	5	6.0	3.8	16	381
Cheese, blue (1 oz)	100	1	6	8.2	5.3	21	396
Cheese, Cheddar (1 oz)	114	0	7	9.4	6.0	30	176
Cheese, Colby (1 oz)	112	1	7	9.1	5.7	27	171
Cheese, fat-free (1 oz)	41	3	7	0.3	0.2	1	439
Cheese, feta (1 oz)	75	4	4	6.0	4.2	25	316
Cheese, goat (1 oz)	76	0	5	6.0	4.1	13	104
Cheese, low-fat (1 oz)	79	1	8	4.9	3.1	15	150
Cheese, low-fat & low-sodium (1 oz)	71	3	7	4.3	2.7	18	88
Cheese, Monterey Jack (1 oz)	104	0	7	8.5	5.4	27	178
Cheese, mozzarella, part-skim-milk (1 oz)	72	1	7	4.5	2.9	16	132
Cheese, Muenster (1 oz)	104	0	7	8.5	5.4	27	178
Cheese, Parmesan, grated (1 tbsp)	23	0	2	1.5	1.0	4	93

fl oz = fluid ounce; tbsp = tablespoon; tsp = teaspoon

NUTRIENT CONTENT OF COMMON FOODS (cont.)

Food	Calories	Carbohydrate g	Protein g	Fat g	Saturated Fat g	Cholesterol mg	Sodium mg
Cheese, pimiento (1 oz)	106	0	6	8.8	5.6	27	405
Cheese, provolone (1 oz)	100	1	7	7.6	4.8	20	248
Cheese, ricotta, part-skim-milk (1 oz)	39	4	10	2.2	1.4	9	35
Cheese, ricotta, whole-milk (1 oz)	49	3	10	3.7	2.4	14	24
Cheese, Romano (1 oz)	101	0	7	7.9	5.0	25	274
Cheese, Swiss (1 oz)	107	1	8	7.8	5.0	26	74
Cheese-flavored twists or puffs (1 oz)	157	15	2	9.7	1.9	1	298
Cheesecake, plain, prepared w/ cream cheese, sugar, eggs, margarine ($\frac{1}{12}$ of 9" diameter)	456	32	9	33.3	18.4	155	362
Cherries, fresh (10)	49	11	1	0.7	0.1	0	0
Cherries, sweet, canned, in heavy syrup ($\frac{1}{2}$ cup)	107	27	1	0.2	0.0	0	3
Cherries, sweet, canned, in juice ($\frac{1}{2}$ cup)	68	17	1	0.0	0.0	0	3
Cherries, sweet, canned, in light syrup ($\frac{1}{2}$ cup)	85	22	1	0.2	0.0	0	3
Cherries, sweet, canned, in water ($\frac{1}{2}$ cup)	57	15	1	0.2	0.0	0	2
Chestnuts, roasted (6 chestnuts)	117	24	2	1.4	0.3	0	12
Chicken, boneless, canned, in broth (3 oz)	140	0	19	6.8	1.9	53	428
Chicken, breast meat w/ skin, fried, w/ batter (4 oz, or 1 piece)	427	21	30	24.2	6.4	74	909
Chicken, breast meat w/ skin, roasted (3 oz)	167	0	25	6.6	1.9	72	60
Chicken, breast meat w/ skin, stewed (3 oz)	156	0	23	6.3	1.8	64	53
Chicken, breast meat w/o skin, roasted (3 oz)	142	0	27	3.1	0.9	73	63
Chicken, breast meat w/o skin, stewed (3 oz)	129	0	25	2.6	0.7	65	52
Chicken, dark meat w/ skin, stewed (3 oz)	198	0	20	12.6	4.8	69	60
Chicken, dark meat w/o skin, roasted (3 oz)	174	0	23	8.3	2.3	79	79
Chicken, dark meat w/o skin, stewed (3 oz)	163	0	22	7.6	2.1	75	63
Chicken, drumstick meat w/ skin, fried, w/ batter ($2\frac{1}{2}$ oz, or 1 piece)	193	6	16	11.3	3.0	62	194
Chicken, drumstick meat w/ skin, stewed (2 oz, or 1 piece)	116	0	9	6.1	1.7	48	43
Chicken, drumstick meat w/o skin, roasted (1.6 oz, or 1 piece)	76	0	12	2.5	0.7	41	42
Chicken, drumstick meat w/o skin, stewed (1.6 oz, or 1 piece)	78	0	13	2.6	0.7	40	37
Chicken, giblets (1 each gizzard, heart, liver) ($2\frac{1}{2}$ oz)	112	1	18	3.6	1.1	243	40
Chicken, light meat w/ skin, stewed (3 oz)	171	0	22	8.4	2.4	63	54
Chicken, light meat w/o skin, roasted (3 oz)	147	0	25	3.8	1.1	72	66
Chicken, light meat w/o skin, stewed (3 oz)	135	0	25	3.4	1.0	65	55
Chicken, roll, light meat (3 oz)	136	2	17	6.3	1.8	43	496
Chicken, thigh meat w/ skin, fried, with batter (3 oz, or 1 piece)	238	8	19	14.2	3.8	80	248
Chicken, thigh meat w/ skin, stewed ($2\frac{1}{2}$ oz, or 1 piece)	158	0	16	10.0	2.8	57	49
Chicken, thigh meat w/o skin, stewed (2 oz, or 1 piece)	107	0	14	5.4	1.5	49	41

fl oz = fluid ounce; tbsp = tablespoon; tsp = teaspoon

NUTRIENT CONTENT OF COMMON FOODS (cont.)

Food	Calories	Carbohydrate g	Protein g	Fat g	Saturated Fat g	Cholesterol mg	Sodium mg
Chicken, wing meat w/ skin, fried, w/ batter (1¾ oz, or 1 piece)	159	5	10	10.7	2.9	39	157
Chicken, wing meat w/ skin, stewed (1½ oz)	100	0	7	6.7	1.9	28	27
Chicken, wing meat w/o skin, roasted (¾ oz, or 1 piece)	43	0	6	1.7	0.5	18	19
Chicken, wing meat w/o skin, stewed (1 oz)	50	0	8	2.0	0.6	21	21
Chicken & dumplings, prepared in restaurant (1 cup)	290	19	23	13.2	3.3	64	288
Chicken fat (1 tbsp)	115	0	0	12.8	3.8	11	7
Chicken-fried steak, prepared in restaurant (12 oz)	928	45	65	52.5	15.2	155	1,986
Chicken tetrazzini, prepared in restaurant (1 cup)	351	28	20	17.1	6.2	48	918
Chickpeas (garbanzo beans), boiled (½ cup)	134	22	7	2.1	0.2	0	6
Chickpeas (garbanzo beans), canned, undrained (½ cup)	143	27	6	1.4	0.1	0	359
Chili w/ beans (meatless), canned (1 cup)	113	23	6	0.9	0.1	0	804
Chili w/ beans and beef (1 cup)	249	22	17	11.3	4.2	41	803
Chili w/ beef (no beans) (1 cup)	243	15	17	13.8	5.2	51	740
Chinese food, prepared in restaurant:							
Beef and broccoli stir-fry (1 serving)	233	3	12	19.6	3.8	29	444
Egg rolls (2 large)	263	22	6	17.3	4.9	79	909
Egg-drop soup (1 cup)	103	6	9	4.3	1.3	106	999
Fried rice (1 serving)	370	45	16	13.5	3.2	128	1,112
Fried wonton (6)	408	50	13	17.1	3.0	147	156
Hot/sour soup (1 cup)	226	11	17	12.3	2.7	83	1,134
Moo goo gai pan (1 serving)	380	12	29	24.4	4.1	62	2,146
Pepper steak (1 cup)	435	9	34	28.6	5.2	86	1,849
Pork lo mein (1 cup)	235	31	8	8.9	1.7	15	499
Sweet/sour chicken (1 serving)	625	58	38	27.0	4.7	83	2,951
Sweet/sour pork (1 serving)	735	67	34	37.3	8.4	95	2,932
Wonton soup (1 cup w/ 4–5 wontons)	326	42	17	9.0	2.7	60	1,078
Chitterlings, simmered (3 oz)	258	0	9	24.4	8.6	122	33
Chow chow, sour (1 tbsp)	4	1	0	0.2	0.0	0	201
Chow chow, sweet (1 tbsp)	18	0	0	0.1	0.0	0	81
Chutney (1 tbsp)	21	5	0	0.1	0.0	0	9
Clams, cooked, moist heat (3 oz)	126	4	22	1.7	0.2	57	95
Clams, raw, drained solids (3 oz)	126	4	22	1.7	0.2	57	95
Club soda (12 fl oz)	0	0	0	0.0	0.0	0	75
Cocktails, see page 370							
Cocoa mix, low-calorie w/ aspartame, prepared w/ water (1 package, or 6 fl oz)	48	9	4	0.5	0.3	1	168
Cocoa mix, prepared w/ water (1 package, or 6 fl oz)	103	24	1	1.1	0.4	0	122
Cocoa powder, unsweetened (1 tbsp)	11	3	1	0.7	0.4	0	1

fl oz = fluid ounce; tbsp = tablespoon; tsp = teaspoon

NUTRIENT CONTENT OF COMMON FOODS (cont.)

Food	Calories	Carbohydrate g	Protein g	Fat g	Saturated Fat g	Cholesterol mg	Sodium mg
Coconut, canned, dried, flaked, sweetened (3 tbsp)	66	6	1	4.8	4.2	0	3
Coconut cream, canned (1 tbsp)	36	2	1	3.4	3.0	0	149
Cod, Atlantic, cooked, dry heat (3 oz)	89	0	19	0.7	0.1	47	66
Cod, Pacific, cooked, dry heat (3 oz)	89	0	20	0.7	0.1	40	77
Coffee, brewed, regular or decaffeinated, unsweetened (1 cup)	5	1	0	0.0	0.0	0	5
Coffee, instant, regular or decaffeinated, unsweetened, prepared w/ water (1 cup)	5	1	0	0.0	0.0	0	8
Cola (12 fl oz)	151	39	0	0.0	0.0	0	14
Cola, diet, sweetened w/ aspartame (12 fl oz)	2	0	0	0.0	0.0	0	21
Cookie, butter, commercial (1 medium)	75	10	1	3.6	0.9	3	68
Cookie, chocolate chip, commercial, 2¼" diameter (1)	46	6	1	2.1	0.7	0	32
Cookie, chocolate sandwich w/ creme filling, commercial (1)	47	7	1	2.1	0.4	0	60
Cookie, fig bars, commercial (1)	56	11	1	1.2	0.2	0	56
Cookie, fortune, commercial (1)	30	7	0	0.2	0.1	0	22
Cookie, gingersnaps, commercial (1)	29	5	0	0.7	0.1	0	185
Cookie, oatmeal, commercial (1)	81	12	1	3.3	0.6	0	69
Cookie, peanut butter, commercial (1)	71	9	1	3.5	0.8	0	62
Cookie, peanut butter sandwich, commercial (1)	67	9	1	3.0	0.8	0	52
Cookie, shortbread, commercial, 1⅝" square (1)	40	5	1	1.9	0.5	2	36
Cookie, sugar, commercial (1)	72	10	1	3.2	0.8	8	53
Cookie, vanilla wafer, commercial (1)	18	3	1	0.6	0.1	0	12
Corn, cream-style, canned (½ cup)	93	23	2	0.5	0.1	0	365
Corn, cream-style, canned, no salt added (½ cup)	93	23	2	1.0	0.1	0	4
Corn, whole-kernel, boiled, prepared w/ margarine & salt (½ cup)	83	17	3	2.0	0.4	0	197
Corn, whole-kernel, canned, drained (½ cup)	66	15	2	0.8	0.1	0	265
Corn, whole-kernel, canned, drained, no salt added (½ cup)	66	15	2	0.8	0.1	0	4
Corn, whole-kernel, frozen, boiled (½ cup)	67	17	2	0.1	0.0	0	4
Cornbread, prepared w/ whole milk, eggs, oil, 2½" × 3" (1 piece)	352	56	8	10.0	2.6	56	856
Corn chips (1 oz)	153	16	2	9.5	1.3	0	179
Cornmeal, degermed (¼ cup)	125	26	3	0.6	0.1	0	1
Cornmeal, self-rising (¼ cup)	100	0	0	1.0	0.1	0	374
Cornmeal, whole-grain (¼ cup)	109	0	0	1.1	0.2	0	11
Corn pudding, prepared w/ whole milk, eggs, butter (½ cup)	136	16	5	6.6	3.2	115	69
Cornstarch (1 tbsp)	30	7	0	0.0	0.0	0	5
Cottage cheese, creamed (½ cup)	109	3	13	4.7	3.0	16	425
Cottage cheese, dry curd (½ cup)	62	1	13	0.3	0.2	5	10

fl oz = fluid ounce; tbsp = tablespoon; tsp = teaspoon

NUTRIENT CONTENT OF COMMON FOODS (cont.)

Food	Calories	Carbohydrate g	Protein g	Fat g	Saturated Fat g	Cholesterol mg	Sodium mg
Cottage cheese, 1% fat (1/2 cup)	82	3	14	1.2	0.7	5	459
Cottage cheese, 2% fat (1/2 cup)	101	4	16	2.2	1.4	9	459
Couscous, cooked (1 cup)	201	42	7	0.3	0.1	0	9
Crab, Alaska king, cooked, moist heat (3 oz)	82	0	16	1.3	0.1	45	911
Crab, Alaska king, imitation, made from surimi (3 oz)	84	6	13	0.8	0.2	26	735
Crab, blue, cooked, moist heat (3 oz)	87	0	17	1.5	0.2	85	237
Crabapple, fresh, sliced (1/2 cup)	42	11	0	0.2	0.1	0	1
Crab cakes, prepared w/ eggs, fried in margarine (2 oz)	93	0	12	4.5	0.9	90	198
Cracker, cheese, 1" squares (1/2 oz, or 14 crackers)	71	8	1	3.6	1.3	2	141
Cracker, graham, 2 1/2" square (1)	30	5	1	0.7	0.2	0	42
Cracker, matzo, plain (1)	112	24	3	0.4	0.1	0	0
Cracker, melba toast, plain (1)	19	4	1	0.2	0.0	0	41
Cracker, saltine (1)	13	2	1	0.4	0.0	0	39
Cracker, sandwich-type, cheese crackers w/ peanut butter (1/2 oz, or 2 crackers)	68	8	2	3.3	0.7	1	141
Cracker, snack type (1 round)	15	2	0	0.8	0.1	0	25
Cracker, wheat (1 thin square)	9	1	0	0.4	0.1	0	16
Cracker, zwieback (1)	30	5	1	0.7	0.3	2	16
Cranberries, chopped, fresh, unsweetened (1/2 cup)	27	7	0	0.1	0.0	0	1
Cranberry juice cocktail (6 fl oz)	102	27	0	0.0	0.0	0	6
Cranberry sauce, canned, sweetened (1/2 cup)	209	54	0	0.2	0.0	0	40
Crayfish, cooked, moist heat (3 oz)	75	0	14	1.0	0.2	113	80
Cream, half-&-half (2 tbsp)	40	1	1	3.4	2.2	12	12
Cream, sour (2 tbsp)	52	1	1	5.0	3.2	10	12
Cream, whipped topping, nondairy, frozen (2 tbsp)	26	2	0	2.0	1.8	0	2
Cream, whipped, pressurized (2 tbsp)	16	1	0	1.4	0.8	4	8
Cream, whipping, heavy, fluid (2 tbsp)	104	1	1	11.2	7.0	42	12
Cream cheese, fat-free (2 tbsp)	24	1	4	0.1	0.1	0	177
Cream cheese, light, whipped (2 tbsp)	44	1	2	3.7	2.3	12	111
Cream cheese, low-fat (2 tbsp)	64	1	3	5.4	3.4	17	163
Cream cheese, Neufchâtel (2 tbsp)	75	1	3	6.8	4.3	22	116
Cream cheese, regular (1 oz)	99	1	2	9.9	6.2	31	84
Cream cheese, whipped (2 tbsp)	70	1	2	7.0	4.4	22	59
Creamer, nondairy, liquid (2 tbsp)	40	2	0	3.0	0.6	0	24
Creamer, nondairy, powder (2 tsp)	22	2	0	1.4	1.4	0	8
Cream soda (12 fl oz)	191	49	0	0.0	0.0	0	43
Croissant, butter, 4 1/2" × 4" × 1 3/4" (1)	265	27	5	15.3	9.2	61	72
Croutons, plain (1/2 oz)	58	10	2	0.9	0.2	0	99
Cucumber, raw, chopped (1/2 cup)	7	2	0	0.1	0.0	0	1
Currants, red or white, fresh (1/2 cup)	31	8	1	0.1	0.0	0	1
Dates (10)	228	61	2	0.4	0.0	0	2

fl oz = fluid ounce; tbsp = tablespoon; tsp = teaspoon

NUTRIENT CONTENT OF COMMON FOODS (cont.)

Food	Calories	Carbohydrate g	Protein g	Fat g	Saturated Fat g	Cholesterol mg	Sodium mg
Dill, fresh (5 sprigs)	0	0	0	0.0	0.0	0	1
Doughnut, cake-type, plain, 4″ diameter (1)	198	23	2	10.8	1.8	18	257
Doughnut, yeast-type, plain, 3¾″ diameter (1)	242	27	4	13.7	3.5	4	205
Eclair, custard-filled w/ chocolate glaze, 5″ × 2″ × 1¾″ (1)	262	24	6	15.7	4.1	127	337
Egg, fried, prepared w/ margarine (1)	91	1	6	6.9	1.9	211	162
Egg, omelet, prepared w/ butter & whole milk (1 egg)	95	1	6	7.1	2.8	225	155
Egg, scrambled, prepared w/ butter & whole milk (1 egg)	95	1	6	7.1	2.8	213	155
Egg, white, cooked (1 medium)	14	0	3	0.0	0.0	0	48
Egg, whole, cooked, hard (1 medium)	79	1	6	5.6	1.7	213	69
Egg, yolk, cooked (1 medium)	54	0	3	4.6	1.4	192	6
Eggnog (1 cup)	342	34	10	19.0	11.3	149	138
Eggplant, boiled, cubed (½ cup)	13	3	0	0.1	0.0	0	2
Eggplant, raw, cubed (½ cup)	11	2	0	0.1	0.0	0	1
Egg substitute, fat-free (¼ cup)	26	1	5	0.0	0.0	0	82
Egg substitute, low-fat (¼ cup)	70	3	7	3.0	1.0	0	114
Elk, roasted (3 oz)	124	0	26	1.6	0.6	62	52
Endive, raw, chopped (½ cup)	4	1	0	0.1	0.0	0	6
English muffin, plain (1)	134	26	4	1.0	0.1	0	265
Fast food:							
Bacon cheeseburger, single meat patty (4 oz raw) w/ catsup, mustard, pickles, onions (1)	609	37	32	36.8	16.3	112	1,044
Burrito w/ beans (2)	448	71	14	13.5	6.9	5	986
Burrito w/ beans, cheese, beef (2)	331	40	15	13.3	7.2	125	990
Cheeseburger, large, single meat patty (4 oz raw) w/ catsup, lettuce, onions, mayonnaise, mustard, tomatoes (1)	665	44	31	40.4	14.6	100	1,540
Cheeseburger, large, single meat patty (4 oz raw), plain (1)	531	36	30	29.0	12.9	92	1,048
Cheeseburger, regular, single meat patty (2 oz raw) w/ catsup, mustard, onions, pickles (1)	354	35	17	15.9	6.7	46	1,033
Chicken, breaded & fried, breast & wing (2 pieces)	494	20	36	29.5	7.8	149	975
Chicken fillet sandwich, plain (1)	515	39	24	29.5	8.5	60	957
Chimichanga w/ beef (1)	425	43	20	19.7	8.5	9	910
Cookies, animal crackers (2.4 oz, or 1 box)	299	50	4	9.0	3.5	11	274
Corn dog (1)	341	22	8	24.5	7.6	45	597
Eggs, scrambled (2)	200	2	13	15.2	5.8	400	211
Enchilada w/ cheese & beef (1)	324	30	12	17.6	9.1	40	1,320
English muffin sandwich w/ egg, cheese, Canadian bacon (1)	383	31	20	19.8	9.1	234	785
Fish sandwich w/ tartar sauce (1)	431	41	17	22.8	5.2	55	615

fl oz = fluid ounce; tbsp = tablespoon; tsp = teaspoon

NUTRIENT CONTENT OF COMMON FOODS (cont.)

Food	Calories	Carbohydrate g	Protein g	Fat g	Saturated Fat g	Cholesterol mg	Sodium mg
Fast-food, *continued*							
Fish sandwich w/ tartar sauce & cheese (1)	524	48	21	28.6	8.1	68	939
French-fried potatoes in beef tallow & vegetable oil (4 oz)	358	29	3	18.5	7.6	16	187
French-fried potatoes in vegetable oil (1 regular order)	235	29	3	12.2	3.8	0	124
Fried pie, apple, cherry, or lemon (1)	266	33	2	14.4	6.5	13	325
Ham & cheese sandwich (1)	353	33	21	15.5	6.4	58	772
Hamburger, regular, double meat patty (each 2 oz raw) w/ catsup, onions, mustard, pickles (1)	454	42	24	20.6	7.4	66	1,059
Hamburger, large, single meat patty (4 oz raw) w/ catsup, onions, lettuce, mayonnaise, mustard, tomatoes (1)	559	43	25	36.6	9.0	74	1,140
Hamburger, regular, single meat patty (2 oz raw), plain (1)	273	28	14	11.2	3.9	33	422
Hamburger, regular, single meat patty (2 oz raw) w/ catsup, lettuce, mayonnaise, mustard, onions, pickles, tomatoes (1)	407	36	15	22.6	5.6	41	914
Hot dog (1)	242	18	10	14.5	5.1	44	671
Hot-fudge sundae (1)	284	48	6	8.6	5.0	21	182
Hush puppies (5 pieces)	256	35	5	11.6	2.7	135	965
Onion rings (8 rings or 1 order)	339	36	5	19.6	2.9	0	630
Pancakes w/ butter & syrup (3)	519	91	8	14.0	5.9	57	1,103
Pizza, see Pizza							
Roast beef on bun (1)	346	33	22	13.8	3.6	52	792
Shake, chocolate (10 fl oz)	360	58	10	10.5	6.5	37	273
Taco, small (1)	370	27	21	20.6	11.4	57	802
Tuna salad sub (1)	584	55	27	28.0	5.3	47	1,294
Fig, fresh (1 medium)	37	10	0	0.2	0.0	0	1
Figs, canned, in heavy syrup (3)	75	19	0	0.1	0.0	0	1
Figs, canned, in light syrup (3)	58	15	0	0.1	0.0	0	1
Figs, canned, in water (3)	42	11	0	0.1	0.0	0	1
Figs, dried (2)	95	24	1	0.4	0.1	0	4
Filberts, see Hazelnuts							
Fish sticks, frozen, heated (3 oz, or 3 sticks)	228	20	13	10.3	2.6	93	489
Flan, prepared w/ whole milk & eggs (1/2 cup)	220	35	7	6.3	3.0	140	86
Flounder, cooked, dry heat (3 oz)	99	0	21	1.3	0.3	58	89
Flour, all-purpose (1/2 cup)	226	47	6	0.6	0.1	0	1
Flour, self-rising, wheat or white (1/2 cup)	219	46	6	0.6	0.1	0	787
Flour, whole-grain, wheat (1/2 cup)	203	44	8	1.1	0.2	0	3
Frankfurter, beef & pork (10 per pound) (1)	144	1	5	13.1	4.8	22	504
Frankfurter, chicken (1)	116	3	6	8.8	2.5	45	617
French fries, cottage-cut, baked, (10)	109	17	2	4.1	1.9	0	23

fl oz = fluid ounce; tbsp = tablespoon; tsp = teaspoon

Nutrient Content of Common Foods (cont.)

Food	Calories	Carbohydrate g	Protein g	Fat g	Saturated Fat g	Cholesterol mg	Sodium mg
French fries, fried, prepared w/ animal & vegetable fat (10)	158	20	2	8.3	3.4	6	108
French toast, fried, prepared w/ milk & margarine (1 slice)	151	16	5	7.3	2.0	76	311
Frosting, chocolate, ready-to-eat, creamy (¹⁄₁₂ of package)	151	24	0	6.7	2.1	0	70
Frosting, coconut-nut, ready-to-eat (¹⁄₁₂ of package)	157	20	1	9.1	2.7	0	74
Frosting, cream-cheese flavor, ready-to-eat (¹⁄₁₂ of package)	157	25	0	6.6	1.9	0	90
Frosting, vanilla, ready-to-eat, creamy (¹⁄₁₂ of package)	159	26	0	6.4	1.9	0	34
Frozen dessert, fruit & juice bar (2.5 fl oz, or 1 bar)	53	14	0	0.0	0.0	0	9
Frozen dessert, gelatin pop (1)	31	7	1	0.0	0.0	0	20
Frozen dessert, pudding pop, chocolate (1)	63	11	1	1.9	0.3	1	61
Frozen dessert, water ice, lime (½ cup)	120	31	0	0.0	0.0	0	14
Frozen dessert, water ice, pineapple-coconut (½ cup)	109	23	0	2.5	2.2	0	34
Frozen yogurt, fat-free (1 cup)	199	46	5	0.3	0.2	3	100
Frozen yogurt, fat-free & sugar-free (1 cup)	152	30	7	0.4	0.2	2	76
Frozen yogurt, low-fat, chocolate (1 cup)	200	38	10	2.8	1.8	8	110
Frozen yogurt, low-fat, vanilla (1 cup)	98	18	4	1.0	0.7	4	56
Fruitcake, prepared w/ eggs, oil, nuts (¹⁄₃₆ of 10″ diameter)	307	54	3	9.6	1.2	24	121
Fruit cocktail, canned, in heavy syrup (½ cup)	93	24	1	0.1	0.0	0	7
Fruit cocktail, canned, in juice (½ cup)	56	15	0	0.0	0.0	0	4
Fruit cocktail, canned, in light syrup (½ cup)	72	19	1	0.1	0.0	0	7
Fruit cocktail, canned, in water (½ cup)	40	10	1	0.1	0.0	0	5
Fruit leather (³⁄₄ oz, or 1 large roll)	73	18	0	0.6	0.1	0	13
Garlic, raw (1 clove)	4	1	0	0.0	0.0	0	1
Gelatin, all flavors, sweetened w/ sugar, prepared w/ water (½ cup)	80	19	2	0.0	0.0	0	57
Gelatin, all flavors, sweetened w/ sugar substitute, prepared w/ water (½ cup)	8	1	1	0.0	0.0	0	56
Gin, see page 370							
Ginger ale (12 fl oz)	124	32	0	0.0	0.0	0	25
Ginger root, raw, ⅛″ × 1″ pieces (5 pieces)	8	2	0	0.1	0.0	0	1
Goat, roasted (3 oz)	122	0	23	2.6	0.8	64	73
Goose, domesticated, meat only, roasted (3 oz)	202	0	25	10.8	3.9	82	65
Goose, domesticated, w/ skin, roasted (3 oz)	259	0	21	18.6	5.8	77	60
Gooseberries, fresh (½ cup)	34	8	1	0.9	0.1	0	1
Graham cracker crumbs (½ cup)	178	32	3	4.2	1.0	0	254

fl oz = fluid ounce; tbsp = tablespoon; tsp = teaspoon

NUTRIENT CONTENT OF COMMON FOODS (cont.)

Food	Calories	Carbohydrate g	Protein g	Fat g	Saturated Fat g	Cholesterol mg	Sodium mg
Granola bar, hard, peanut (1 bar)	113	15	3	5.0	0.6	0	66
Granola bar, hard, plain (1 bar)	115	16	3	4.9	0.6	0	72
Granola bar, soft, milk-chocolate-coated, peanut butter (1 bar)	187	20	4	11.4	6.2	4	71
Grape juice (6 fl oz)	114	28	1	0.1	0.0	0	6
Grapes, fresh (10)	15	4	0	0.1	0.0	0	0
Grape soda (12 fl oz)	161	42	0	0.0	0.0	0	57
Grapefruit, canned, in juice (½ cup)	46	11	1	0.1	0.0	0	9
Grapefruit, canned, in light syrup (½ cup)	76	20	1	0.1	0.0	0	2
Grapefruit, canned, in water (½ cup)	44	11	1	0.1	0.0	0	2
Grapefruit, fresh (½)	38	10	1	0.1	0.0	0	0
Grapefruit juice, sweetened (6 fl oz)	87	21	1	0.2	0.0	0	3
Grapefruit juice, unsweetened (6 fl oz)	72	17	1	0.2	0.0	0	2
Gravy, au jus, canned (½ cup)	20	3	2	0.3	0.1	0	531
Gravy, au jus, mix, prepared w/ water (½ cup)	10	1	0	0.4	0.2	0	290
Gravy, beef, canned (½ cup)	62	6	4	2.7	1.4	4	59
Gravy, brown, mix, prepared w/ water (½ cup)	5	1	0	0.2	0.0	0	63
Gravy, chicken, canned (½ cup)	95	6	2	6.8	1.7	3	688
Gravy, chicken, mix, prepared w/ water (½ cup)	42	7	1	1.0	0.3	2	567
Gravy, mushroom, canned (½ cup)	60	7	2	3.2	0.5	0	680
Gravy, mushroom, mix, prepared w/ water (½ cup)	35	7	1	0.4	0.3	1	701
Gravy, onion, mix, prepared w/ water (½ cup)	40	8	1	0.4	0.2	1	518
Gravy, pork, mix, prepared w/ water (½ cup)	38	7	1	1.0	0.4	2	618
Gravy, turkey, canned (½ cup)	62	6	4	2.8	1.3	3	652
Gravy, turkey, mix, prepared w/ water (½ cup)	44	8	1	0.9	0.3	2	749
Green bean casserole, prepared w/ mushroom soup, milk, margarine, fried onions (½ cup)	104	8	2	7.7	2.9	9	325
Greens, beet, boiled, pieces (½ cup)	20	4	2	0.1	0.0	0	173
Greens, dandelion, boiled, chopped (½ cup)	17	3	1	0.3	0.0	0	23
Greens, mustard, boiled, chopped (½ cup)	11	2	1	0.2	0.0	0	11
Greens, mustard, frozen, boiled (½ cup)	14	2	2	0.2	0.0	0	19
Greens, turnip, boiled, chopped (½ cup)	15	3	1	0.2	0.0	0	21
Greens, turnip, canned, undrained (½ cup)	17	3	2	0.4	0.1	0	325
Greens, turnip, frozen, boiled (½ cup)	24	4	3	0.4	0.1	0	12
Grouper, cooked, dry heat (3 oz)	100	0	21	1.1	0.3	40	45
Guacamole, see Mexican food							
Guava, fresh (1)	45	11	1	0.5	0.2	0	2
Haddock, cooked, dry heat (3 oz)	95	0	21	0.8	0.1	63	74
Halibut, cooked, dry heat (3 oz)	119	0	23	2.5	0.4	35	59
Ham, boneless, canned, extra-lean, roasted (3 oz)	116	0	18	4.1	1.4	25	965
Ham, boneless, canned, regular, roasted (3 oz)	192	0	17	12.9	4.2	52	800
Ham, boneless, extra-lean, roasted (3 oz)	123	1	18	4.7	1.5	45	1,023
Hash, corned beef (1 cup)	454	23	18	32.0	9.5	85	1,323

fl oz = fluid ounce; tbsp = tablespoon; tsp = teaspoon

NUTRIENT CONTENT OF COMMON FOODS (cont.)

Food	Calories	Carbohydrate g	Protein g	Fat g	Saturated Fat g	Cholesterol mg	Sodium mg
Hazelnuts or filberts, oil-roasted, salted (1 oz)	187	5	4	18.1	1.3	0	220
Hazelnuts or filberts, oil-roasted, unsalted (1 oz)	187	5	4	18.1	1.3	0	1
Herring, pickled (3 oz)	223	8	12	15.3	2.0	11	740
Honey (1 tbsp)	64	17	0	0.0	0.0	0	1
Hush puppy, prepared w/ eggs & oil, 2¼″ × 1¼″ (1)	74	10	2	3.0	0.5	10	147
Ice cream, regular, 10% fat (1 cup)	264	32	4	14.6	9.0	58	106
Ice cream, rich, 16% fat (1 cup)	356	34	6	24.0	14.8	90	82
Ice cream cone, sugar, rolled type (1 cone)	40	8	1	0.4	0.1	0	32
Ice cream sundae, prepared w/ fudge, nuts, whipped topping (1 cup)	702	88	8	39.0	22.2	218	194
Ice milk, regular (1 cup)	184	30	6	5.6	3.4	18	112
Ice milk, soft-serve (1 cup)	222	38	8	4.6	2.8	20	124
Italian food, prepared in restaurant:							
Calzone w/ cheese (1)	1,416	139	69	63.0	28.7	184	2,383
Cheese ravioli w/ tomato sauce, 1¾″ square (6)	296	27	15	14.3	5.3	132	1,352
Chicken parmigiana (1 breast w/ sauce)	320	16	30	14.9	5.0	123	841
Fettuccine Alfredo (1¾ cups pasta & ½ cup sauce)	697	65	20	39.8	23.3	197	841
Garlic bread, 5″ × 2½″ × 1″ (1 slice)	138	20	3	4.8	0.9	0	260
Lasagna, beef (1 serving)	697	19	44	35.8	15.5	145	1,692
Manicotti, filled w/ cheese & tomato-meat sauce (6″ long) (2)	284	32	18	9.1	4.4	79	1,232
Meat ravioli, w/ tomato sauce, 1¾″ square (6)	405	51	21	13.4	5.0	216	1,996
Spaghetti, w/ marinara sauce (2 cups spaghetti & 1 cup sauce)	549	96	16	11.6	1.7	0	1,096
Spaghetti, w/ meat sauce (2 cups spaghetti & 1 cup sauce)	691	93	34	19.7	7.2	69	1,033
Veal Parmigiana (1 cutlet w/ sauce)	514	23	33	32.3	13.8	138	1,408
Jams or preserves, all flavors (1 tbsp)	48	13	0	0.0	0.0	0	6
Jelly (1 tbsp)	52	14	0	0.0	0.0	0	7
Jicama, raw, slices (1 cup)	46	11	1	0.1	0.0	0	5
Kale, boiled, chopped (½ cup)	21	4	1	0.3	0.0	0	15
Kale, raw, chopped (½ cup)	17	3	1	0.2	0.0	0	15
Kiwifruit, fresh (1 medium)	46	11	1	0.3	0.0	0	4
Kohlrabi, boiled, slices (½ cup)	24	5	1	0.1	0.0	0	17
Kohlrabi, raw, slices (½ cup)	19	4	1	0.1	0.0	0	14
Kumquat, fresh (1)	12	3	0	0.0	0.0	0	1
Lamb, cubed for stew or kabob, leg & shoulder, lean only, broiled (3 oz)	158	0	24	6.2	2.2	77	65
Lamb, foreshank, lean only, braised (3 oz)	159	0	26	5.1	1.8	89	63
Lamb, lean only, average all grades, cooked (3 oz)	175	0	24	8.1	2.9	78	64

fl oz = fluid ounce; tbsp = tablespoon; tsp = teaspoon

NUTRIENT CONTENT OF COMMON FOODS (cont.)

Food	Calories	Carbohydrate g	Protein g	Fat g	Saturated Fat g	Cholesterol mg	Sodium mg
Lamb, leg, shank half, Choice, lean only, roasted (3 oz)	153	0	24	5.7	2.0	74	56
Lamb, loin, Choice, lean only, roasted (3 oz)	171	0	23	8.3	3.2	74	56
Lamb, rack, rib, lean only, roasted (3 oz)	197	0	22	11.3	4.0	74	69
Lamb, shoulder, arm, Choice, lean only, broiled (3 oz)	170	0	24	7.7	2.9	78	70
Lamb, shoulder, arm, Choice, lean only, roasted (3 oz)	163	0	22	7.9	3.1	73	57
Lard (1 tbsp)	116	0	0	12.8	5.0	12	0
Lasagna, see Italian food							
Leeks, boiled, chopped (¼ cup)	8	2	0	0.1	0.0	0	3
Leeks, raw, chopped (¼ cup)	16	4	0	0.1	0.0	0	5
Lemon, fresh (1 medium)	17	5	1	0.2	0.0	0	1
Lemon juice (1 tbsp)	3	1	0	0.0	0.0	0	3
Lemon-lime soda (12 fl oz)	149	38	0	0.0	0.0	0	41
Lentils, boiled (½ cup)	115	20	9	0.4	0.1	0	2
Lettuce, iceberg (¼ head)	18	3	2	0.3	0.0	0	12
Lime, fresh (1)	20	7	0	0.1	0.0	0	1
Lime juice (1 tbsp)	3	1	0	0.0	0.0	0	2
Liqueurs, see page 370							
Lobster, Northern, cooked, moist heat (3 oz)	83	1	17	0.5	0.1	61	323
Loganberries, frozen (½ cup)	40	10	1	0.2	0.0	0	1
Loquat, fresh (1)	5	1	0	0.0	0.0	0	0
Luncheon meat, olive loaf (1 oz)	67	3	3	4.7	1.7	11	421
Luncheon meat, pickle & pimento loaf (1 oz)	74	2	3	6.0	2.2	10	394
Lychee, fresh (1)	6	2	0	0.0	0.0	0	0
Macadamia nuts, salted (1 oz, or 10–12 whole nuts)	204	4	2	21.7	3.3	0	73
Macaroni, plain, cooked (1 cup)	197	40	7	0.9	0.1	0	1
Macaroni & cheese, prepared w/ whole milk (1 cup)	402	44	12	18.6	4.8	8	484
Mackerel, canned, drained (3 oz)	132	0	20	5.4	1.5	67	322
Malted milk beverage (1 cup whole milk & 4–5 heaping tsp powder)	225	29	9	8.9	5.5	33	244
Mango, fresh (1)	135	35	1	0.6	0.1	0	4
Margarine, corn oil, stick, salted (1 tsp)	34	0	0	3.8	0.6	0	44
Margarine, corn oil, tub (1 tsp)	34	0	0	3.8	0.7	0	51
Margarine, safflower oil, tub (1 tsp)	34	0	0	3.8	0.4	0	51
Margarine, soybean & cottonseed oil, squeeze (1 tsp)	34	0	0	3.8	0.6	0	37
Margarine, soybean oil, stick (1 tsp)	34	0	0	3.8	0.8	0	44
Margarine, soybean oil, tub (1 tsp)	34	0	0	3.8	0.6	0	51
Marmalade (1 tbsp)	49	13	0	0.0	0.0	0	11
Marshmallows, miniature (1 cup)	146	37	1	0.0	0.0	0	22
Mayonnaise, see Salad dressing							

fl oz = fluid ounce; tbsp = tablespoon; tsp = teaspoon

NUTRIENT CONTENT OF COMMON FOODS (cont.)

Food	Calories	Carbohydrate g	Protein g	Fat g	Saturated Fat g	Cholesterol mg	Sodium mg
Meat loaf (8 oz)	574	26	39	33.6	13.3	181	1,302
Meatballs, w/o sauce, 1⅖″ diameter (4)	236	12	22	17.4	6.8	68	647
Melon, cantaloupe, fresh (½ of 5″ diameter)	94	22	2	0.7	0.0	0	23
Melon, casaba, fresh, cubed (½ cup)	23	6	1	0.1	0.0	0	10
Melon, honeydew, fresh, cubed (½ cup)	30	8	0	0.1	0.0	0	9
Melon balls, frozen (½ cup)	28	7	1	0.2	0.0	0	27
Mexican food prepared in restaurant:							
Bean burrito smothered in sauce, 6″ long (1)	404	48	18	17.1	7.3	30	1,521
Beef burrito w/o beans or cheese, 6″ long (1)	221	25	10	8.7	2.7	22	377
Enchilada w/ beef & cheese sauce (1)	320	10	18	23.1	10.7	67	592
Fajita, beef w/ onions (no tortillas) (8 oz)	558	11	43	37.8	13.2	127	780
Fajita, chicken w/ onions (no tortillas) (8 oz)	362	11	50	12.2	3.3	124	792
Guacamole (½ cup)	164	12	3	13.5	2.1	0	547
Nachos w/ meat, beans, guacamole, cheese, lettuce, tomatoes (3)	316	12	16	22.8	10.7	59	450
Refried beans (1 cup)	515	53	17	26.7	10.3	24	493
Spanish rice (1 cup)	233	46	5	3.5	0.8	0	846
Tacos (2)	487	22	29	32.2	14.0	95	834
Tortilla, see Tortilla							
Milk, ½% fat (1 cup)	94	12	8	1.0	1.0	7	125
Milk, 1% fat (1 cup)	102	12	8	2.6	1.6	10	123
Milk, buttermilk, cultured (1 cup)	99	12	8	2.2	1.3	9	257
Milk, evaporated, skim, canned (½ cup)	99	14	10	0.3	0.2	5	147
Milk, evaporated, whole, canned (½ cup)	169	13	9	9.5	5.8	37	133
Milk, fat-free, dry (¼ cup)	109	16	11	0.2	0.0	0	161
Milk, skim (1 cup)	86	12	8	0.4	0.3	4	126
Milk, sweetened condensed, canned (1 cup)	982	27	24	24.2	16.8	104	389
Milk, whole (1 cup)	150	11	8	8.2	5.1	33	120
Milk, whole, chocolate (1 cup)	208	26	8	8.5	5.3	30	149
Milkshake, vanilla, thick (11 fl oz)	350	56	12	9.5	5.9	37	299
Mixed drinks, see pages 370–71							
Mixed nuts, w/ peanuts, salted (1 oz)	169	7	5	14.6	2.0	0	190
Mixed nuts, w/ peanuts, unsalted (1 oz)	169	7	5	14.6	2.0	0	3
Mixed nuts, w/o peanuts, salted (1 oz)	175	6	4	16.0	2.6	0	198
Mixed nuts, w/o peanuts, unsalted (1 oz)	175	6	4	16.0	2.6	0	3
Mixed vegetables, canned, drained (½ cup)	39	8	2	0.4	0.0	0	122
Mixed vegetables, frozen (½ cup)	54	12	3	0.1	0.0	0	32
Molasses (1 tbsp)	53	14	0	0.0	0.0	0	7
Molasses, blackstrap (1 tbsp)	47	12	0	0.0	0.0	0	11
Moose, roasted (3 oz)	114	0	24	0.8	0.3	66	58
Mousse, chocolate, prepared w/ whole milk, heavy cream, chocolate, egg yolks (½ cup)	447	33	9	32.9	18.6	299	87

fl oz = fluid ounce; tbsp = tablespoon; tsp = teaspoon

NUTRIENT CONTENT OF COMMON FOODS (cont.)

Food	Calories	Carbohydrate g	Protein g	Fat g	Saturated Fat g	Cholesterol mg	Sodium mg
Muffin, blueberry, commercial, 2½″ diameter × 2¼″ (1)	230	36	4	7.8	2.2	39	305
Muffin, oat bran, commercial, 2½″ diameter × 2¼″ (1)	216	30	5	8.4	3.6	33	212
Mulberries, fresh (½ cup)	31	7	1	0.6	0.0	0	7
Mushrooms, canned, pieces, drained (½ cup)	19	4	2	0.2	0.0	0	332
Mushrooms, fried, w/ batter (6)	314	35	8	15.5	2.7	98	523
Mushrooms, cooked, pieces (½ cup)	21	4	2	0.4	0.1	0	2
Mushrooms, raw, pieces (½ cup)	9	2	1	0.2	0.0	0	1
Mustard, Chinese, horseradish or regular (1 tsp)	4	0	0	0.2	0.0	0	63
Nectarine, fresh, 2½″ diameter (1)	67	16	1	0.6	0.0	0	0
Noodles, chow mein (1 cup)	237	26	4	13.8	2.0	0	197
Noodles, egg, cooked, w/o salt (1 cup)	212	40	8	2.4	0.5	53	11
Noodles, Japanese, soba, boiled (1 cup)	113	24	6	0.1	0.0	0	68
Noodles, Japanese, somen, boiled (1 cup)	230	48	7	0.3	0.0	0	284
Ocean perch, cooked, dry heat (3 oz)	103	0	20	1.8	0.3	46	82
Octopus, common, cooked, moist heat (3 oz)	139	4	25	1.8	0.4	82	391
Oil, canola (1 tbsp)	120	0	0	13.6	0.8	0	0
Oil, corn (1 tbsp)	120	0	0	13.6	1.7	0	0
Oil, olive (1 tbsp)	119	0	0	13.5	1.8	0	0
Oil, peanut (1 tbsp)	119	0	0	13.5	2.3	0	0
Oil, safflower (1 tbsp)	120	0	0	13.6	1.2	0	0
Oil, sesame (1 tbsp)	120	0	0	13.6	1.9	0	0
Oil, soybean (partially hydrogenated) (1 tbsp)	120	0	0	13.6	2.0	0	0
Oil, soybean (partially hydrogenated) & cottonseed (1 tbsp)	120	0	0	13.6	2.4	0	0
Oil, sunflower (1 tbsp)	120	0	0	13.6	1.4	0	0
Okra, cooked, slices (½ cup)	25	6	2	0.1	0.0	0	4
Okra, fried, in cornmeal (½ cup)	84	9	2	4.0	0.7	25	135
Okra, frozen, boiled (½ cup)	34	8	2	0.3	0.1	0	3
Olives, green (10 small)	33	0	0	3.6	0.4	0	686
Olives, ripe (10 extra large)	61	1	1	6.5	0.7	0	385
Onion, boiled, chopped (½ cup)	29	7	1	0.2	0.0	0	8
Onion, pickled, cocktail (1 onion)	1	0	0	0.0	0.0	0	5
Onion, raw, chopped (½ cup)	27	6	1	0.2	0.0	0	2
Onion rings, frozen, baked (7 rings)	285	27	4	18.7	6.0	0	263
Orange, fresh, 2⅝″ diameter (1)	62	15	1	0.2	0.0	0	0
Orange & grapefruit juice (6 fl oz)	78	19	1	0.2	0.0	0	6
Orange juice (6 fl oz)	78	18	1	0.3	0.0	0	5
Orange juice, reconstituted from frozen (6 fl oz)	84	20	1	0.1	0.0	0	2
Orange roughy, cooked, dry heat (3 oz)	75	0	16	0.8	0.0	22	69
Orange soda (12 fl oz)	177	46	0	0.0	0.0	0	46
Oysters, breaded, fried (3 oz)	167	10	7	10.7	2.7	69	355

fl oz = fluid ounce; tbsp = tablespoon; tsp = teaspoon

NUTRIENT CONTENT OF COMMON FOODS (cont.)

Food	Calories	Carbohydrate g	Protein g	Fat g	Saturated Fat g	Cholesterol mg	Sodium mg
Oysters, canned (3 oz)	58	3	6	2.1	0.5	46	95
Pancake, prepared w/ egg & milk, 4″ diameter (1)	86	11	2	3.7	0.8	23	167
Papaya, fresh, cubed (½ cup)	27	7	0	0.1	0.1	0	2
Papaya nectar (6 fl oz)	108	27	0	0.3	0.0	0	12
Parsnip, sliced, boiled (½ cup)	63	15	1	0.2	0.0	0	8
Parsnip, sliced, raw (½ cup)	50	12	1	0.4	0.0	0	7
Passion fruit, fresh (1)	18	2	0	0.1	0.0	0	5
Passion fruit juice, purple, unsweetened (6 fl oz)	96	25	1	0.1	0.0	0	12
Passion fruit juice, yellow, unsweetened (6 fl oz)	114	27	1	0.3	0.0	0	12
Pasta, plain, cooked (1 cup)	197	40	7	0.9	0.1	0	1
Pasta, spinach, cooked (1 cup)	183	37	6	0.9	0.1	0	20
Pastrami, beef (1 oz)	99	1	5	8.3	3.0	26	348
Pastrami, turkey (1 oz)	40	0	5	1.8	0.5	15	297
Pastry, Danish, plain, 4¾″ diameter × 1″ thick (1)	381	36	6	23.3	8.2	43	167
Pastry, toaster, commercial (1)	204	37	2	5.3	0.8	0	218
Peach, fresh, 2½″ diameter (1)	37	5	0	0.1	0.0	0	0
Peaches, canned, in heavy syrup (½ cup)	95	26	1	0.1	0.0	0	8
Peaches, canned, in juice (½ cup)	55	14	1	0.0	0.0	0	6
Peaches, canned, in light syrup (½ cup)	68	18	1	0.0	0.0	0	7
Peaches, canned, in water (½ cup)	29	7	1	0.1	0.0	0	4
Peaches, dried (10 halves)	311	80	5	1.0	0.1	0	9
Peaches, dried, cooked w/o sugar (½ cup)	99	25	1	0.3	0.0	0	3
Peaches, frozen, sliced, sweetened (½ cup)	118	30	1	0.1	0.0	0	8
Peaches, spiced, canned, in heavy syrup (½ cup)	90	24	1	0.1	0.0	0	5
Peach nectar (6 fl oz)	102	26	1	0.0	0.0	0	12
Peanut butter, chunk-style (1 tbsp)	94	3	4	8.0	1.5	0	78
Peanut butter, fat reduced by 25% (1 tbsp)	94	7	5	6.0	0.9	0	101
Peanut butter, smooth-style (1 tbsp)	95	3	4	8.1	3.1	0	75
Peanuts, all types, salted, dry-roasted (1 oz, or 28 nuts)	164	6	7	13.9	1.9	0	228
Peanuts, all types, salted, oil-roasted (1 oz, or 32 nuts)	163	14	7	13.8	1.9	0	121
Pear, Asian, fresh, 2¼″ × 2½″ diameter (1)	51	13	1	0.3	0.0	0	0
Pear, canned, in heavy syrup (1 half)	58	24	0	0.1	0.0	0	4
Pear, canned, in juice (1 half)	38	16	0	0.1	0.0	0	3
Pear, canned, in light syrup (1 half)	45	10	0	0.0	0.0	0	4
Pear, canned, in water (1 half)	22	6	0	0.0	0.0	0	2
Pear, fresh, 2½″ × 3½″ diameter (1)	98	13	1	0.7	0.0	0	1
Pear nectar, canned (6 fl oz)	114	30	0	0.0	0.0	0	6
Pears, dried, cooked w/o sugar (½ cup)	163	43	1	0.4	0.0	0	4
Pears, dried, uncooked (5 halves)	230	61	2	0.6	0.0	0	5

fl oz = fluid ounce; tbsp = tablespoon; tsp = teaspoon

NUTRIENT CONTENT OF COMMON FOODS (cont.)

Food	Calories	Carbohydrate g	Protein g	Fat g	Saturated Fat g	Cholesterol mg	Sodium mg
Peas, green, boiled, plain (½ cup)	67	13	4	0.2	0.0	0	2
Peas, green, boiled, prepared w/ margarine & salt (½ cup)	79	11	4	2.1	0.4	0	262
Peas, green, canned, drained (½ cup)	59	11	4	0.3	0.1	0	186
Peas, green, canned, drained, no salt added (½ cup)	59	11	4	0.3	0.1	0	2
Peas, green, frozen, boiled (½ cup)	63	11	4	0.2	0.0	0	70
Peas, split, boiled (½ cup)	116	21	8	0.4	0.1	0	2
Peas & carrots, canned, undrained (½ cup)	48	11	3	0.4	0.1	0	332
Peas & carrots, canned, undrained, no salt added (½ cup)	48	11	3	0.4	0.1	0	5
Peas & carrots, frozen, boiled (½ cup)	38	8	2	0.3	0.1	0	55
Peas and onions, canned, undrained (½ cup)	30	0	0	0.2	0.0	0	265
Peas and onions, frozen, boiled (½ cup)	40	8	2	0.2	0.0	0	40
Pecans, unsalted (1 oz, or 15 halves)	187	6	2	18.4	1.5	0	0
Pepper, hot chili, canned, drained (1 pepper)	10	2	0	0.0	0.0	0	472
Pepper, hot chili, raw (1 pepper)	18	4	1	0.1	0.0	0	3
Pepper, jalapeño, canned, chopped (½ cup)	17	3	1	0.4	0.0	0	995
Pepper, sweet, bell, green, chopped, raw (½ cup)	12	3	0	0.2	0.0	0	2
Pepper, sweet, bell, yellow, raw, 5″ × 3″ (1)	50	12	2	0.4	0.0	0	3
Pepperoni, pork & beef (1 oz)	141	1	6	12.5	4.6	22	578
Perch, cooked, dry heat (3 oz)	99	0	21	1.0	0.2	98	67
Persimmon, Japanese, fresh, 2½″ × 3½″ (1)	118	31	0	0.3	0.0	0	3
Persimmon, native, fresh (1)	32	8	0	0.1	0.0	0	0
Phyllo dough (1 oz)	85	15	2	1.7	0.2	0	137
Pickle, bread-&-butter (2 slices)	11	3	0	tr	0.0	0	101
Pickle, dill, 3¾″ long (1)	12	3	0	0.1	0.0	0	833
Pickle, dill, low-sodium, 3¾″ long (1)	12	3	0	0.1	0.0	0	12
Pickle, sour, 3¾″ long (1)	4	1	0	0.0	0.0	0	423
Pickle, sour, low-sodium, 3¾″ long (1)	4	1	0	0.0	0.0	0	6
Pickle, sweet, 3″ long (1)	41	11	0	0.0	0.0	0	328
Pickle, sweet, low-sodium, 3″ long (1)	41	11	0	0.0	0.0	0	6
Pie, apple, 2-crust, commercial (⅛ of 9″ diameter)	297	43	2	13.8	2.6	0	333
Pie, Boston cream, 2-layer, prepared w/ low-fat milk, shortening, eggs, margarine, butter, baking chocolate (1/12 of 9″ diameter)	293	43	4	12.2	3.9	43	309
Pie, cherry, 2-crust, commercial (⅛ of 9″ diameter)	325	50	3	13.7	2.6	0	308
Pie, chocolate cream, commercial (⅙ of 8″ diameter)	344	40	3	21.9	6.0	6	153
Pie, coconut cream, commercial (⅙ of 7″ diameter)	191	24	1	10.6	4.8	0	163
Pie, egg custard, commercial (⅙ of 8″ diameter)	220	22	6	12.2	2.9	35	252

fl oz = fluid ounce; tbsp = tablespoon; tsp = teaspoon

NUTRIENT CONTENT OF COMMON FOODS (cont.)

Food	Calories	Carbohydrate g	Protein g	Fat g	Saturated Fat g	Cholesterol mg	Sodium mg
Pie, fried, fruit (4¼ oz, or 1 pie)	379	51	4	19.3	2.9	12	449
Pie, lemon meringue, commercial (⅙ of 8" diameter)	303	53	2	9.8	1.8	51	165
Pie, pecan, commercial (⅙ of 8" diameter)	452	65	5	20.9	4.3	36	480
Pie, pumpkin, commercial (⅙ of 8" diameter)	229	30	4	10.4	2.2	22	308
Pie crust, baked, prepared w/ vegetable shortening (⅛ of 9" diameter)	119	11	1	7.8	1.9	0	122
Pike, Northern, cooked, dry heat (3 oz)	96	0	21	0.8	0.1	43	42
Pineapple, chunks, frozen, sweetened (½ cup)	104	27	0	0.1	0.0	0	2
Pineapple, fresh, diced (½ cup)	39	10	0	0.3	0.1	0	1
Pineapple, tidbits, canned, in heavy syrup (½ cup)	100	26	0	0.1	0.0	0	2
Pineapple, tidbits, canned, in juice (½ cup)	75	20	1	0.1	0.0	0	2
Pineapple, tidbits, canned, in light syrup (½ cup)	66	17	0	0.1	0.0	0	2
Pineapple, tidbits, canned, in water (½ cup)	40	10	0	0.1	0.0	0	2
Pineapple juice (6 fl oz)	102	26	1	0.2	0.0	0	0
Pistachio nuts, salted (1 oz, or 47 nuts)	172	8	4	15.0	1.9	0	218
Pita, white, 6½" diameter (2 oz, or 1 pita)	165	33	5	0.7	0.1	0	322
Pita, white, miniature, 4" diameter (1 oz, or 1 pita)	78	16	3	0.4	0.0	0	152
Pita, whole-wheat or seasoned, 6½" diameter (2¼ oz, or 1 pita)	170	35	6	1.7	0.3	0	340
Pita, whole-wheat or seasoned, miniature, 4" diameter (1 oz, or 1 pita)	76	16	3	0.7	0.1	0	151
Pizza, cheese (⅛ of 12" diameter)	140	21	8	3.2	1.5	9	336
Pizza, cheese & pepperoni (⅛ of 12" diameter)	181	20	10	7.0	2.2	14	267
Plantain, raw (1)	218	57	2	0.7	0.0	0	7
Plum, fresh, 2⅛" diameter (1)	36	9	1	0.4	0.0	0	0
Plums, canned, in heavy syrup (3)	119	31	0	0.1	0.0	0	26
Plums, canned, in juice (3)	55	14	0	0.0	0.0	0	1
Plums, canned, in light syrup (3)	83	22	0	0.1	0.0	0	26
Plums, canned, in water (3)	39	10	0	0.0	0.0	0	1
Pollack, walleye, cooked, dry heat (3 oz)	96	0	20	1.0	0.2	82	98
Pomegranate, fresh, 3⅜" × 3¾" diameter (1)	104	26	1	0.5	0.0	0	5
Pompano, cooked, dry heat (3 oz)	179	0	20	10.3	3.8	54	65
Popcorn, caramel-coated, w/ peanuts (6 cups)	1,026	204	18	19.8	2.4	0	756
Popcorn, cheese-flavor (6 cups popped)	348	36	6	22.2	4.2	0	588
Popcorn, commercially popped in fat, "buttered" & salted (6 cups popped)	660	36	6	57.0	10.2	0	1,098
Popcorn, prepared w/o fat or salt (6 cups popped)	183	37	6	2.0	0.3	0	2
Popcorn cake (1 cake)	38	8	1	0.3	0.0	0	29
Popover, 2¾" diameter × 4" high (1)	90	11	4	3.4	1.1	47	82

fl oz = fluid ounce; tbsp = tablespoon; tsp = teaspoon

NUTRIENT CONTENT OF COMMON FOODS (cont.)

Food	Calories	Carbohydrate g	Protein g	Fat g	Saturated Fat g	Cholesterol mg	Sodium mg
Pork, brains, braised (3 oz)	117	0	10	8.1	1.8	2,169	77
Pork, fresh, boneless loin, chops, lean only, broiled (3 oz)	173	0	26	6.6	2.3	68	55
Pork, fresh, boneless loin, roast, lean only, roasted (3 oz)	165	0	26	6.4	2.4	66	38
Pork, fresh, boneless sirloin, chops, lean & fat, broiled (3 oz)	177	0	26	7.3	2.5	78	47
Pork, fresh, boneless sirloin, chops, lean only, broiled (3 oz)	164	0	26	5.7	1.9	78	48
Pork, fresh, loin chops, lean only, broiled (3 oz)	171	0	26	6.9	2.5	70	51
Pork, fresh, shoulder, arm picnic, lean only, roasted (3 oz)	194	0	23	10.7	3.7	81	68
Pork, fresh, shoulder, blade Boston, lean only, roasted (3 oz)	198	0	21	12.2	4.4	72	60
Pork, fresh, sirloin, lean only, broiled (3 oz)	181	0	24	8.6	3.1	72	61
Pork, fresh, tenderloin, lean only, roasted (3 oz)	139	0	24	4.1	1.4	67	48
Pork, fresh, whole leg, lean only, roasted (3 oz)	179	0	25	8.0	2.8	80	54
Pork, liver, braised (3 oz)	141	3	22	3.7	1.2	302	42
Pork, spareribs, lean & fat, braised (3 oz)	338	0	25	25.8	9.5	103	79
Pork skins, plain (1 oz)	154	0	17	8.9	3.2	27	521
Potpie, beef, double-crust (8 oz)	389	28	12	25.2	9.7	37	512
Potpie, chicken, double-crust (8 oz)	439	37	17	24.2	9.1	46	626
Potato, baked, w/ skin (2⅓″ diameter × 4¾″ long)	220	51	5	0.2	0.1	0	16
Potato chips (1 oz, or about 14 chips)	152	15	2	9.8	3.1	0	168
Potatoes, au gratin, prepared w/ whole milk, butter, cheese (½ cup)	160	14	6	9.3	5.8	29	528
Potatoes, boiled, w/ skin (½ cup)	68	16	2	0.1	0.0	0	3
Potatoes, canned, whole, drained (½ cup)	54	12	1	0.2	0.0	0	234
Potatoes, hash-brown, fried, in vegetable oil (½ cup)	163	17	2	10.9	4.3	0	19
Potatoes, mashed, prepared w/ whole milk & margarine (½ cup)	111	18	2	4.4	1.1	2	309
Potatoes, O'Brien, prepared w/ whole milk & butter (½ cup)	79	15	2	1.2	0.8	4	211
Potatoes, scalloped, prepared w/ whole milk & butter (½ cup)	105	13	4	4.5	2.8	14	409
Potato pancake, prepared w/ eggs & margarine, 3¼″ diameter (1)	101	11	2	5.6	1.1	35	188
Potato puff, prepared w/ vegetable oil (½ cup)	138	19	2	6.7	3.2	0	462
Pretzels (1 oz, or about 5 pretzels)	108	23	3	1.0	0.2	0	486
Pretzels, chocolate-covered (1 oz, or about 3)	138	24	3	3.7	1.9	2	415

fl oz = fluid ounce; tbsp = tablespoon; tsp = teaspoon

Nutrient Content of Common Foods (cont.)

Food	Calories	Carbohydrate g	Protein g	Fat g	Saturated Fat g	Cholesterol mg	Sodium mg
Prickly pear, fresh (1)	42	10	1	0.5	0.0	0	6
Prune juice (6 fl oz)	138	33	1	0.1	0.0	0	6
Prunes, dried (5)	100	26	1	0.2	0.0	0	2
Prunes, canned, in heavy syrup, undrained (5)	90	24	1	0.2	0.0	0	2
Prunes, cooked, w/o sugar (½ cup)	113	30	1	0.3	0.0	0	2
Pudding, chocolate, prepared w/ whole milk (½ cup)	158	26	5	4.8	3.0	17	147
Pudding, rice, prepared w/ whole milk (½ cup)	217	40	6	4.2	2.6	17	85
Pudding, tapioca (½ cup)	109	16	5	3.0	1.4	63	107
Pumpkin, canned (½ cup)	41	10	1	0.3	0.0	0	6
Pumpkin, mashed, cooked (½ cup)	24	6	1	0.9	0.1	0	2
Pumpkin & squash seed kernels, salted (1 tbsp, or 44 seeds)	47	2	2	4.0	0.7	0	161
Pumpkin pie mix, canned (½ cup)	141	36	1	0.2	0.1	0	280
Quiche Lorraine, prepared w/ cheese, heavy cream, bacon (⅐ of 9″ diameter pie)	391	19	15	27.7	12.8	134	468
Quince, fresh (1)	53	14	0	0.1	0.0	0	4
Rabbit, domesticated, stewed (3 oz)	175	0	26	7.2	2.1	73	31
Radicchio, shredded, raw (½ cup)	5	1	0	0.1	0.0	0	4
Radishes, 1″ diameter, raw (10)	7	2	0	0.2	0.0	0	11
Raisins (¼ cup)	127	33	1	0.2	0.1	0	5
Raspberries, canned, in heavy syrup (½ cup)	117	30	1	0.2	0.0	0	4
Raspberries, fresh (½ cup)	31	17	1	0.3	0.0	0	0
Raspberries, frozen, sweetened (½ cup)	128	33	1	0.2	0.0	0	1
Relish, corn (1 tbsp)	13	3	0	0.1	0.0	0	59
Relish, cranberry-orange, canned (½ cup)	246	64	0	0.1	0.0	0	44
Relish, hot dog (1 tbsp)	14	4	0	0.1	0.0	0	164
Relish, pickle, sour (1 tbsp)	3	1	0	0.0	0.0	0	192
Relish, pickle, sweet (1 tbsp)	19	5	0	0.1	0.0	0	122
Reuben sandwich w/ corned beef, sauerkraut, cheese, dressing on rye bread (1)	543	30	23	36.8	12.3	79	1,516
Rhubarb, fresh, cooked, w/ sugar (½ cup)	139	37	1	0.1	0.0	0	1
Rice, brown, long-grain, cooked, w/o salt (1 cup)	216	45	5	1.8	0.4	0	9
Rice, seasoned mixes, prepared w/ margarine as directed (1 cup)	247	43	5	5.7	1.1	1	1,147
Rice, white, long-grain, parboiled, cooked, w/o salt (1 cup)	199	43	4	0.5	0.1	0	6
Rice, white, long-grain, precooked or instant, cooked, w/o salt (1 cup)	161	35	3	0.3	0.1	0	4
Rice, white, long-grain, regular, cooked, w/o salt (1 cup)	205	45	4	0.5	0.1	0	1
Rice, wild, cooked, w/o salt (1 cup)	166	35	7	0.6	0.1	0	6
Rice cake, plain (1 cake)	35	7	1	0.3	0.1	0	29

fl oz = fluid ounce; tbsp = tablespoon; tsp = teaspoon

NUTRIENT CONTENT OF COMMON FOODS (cont.)

Food	Calories	Carbohydrate g	Protein g	Fat g	Saturated Fat g	Cholesterol mg	Sodium mg
Rice pilaf, prepared w/ margarine (1 cup)	321	53	7	8.4	2.4	5	1,507
Rockfish, cooked, dry heat (3 oz)	103	0	20	1.7	0.4	38	65
Roll, dinner (1)	85	14	2	2.1	0.5	0	148
Roll, hard, 3½″ diameter (1)	167	30	6	2.4	0.3	0	310
Root beer (12 fl oz)	152	39	0	0.0	0.0	0	49
Rum, see pages 370–71							
Rutabaga, cubed, boiled (½ cup)	29	7	1	0.2	0.0	0	15
Rutabaga, cubed, raw (½ cup)	25	6	1	0.1	0.0	0	14
Salad, ambrosia, prepared w/ sour cream & coconut (½ cup)	127	16	1	7.1	5.1	15	33
Salad, Caesar, prepared w/ egg & oil (1 cup)	209	8	5	17.6	3.6	47	390
Salad, carrot & raisin, prepared w/ mayonnaise (1 cup)	180	14	1	14.3	2.1	10	235
Salad, chef's, w/ 1 oz turkey, 1 oz ham, 1 oz cheese, ½ egg, no dressing (1)	245	7	23	13.6	6.8	158	848
Salad, chicken, prepared w/ mayonnaise (½ cup)	352	2	14	32.2	5.2	61	441
Salad, coleslaw, prepared w/ mayonnaise (½ cup)	142	3	1	14.7	2.2	11	121
Salad, egg, prepared w/ mayonnaise (½ cup)	271	3	9	25.3	4.8	288	456
Salad, macaroni, prepared w/ mayonnaise (½ cup)	222	19	3	15.0	2.2	11	410
Salad, potato, prepared w/ mayonnaise (½ cup)	212	19	2	14.8	2.2	11	544
Salad, tuna, prepared w/ mayonnaise (½ cup)	279	2	15	23.7	3.7	24	338
Salad, Waldorf, prepared w/ mayonnaise (½ cup)	205	9	1	18.9	2.6	11	123
Salad dressing, blue cheese (1 tbsp)	77	1	1	8.0	1.5	3	167
Salad dressing, French (1 tbsp)	67	3	0	6.4	1.5	9	214
Salad dressing, French, low-calorie (1 tbsp)	34	3	0	2.7	0.4	2	143
Salad dressing, Italian (1 tbsp)	69	2	0	7.1	1.0	0	116
Salad dressing, Italian, low-calorie (1 tbsp)	16	1	0	1.5	0.2	1	118
Salad dressing, mayonnaise (1 tbsp)	99	0	0	11.0	1.6	8	78
Salad dressing, mayonnaise, fat-free (1 tbsp)	16	4	0	0	0	0	148
Salad dressing, mayonnaise, reduced-fat (1 tbsp)	49	2	0	4.8	0.7	4	98
Salad dressing, mayonnaise type (1 tbsp)	57	4	0	4.9	0.7	4	105
Salad dressing, oil & vinegar (1 tbsp)	69	2	0	7.0	1.0	0	116
Salad dressing, Thousand Island (1 tbsp)	59	2	0	5.6	0.9	4	109
Salad dressing, Thousand Island, low-calorie (1 tbsp)	24	3	0	1.6	0.2	2	153
Salami, dry, pork & beef (3 oz)	355	2	19	29.2	10.4	67	1,581
Salisbury steak w/ gravy (1 steak)	331	13	25	19.2	7.4	122	887
Salmon, Atlantic, cooked, dry heat (3 oz)	155	0	22	6.9	1.1	60	48
Salmon, chinook, smoked (3 oz)	99	0	16	3.7	0.8	20	666

fl oz = fluid ounce; tbsp = tablespoon; tsp = teaspoon

NUTRIENT CONTENT OF COMMON FOODS (cont.)

Food	Calories	Carbohydrate g	Protein g	Fat g	Saturated Fat g	Cholesterol mg	Sodium mg
Salmon, chum, canned, w/ bones, drained (3 oz)	120	0	18	4.7	1.3	33	414
Salmon, chum, cooked, dry heat (3 oz)	131	0	22	4.1	0.9	81	54
Salmon, coho, cooked, moist heat (3 oz)	157	0	23	6.4	1.2	42	50
Salmon, pink, canned, drained (3 oz)	118	0	17	5.2	1.3	47	471
Salmon, pink, cooked, dry heat (3 oz)	127	0	22	3.8	0.6	57	73
Salmon, sockeye, canned, w/ bones, drained (3 oz)	130	0	17	6.2	1.4	37	458
Salsa, prepared w/ tomatoes, green chili peppers, onions (1/2 cup)	29	6	1	0.3	0.0	0	337
Salt (1 tsp)	0	0	0	0.0	0.0	0	2,325
Salt, celery (1 tsp)	2	0	0	0.2	0.0	0	1,505
Salt, garlic (1 tsp)	4	1	0	0.0	0.0	0	968
Salt, seasoned (1 tsp)	3	1	0	0.1	0.0	0	1,367
Sandwich spread (1 tbsp)	60	3	0	5.2	0.8	12	153
Sardines, Atlantic, canned, in oil, w/ bones, drained (3 oz)	177	0	21	9.7	1.3	121	429
Sardines, Pacific, canned, in tomato sauce, w/ bones, drained (3 oz)	151	0	14	10.2	2.6	52	352
Sauce, béarnaise, prepared w/ milk & butter (1/2 cup)	351	9	4	34.1	20.9	95	633
Sauce, cheese, prepared w/ milk (1/4 cup)	154	12	8	8.6	4.7	27	783
Sauce, hollandaise, prepared w/ milk & butter (1/2 cup)	352	9	4	34.1	20.9	95	567
Sauce, mushroom, prepared w/ milk (1/2 cup)	114	12	6	5.2	2.7	17	767
Sauce, sour cream, prepared w/ milk (1/2 cup)	255	23	10	15.1	8.0	46	504
Sauce, steak (1 tbsp)	10	2	0	0.1	0.0	0	227
Sauce, stroganoff, mix, prepared w/ milk & water (1/2 cup)	136	17	6	5.4	3.4	19	915
Sauce, sweet/sour, prepared w/ water & vinegar (1/2 cup)	147	36	0	0.0	0.0	0	390
Sauce, white, prepared w/ milk (1/2 cup)	121	11	5	6.7	3.2	17	398
Sauce, Worcestershire (1 tsp)	3	1	0	0.0	0.0	0	49
Sauerkraut, canned, undrained (1/2 cup)	22	5	1	0.2	0.0	0	201
Sausage, Italian, pork, cooked (3 oz)	216	1	13	17.2	6.1	52	618
Sausage, knockwurst, pork & beef, 4" link (1)	209	1	8	18.9	6.9	39	687
Sausage, liverwurst, pork (3 oz)	276	2	12	24.3	9.0	135	731
Sausage, pork, fresh, cooked (3 oz)	314	1	17	26.5	9.2	71	2,000
Sausage, pork, Polish (3 oz)	276	1	12	24.4	8.8	60	744
Sausage, pork, smoked, 4" long × 1⅛" diameter (1 link)	265	1	15	21.6	7.7	46	1,020
Sausage, Vienna, beef & pork, canned (4 oz, or 7 links)	315	2	12	28.5	10.5	59	1,077
Scallops, fried, breaded (6 large)	201	9	17	10.2	2.5	57	432
Scallops, imitation, made from surimi (3 oz)	84	9	11	0.4	0.1	18	676

fl oz = fluid ounce; tbsp = tablespoon; tsp = teaspoon

NUTRIENT CONTENT OF COMMON FOODS (cont.)

Food	Calories	Carbohydrate g	Protein g	Fat g	Saturated Fat g	Cholesterol mg	Sodium mg
Scotch, see pages 370–71							
Sea bass, cooked, dry heat (3 oz)	105	0	20	2.2	0.6	45	74
Sesame seeds (1 tbsp)	47	1	2	4.4	0.6	0	3
Shallots, chopped, raw (1 tbsp)	7	2	0	0.0	0.0	0	1
Sherbet, orange (½ cup)	132	29	1	1.9	1.1	5	44
Shortening, soybean & cottonseed (1 tbsp)	113	0	0	12.8	3.2	0	0
Shrimp, breaded, fried (12 large)	219	10	19	11.0	1.9	159	309
Shrimp, cooked (3 oz)	84	0	18	0.9	0.2	166	190
Shrimp, imitation, made from surimi (3 oz)	86	8	11	1.3	0.3	31	599
Snack cake, cream-filled, sponge (1 cake)	155	27	1	4.9	1.2	7	155
Snapper, cooked, dry heat (3 oz)	109	0	22	1.5	0.3	40	48
Snow peas, boiled (½ cup)	34	6	3	0.2	0.0	0	3
Snow peas, frozen, boiled (½ cup)	42	7	3	0.3	0.1	0	4
Snow peas, raw (½ cup)	30	5	2	0.1	0.0	0	3
Soup, bean w/ bacon, prepared w/ water (1 cup)	173	23	8	5.9	1.5	3	952
Soup, beef, broth or bouillon, ready-to-serve (1 cup)	16	1	3	0.5	0.3	0	782
Soup, beef, chunky-style, ready-to-serve (1 cup)	171	20	12	5.1	2.6	14	867
Soup, cheese, prepared w/ water (1 cup)	155	11	5	10.5	6.7	30	959
Soup, chicken, chunky-style, ready-to-serve (1 cup)	178	17	13	6.6	2.0	30	887
Soup, chicken broth, prepared w/ water (1 cup)	39	1	5	1.4	0.4	1	776
Soup, chicken noodle, prepared w/ water (1 cup)	75	9	4	2.5	0.7	7	1,107
Soup, chicken rice, chunky-style, ready-to-serve (1 cup)	127	13	12	3.2	1.0	12	888
Soup, chicken rice, prepared w/ water (1 cup)	60	7	4	1.9	0.5	7	814
Soup, chicken vegetable, prepared w/ water (1 cup)	74	9	4	2.8	0.9	10	944
Soup, chili, see Chili							
Soup, clam chowder, Manhattan, prepared w/ water (1 cup)	78	12	4	2.3	0.4	2	1,808
Soup, clam chowder, New England, prepared w/ whole milk (1 cup)	163	17	9	6.6	3.0	22	992
Soup, cream of asparagus, prepared w/ water (1 cup)	87	11	2	4.1	1.0	5	981
Soup, cream of celery, prepared w/ water (1 cup)	90	9	2	5.6	1.4	15	949
Soup, cream of chicken, prepared w/ water (1 cup)	116	9	3	7.4	2.1	10	986
Soup, cream of mushroom, prepared w/ water (1 cup)	129	9	2	9.0	2.4	2	1,031

fl oz = fluid ounce; tbsp = tablespoon; tsp = teaspoon

NUTRIENT CONTENT OF COMMON FOODS (cont.)

Food	Calories	Carbohydrate g	Protein g	Fat g	Saturated Fat g	Cholesterol mg	Sodium mg
Soup, cream of potato, prepared w/ water (1 cup)	73	11	2	2.4	1.2	5	1,000
Soup, gazpacho, ready-to-serve (1 cup)	57	1	9	2.2	0.3	0	1,183
Soup, minestrone, chunky-style, ready-to-serve (1 cup)	127	21	5	2.8	1.5	5	864
Soup, minestrone, prepared w/ water (1 cup)	83	11	4	2.5	0.5	2	911
Soup, onion, prepared w/ water (1 cup)	57	8	4	1.7	0.3	0	1,053
Soup, oyster stew, prepared w/ whole milk (1 cup)	134	10	6	7.9	5.1	32	1,040
Soup, oyster stew, prepared w/ water (1 cup)	59	4	4	3.8	2.5	14	980
Soup, split pea w/ ham, prepared w/ water (1 cup)	189	28	10	4.4	1.8	8	1,008
Soup, tomato, prepared w/ water (1 cup)	86	17	2	1.9	0.4	0	872
Soup, tomato rice, prepared w/ water (1 cup)	120	22	2	2.7	0.5	2	815
Soup, vegetarian vegetable, prepared w/ water (1 cup)	72	12	2	1.9	0.3	0	823
Soy sauce (1 tbsp)	9	2	1	0.0	0.0	0	1,029
Spaghetti, plain, cooked (1 cup)	197	40	7	0.9	0.1	0	1
Spaghetti, spinach, cooked (1 cup)	183	37	6	0.9	0.1	0	20
Spaghetti, whole-wheat, cooked (1 cup)	174	37	7	0.8	0.1	0	4
Spaghetti w/ sauce, see Italian food							
Spices, all varieties w/o salt (1 tsp)	0	0	0	0.0	0.0	0	0
Spinach, boiled, plain (1/2 cup)	21	4	3	0.2	0.0	0	63
Spinach, boiled, prepared w/ margarine & salt (1/2 cup)	42	5	3	2.1	0.4	0	270
Spinach, canned, drained (1/2 cup)	25	4	3	0.5	0.1	0	373
Spinach, canned, drained, no salt added (1/2 cup)	25	4	3	0.5	0.1	0	29
Spinach, chopped, raw (1/2 cup)	6	1	1	0.1	0.0	0	22
Spinach, frozen, boiled (1/4 cup)	27	5	3	0.2	0.0	0	82
Squash, summer, all varieties, sliced, boiled (1/2 cup)	18	4	1	0.3	0.1	0	1
Squash, summer, all varieties, sliced, raw (1/2 cup)	13	3	1	0.1	0.0	0	1
Squash, winter, all varieties, cubed, boiled (1/2 cup)	39	9	1	0.6	trace	0	1
Squash, winter, all varieties, cubed, raw (1/2 cup)	21	5	1	0.1	0.0	0	2
Squash, zucchini, cooked, prepared w/ margarine & salt (1/2 cup)	31	4	1	2.0	0.4	0	196
Squash, zucchini, fried, prepared in restaurant (6 pieces)	126	13	3	6.8	1.9	44	180
Squash, zucchini, Italian-style, canned, undrained (1/2 cup)	33	1	1	0.1	0.0	0	427
Squash, zucchini, sliced, boiled (1/2 cup)	14	4	1	0.1	0.0	0	2
Squash casserole, prepared w/ eggs, cheese, milk, margarine (1/2 cup)	290	17	9	20.9	7.6	71	667

fl oz = fluid ounce; tbsp = tablespoon; tsp = teaspoon

NUTRIENT CONTENT OF COMMON FOODS (cont.)

Food	Calories	Carbohydrate g	Protein g	Fat g	Saturated Fat g	Cholesterol mg	Sodium mg
Squirrel, roasted (3 oz)	116	0	21	3.1	0.4	80	80
Steak, see Beef							
Strawberries, canned, in heavy syrup (½ cup)	117	30	1	0.3	0.0	0	5
Strawberries, fresh (½ cup)	23	5	0	0.3	0.0	0	1
Strawberries, frozen, sweetened (½ cup)	100	25	0	0.0	0.0	0	2
Strawberries, frozen, unsweetened (½ cup)	26	7	0	0.0	0.0	0	2
Strawberry shortcake, 3″ diameter cake, ½ cup fruit, 3 tbsp whipped topping (1)	137	22	2	4.8	3.4	40	65
Stuffing mix, bread, prepared w/ margarine (½ cup)	178	22	3	8.6	1.7	0	543
Succotash, boiled (½ cup)	111	23	5	0.8	0.1	0	16
Succotash, frozen, boiled (½ cup)	79	17	4	0.8	0.1	0	38
Succotash, canned, undrained (½ cup)	81	18	3	0.6	0.1	0	283
Succotash, w/ cream-style corn, canned (½ cup)	102	23	4	0.7	0.1	0	325
Sugar, brown, packed (1 tsp)	17	4	0	0.0	0.0	0	2
Sugar, confectioners' (powdered) (1 tsp)	10	3	0	0.0	0.0	0	0
Sugar, white (1 tsp)	15	4	0	0.0	0.0	0	0
Sunflower seed kernels, salted (1 oz)	176	6	5	16.1	1.7	0	172
Swedish meatballs, w/ cream sauce, prepared in restaurant (8 oz)	426	15	26	28.6	12.5	147	1,054
Sweet potatoes, boiled, mashed (½ cup)	103	24	2	0.1	0.0	0	10
Sweet potatoes, candied, prepared w/ brown sugar & butter, 2½″ × 2″ piece (1)	144	29	1	3.4	1.4	8	73
Sweet potatoes, canned, in syrup, drained (½ cup)	106	24	1	0.3	0.1	0	38
Sweet potatoes, canned, mashed (½ cup)	129	59	5	0.3	0.1	0	96
Sweet potatoes, frozen, cubed, boiled (½ cup)	88	21	2	0.1	0.0	0	7
Swiss steak, prepared in restaurant (8 oz)	222	9	26	8.6	2.0	66	537
Swordfish, cooked, dry heat (3 oz)	132	0	22	4.4	1.2	43	98
Syrup, chocolate (2 tbsp)	82	22	1	0.3	0.2	0	36
Syrup, maple (1 tbsp)	50	13	0	0.0	0.0	0	2
Syrup, pancake (1 tbsp)	57	15	0	0.0	0.0	0	17
Syrup, pancake, w/ butter (1 tbsp)	59	15	0	0.3	0.2	1	20
Taco shell, 5″ diameter (1)	61	8	1	2.9	0.4	0	48
Tamarind, fresh, 3″ long × 1″ wide (1)	5	1	0	0.0	0.0	0	1
Tangerine, fresh, 2⅜″ diameter (1)	37	9	1	0.2	0.0	0	1
Tofu, raw, regular (½ cup)	94	2	10	5.9	0.9	0	9
Tomatillo, raw, 1⅝″ diameter (1)	11	2	0	0.4	0.0	0	0
Tomato, red, fresh, 2¾″ diameter (1)	31	7	1	0.5	0.1	0	13
Tomatoes, red, boiled (½ cup)	30	7	1	0.3	0.0	0	13
Tomatoes, red, canned, stewed (½ cup)	34	8	0	0.2	0.0	0	325
Tomatoes, red, canned, w/ green chilies (½ cup)	18	4	1	0.0	0.0	0	481

fl oz = fluid ounce; tbsp = tablespoon; tsp = teaspoon

NUTRIENT CONTENT OF COMMON FOODS (cont.)

Food	Calories	Carbohydrate g	Protein g	Fat g	Saturated Fat g	Cholesterol mg	Sodium mg
Tomatoes, red, canned, whole (½ cup)	24	5	1	0.3	0.0	0	195
Tomatoes, red, canned, whole, no salt added (½ cup)	24	5	1	0.3	0.0	0	16
Tomatoes, sun-dried, chopped (1 tbsp)	9	2	0	0.1	0.0	0	71
Tomato juice, canned (6 fl oz)	32	8	1	0.1	0.0	0	658
Tomato juice, canned, no salt added (6 fl oz)	32	8	1	0.1	0.0	0	18
Tomato paste, canned (½ cup)	110	25	5	1.2	0.2	0	1,035
Tomato paste, canned, no salt added (½ cup)	110	25	5	1.2	0.2	0	86
Tomato puree, canned (½ cup)	51	13	2	0.1	0.0	0	499
Tomato puree, canned, no salt added (½ cup)	51	13	2	0.1	0.0	0	25
Tonic water (12 fl oz)	125	32	0	0.0	0.0	0	15
Topping, butterscotch or caramel (2 tbsp)	104	27	1	0.0	0.0	0	144
Topping, chocolate fudge (2 tbsp)	148	26	2	5.8	2.4	6	56
Topping, pineapple (2 tbsp)	102	27	0	0.0	0.0	0	16
Topping, strawberry (2 tbsp)	102	27	0	0.1	0.0	0	16
Tortilla, corn, 6"–7" diameter (1)	56	12	1	0.6	0.1	0	40
Tortilla, flour, 7" diameter (1)	114	20	3	2.5	0.4	0	167
Tortilla chips (1 oz)	142	18	2	7.4	1.4	0	150
Trail mix (1 cup)	693	67	21	44.1	8.3	0	343
Trout, rainbow, cooked, dry heat (3 oz)	129	0	22	3.7	0.7	62	29
Tuna, bluefin, fresh, cooked, dry heat (3 oz)	157	0	25	5.3	1.4	42	43
Tuna, light, canned, in oil, drained (3 oz)	169	0	25	7.0	1.3	15	301
Tuna, light, canned, in water, drained (3 oz)	99	0	22	0.7	0.2	26	287
Tuna, white, canned, in oil, drained (3 oz)	158	0	23	6.9	1.3	26	336
Tuna, white, canned, in water, drained (3 oz)	116	0	23	2.1	0.6	35	333
Tuna, yellowfin, fresh, cooked, dry heat (3 oz)	118	0	25	1.0	0.3	49	40
Turkey, dark meat w/ skin, roasted (3 oz)	188	0	23	9.9	3.0	76	65
Turkey, dark meat w/o skin, roasted (3 oz)	159	0	24	6.1	2.1	72	67
Turkey, giblets (3 oz)	141	2	23	4.3	1.3	355	50
Turkey, giblets, 1 each gizzard, heart, liver (5½ oz)	264	3	42	8.0	2.4	660	93
Turkey, ground, cooked (3 oz)	200	0	23	11.2	2.9	87	91
Turkey, light meat w/ skin, roasted (3 oz)	167	0	24	7.1	2.0	65	54
Turkey, light meat w/o skin, roasted (3 oz)	133	0	25	2.7	0.9	59	54
Turkey, roll, light & dark meat (3 oz)	126	2	15	5.9	1.7	47	498
Turkey, w/ gravy, frozen (3 oz)	57	4	5	2.2	0.7	NA	471
Turkey, young tom, dark meat w/ skin, roasted (3 oz)	158	0	24	5.9	2.0	75	70
Turkey, young tom, light meat w/ skin, roasted (3 oz)	163	0	24	6.5	1.8	64	57
Turkey, young tom, light meat w/o skin, roasted (3 oz)	129	0	25	2.5	0.8	59	58
Turkey, young tom, meat only w/o skin, roasted (3 oz)	143	0	25	4.0	1.3	66	63
Turkey ham, thigh meat, cured (3 oz)	110	0	16	4.3	1.5	48	848

fl oz = fluid ounce; tbsp = tablespoon; tsp = teaspoon

NUTRIENT CONTENT OF COMMON FOODS (cont.)

Food	Calories	Carbohydrate g	Protein g	Fat g	Saturated Fat g	Cholesterol mg	Sodium mg
Turkey pastrami (1 oz)	40	1	5	1.8	0.5	15	297
Turnips, cubed, boiled (½ cup)	14	4	1	0.1	0.0	0	39
Turnips, cubed, raw (½ cup)	18	4	1	0.1	0.0	0	44
Vanilla extract (1 tsp)	12	1	0	0.0	0.0	0	0
Veal, arm steak, lean only, braised (3 oz)	171	0	30	4.5	1.2	132	76
Veal, blade steak, lean only, braised (3 oz)	168	0	28	5.5	1.5	135	86
Veal, lean only, average all grades, cooked (3 oz)	166	0	27	5.7	1.5	99	76
Veal, loin chop, lean only, braised (3 oz)	192	0	28	7.8	2.1	107	71
Veal, rib roast, lean only, cooked (3 oz)	151	0	22	6.3	1.8	97	81
Veal, sweetbreads (thymus), braised (3 oz)	148	0	27	3.7	1.3	399	56
Veal parmigiana, see Italian food							
Vegetable juice cocktail (6 fl oz)	34	8	1	0.2	0.0	0	664
Venison, roasted (3 oz)	134	0	26	2.7	1.1	95	46
Vinegar (1 tbsp)	2	1	0	0.0	0.0	0	0
Vodka, see pages 370–71							
Waffle, frozen, 4″ square (1)	82	13	2	2.6	0.6	9	245
Walnuts (1 oz, or 14 halves)	172	3	7	16.1	1.0	0	0
Water chestnuts, canned, sliced, undrained (½ cup)	35	9	1	0.0	0.0	0	6
Water chestnuts, raw (½ cup)	66	15	1	0.1	0.0	0	9
Watercress, chopped, fresh (½ cup)	2	0	0	0.0	0.0	0	7
Watermelon, diced, fresh (½ cup)	25	6	0	0.3	0.0	0	2
Whiskey, see pages 370–71							
Whitefish, smoked (3 oz)	92	0	20	0.8	0.2	28	866
Whiting, cooked, dry heat (3 oz)	98	0	20	1.4	0.3	71	113
Wine, see pages 370–71							
Yam, cubed, boiled (½ cup)	79	19	1	0.1	0.0	0	6
Yeast, baker's, active, dry (1 packet, or ¼ oz)	21	3	3	0.3	0.0	0	4
Yogurt, fat-free, plain (1 cup)	127	17	13	0.4	0.3	4	174
Yogurt, low-fat, fruit-flavored (8 oz)	225	42	9	2.6	1.7	10	121
Yogurt, low-fat, plain (1 cup)	144	16	12	3.5	2.3	14	159
Zucchini, see Squash							

Adapted from USDA, Composition of Foods, *Agriculture Handbook series no. 8 (Washington, D.C.: USDA, 1976–1992) and Nutrition Data System, University of Minnesota, Minneapolis.*

fl oz = fluid ounce; tbsp = tablespoon; tsp = teaspoon

Subject Index

Recipe Index

Page numbers in **boldprint** refer to low-sodium recipe variations.

Page numbers in **boldprint** refer to low-sodium recipe variations.

Page numbers in **boldprint** refer to low-sodium recipe variations.

Page numbers in **boldprint** refer to low-sodium recipe variations.

Order Form—Books in the Living Heart Series

The Living Heart Guide to Eating Out is a guide to heart-healthy eating away from home. It includes 160 tips on selecting foods lower in fat and sodium in American and ethnic restaurants, as well as fast-food establishments. The book lists the amounts of calories, fat, saturated fat, and cholesterol in 1,630 restaurant foods. Softcover, pocket size.

The Living Heart Brand Name Shopper's Guide—Third Edition lists more than 5,000 supermarket foods low in saturated fat; values are given for calories, fat, saturated fat, carbohydrate, fiber, and sodium. It is designed to aid in the selection of foods to help you (1) lose weight, (2) lower blood cholesterol and triglyceride levels, (3) lower high blood pressure, and (4) reduce cancer risk by eating fiber. Softcover.

The New Living Heart uses easily understood terms to describe how the heart works, how it can fail, and what interventions are available for prevention and treatment of heart disorders. A number of cardiac tests are described, along with how to prepare for them and what to expect. Available October 1996.

Print Name _____

Address _____

City _____ State _____ Zip _____

Please send me the book(s) indicated below:

_____ copy(ies) of *The Living Heart Guide to Eating Out* at $9.95 each   = $_____

_____ copy(ies) of *The Living Heart Brand Name Shopper's Guide* at $14.95 each = $_____

_____ copy(ies) of *The New Living Heart Diet* at $16 each   = $_____

_____ copy(ies) of *The New Living Heart* (call for price)   = $_____

Add $2.00 for postage and handling
for the first book and $1.50
for each additional book $_____

Total Enclosed $_____

Make payment by check or money order payable to Diet Modification Clinic. (We cannot accept credit cards.)

Please return to:

Diet Modification Clinic   Phone: (713) 798-4150
6565 Fannin, F770
Houston, TX 77030-2707